Printed in the United States of America

First Printing, 2025

ISBN 979-8-9858062-1-2

www.placebojournal.com
www.authenticmedicine.com
www.dpcnews.com

# Foreword

## How I met Doug Farrago

I found a life-long partner in laughter on October 25, 2005. I was a 2nd year Family Medicine resident, preparing for a career practicing medicine in rural Kansas. I was living the typical existence of a hard-working resident at the time--very long hours of mostly thankless, underpaid work. One of my attendings approached my desk, laughing at a sarcastic editorial I'd published. (Laughter has always been medicine and therapy for me.) In-between bouts of her famous loud and howling laughter, she asked me: "Why don't you try to write for the Placebo Journal?" My response: "Wait...what is The Placebo Journal?"

She had been a Placebo Journal subscriber ever since she'd gotten a free copy at a conference and was incredulous that I'd never heard of "The Mad magazine of medicine." She ran to her office and loaned me an issue. I read it cover to cover before I slept that night (which is saying something, because in residency sleep is a rare treat.)

I had so many questions. How had I not known about this magazine? How had I not already started it on my own? How had I not been contacted by the editor and offered a highly lucrative 6-figure offer to retire from medicine and exclusively write comedy for them? What time was it? Did I miss dinner?

My course of action was clear. I needed to write for the Placebo Journal--or more accurately, The Placebo Journal needed me to write for them. (It was good- but with my help, could be great--at the time I wasn't aware of the functional mental retardation of the Journal's editor). So, I found the name and e-mail address of the editor and main author- some doc 7,133 miles away in Maine named Douglas Farrago, MD.

Here was a guy I'd never met, never heard of, yet immediately I recognized as a kindred spirit. I had to e-mail him right now. It was 11PM. I know this because I still have that 20-year-old e-mail. The email I sent to Doug was a ridiculous, overconfident introduction and included a few attachments of material I'd written. It was 3,035 words long and was basically 2 pages of me saying "Dude, we need to work together." (But I remained true to my motto "Why use 6 words when 3,000 will do?")

Five hours later (at 4:42 AM!) Doug replied. His reply was 36 words long, which itself could have used some brevity, and could have been the following 7: "Busy now, will read and reply soon. -DF."

"Wait, this dude is reading my e-mail at 4:30 AM. Are you kidding me?" I was elated. I was patient. I figured he'd write me back later that day or something--I get it, he's a busy doctor like me.

Eleven days later he wrote me back. Doug's e-mail was short and sweet. It was in 2 brief parts. Part 1: "I like your stuff. Keep it up and maybe we will get you on staff - no pay but you are listed inside the cover." Part 2: My first assignment. Just 3 sentences outlining an idea for a gag he wanted to work up.

That was it. I was in. I was writing for the Placebo Journal. I got a job that paid no money, required time I didn't have, sacrificed even more sleep I desperately needed, had challenging deadlines, and I got virtually no credit for my work. But you'd have thought I got a job as a writer for SNL or Mad. I was ecstatic.

The rest is the second chapter of our history and will be found in volume 2 of this compendium. Doug has been making obscene profit off my unpaid hard work and brilliance for 2 decades. It's hard to believe that we have been making each other laugh for 20 years. My son (a brilliant college freshman) who grew up reading PJ's I left lying around, idolizes him. I'm proud to call Doug one of my best friends.

**Vance Lassey, MD**
July 2025

# Introduction

Welcome to the best of the Placebo Journal. For those who don't know about this publication, it was described as the "Mad Magazine of Medicine". For those who don't know what Mad Magazine is then let me just state that this book (Vol. 1) and the next (Vol. 2) are the funniest medical humor tomes you will ever read. Period.

The Placebo Journal was a print magazine (yes, actually print) and not online. It went out to as many as 10,000 subscribers bimonthly from 2001-2011. I launched it at the Scientific Assembly as a vendor and was promptly thrown out after two days. The system doesn't like rebels. It didn't help that we broke every rule and probably deserved it, but we persevered and continued.

It was a lot of work for me and Gordon Marshall, who is the illustrator. I also had a lot of help who I'll mention in the acknowledgements. That being said, the stories were mostly sent in by other medical personnel and are all true. Everything else you see is a way to make fun of the medical system. We make fun of patients, doctors, nurses, administrators, drug companies, health insurance companies, and on and on. You may be offended by some stuff. Get over it. The Placebo Journal was irreverent and way ahead of its time. Some of this stuff is gross. Much of it is politically incorrect. I don't care. Get over that, too.

There is no new stuff in these two books. Sorry. We had almost 1700 pages to choose from. These are our greatest hits, and I believe a cure for your medical boredom. It amazes me that all the stuff we made fun of back then is still applicable today.

These books are expensive. Get over that, too. You can afford it. Why so costly? There are tons of full colored pictures for every story. These books are works of art and art is expensive even if you think it sucks.

The format of these books is just like the actual Placebo Journal. They are like big magazines so there no story from start to finish. It was made to sit on the toilet and read and laugh just like the original was.

Here is another little secret and white lie. These two books are really comprised from issues #12 through issue #60. The first two years were published in The Placebo Chronicles by Broadway Books, a division of Random House in 2005. You can buy that if you want to see some more but it wasn't in color nor was it as pretty as these two are.

So, there you have it. I am making this short and sweet because you probably won't read it anyway. The healthcare system is still broken so try to enjoy an attempt to make fun of it otherwise you will just cry. I have always said that writing the Placebo Journal was the psychotherapy my health insurance kept denying me and I was right. Reading this stuff again made me laugh and be happy all over again. I hope it does the same for you.

Enjoy!

Doctor Doug

*King of Medicine*

# DOCTOR BUMPER STICKERS

You Are Unlikely To See.

Be nice to me: my parents made me go into medicine.

Doctors do it in the exam room.

I do NOT determine if you get SSD.

I am a doctor. I am human.
If you cut me do I not need zidovudine, lamivudine, indinavir, and interferon ribavirin prophylaxis?

My other wife is a drug rep.

MEAN PATIENT FREE ZONE

Healthcare is a human right BUT GOOD HEALTHCARE COSTS MONEY.

If you can read this . . . you'll get MRSA!

Will diagnose for food.

MY CHILD IS AN HONOR STUDENT and will go to medical school OVER MY DEAD BODY.

Defibrillate this!

My other car was lost in a malpractice suit.

I haven't washed my hands all day!

*Maybe Hippocrates was wrong?*

WWKD
What would Kevorkian do?

*JCAHO is coming. Look busy.*

ON-CALL PHYSICIAN:
This vehicle makes frequent stops at the liquor store.

If you are going to sell the narcotics I prescribe for you, then the least you can do is give me my cut.

This vehicle does NOT slow down for lawyers.

Will not answer any medical question outside the office without a co-pay.

NEW from PLACEBO Cards

# STD CARDS

Remember last night when I said you have NICE ABS? Well, you do, but now you also HAVE CRABS.

Maybe we will date some more, get married, and have babies, but until then I think you should know that I have a roaring case of scabies.

Don't be mad and get all out of sorts but I thought you should know that I probably gave you genital warts.

I relished our time together,
We frolicked all over the map.
You gave me my first standing O
And also a dose of the clap.

Roses are red,
Violets are blue,
So are the pustules
I gave to you.

**Available now at an adult store near you.**

**For those times you just want to tell that special someone (or just someone) that you may have given them a present he or she wasn't expecting.**

(Also available in text messaging format)

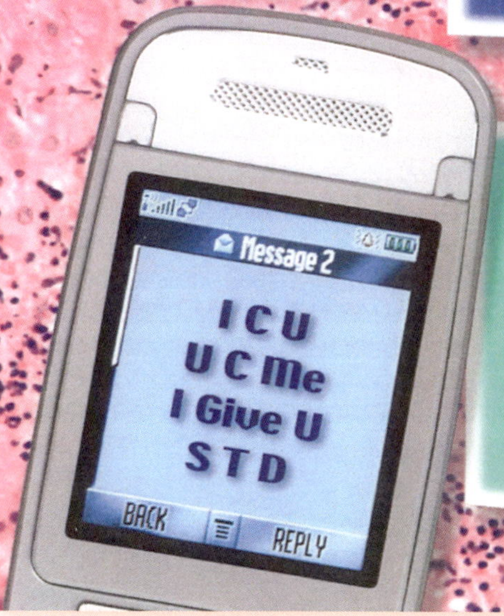


*It was a one night stand and I am glad to GET RID OF YA' but I thought I should tell you that you now have CHLAMYDIA.*

**Our tryst was a frolic to beholden,
Memories of such passions are golden,
But in my urethra was hid,
A bacteria GNID,
Which soon will leave your parts swollen.**

The hot bachelorette party dancer, whose phone calls you chose not to answer,
Would like to at least let you know you've increased, your risk of a cervical cancer.

## A TRUE STORY OF MEDICINE

# MASTER OF CLAY

Life at my hospital is not just a job; often times it is an adventure in crisis and tragedy . . . but when it's neither of these, it is simply one long on-going conquest for fun!

Dr. Vlaud Kreloshki was our medical examiner; or as he called himself 'Master of Clay" in reference to the stiff, pasty, clay-like state his "patients" assumed. Vlaud was not your typical doctor. He was 270 pounds of chiseled Romanian bedrock, sculpted into a six foot four inch tall appropriation of a man. Bald as the day he was born, he looked more like a night club bouncer than a learned man of medicine. The tribal tattoos (acquired as a med student) that ran from his chest to his wrists were often visible under a short-sleeved lab coat. Dr. Kreloshki is scary when he doesn't try to be. When he does try to be, many find themselves on the brink of hydrating their shorts.

Now, there are a rare number of things that bring a medical assistant and a medical examiner together in an adventurous, fruitful friendship. However, the love of f*cking with medical students is one of those very things!

In our hospital, **The Ringer** (my nickname) **& Vlaud Show** was legendary. Revered! Worshipped! And most of all . . . *grin* fully – if secretly – encouraged by our fun-loving administrative demigod *(yes, you read that right . . . 'fun-loving' and 'administrator' in the same sentence)*.

Much like the *Placebo Journal*, a new "episode" of **RVS** would circulate through the hospital as a new crop of cadavar-hungry med students showed up every couple of months. One class of neophytes we took great pleasure in harassing was the SurgStud, the surgery-bound know-it-alls who believed themselves endowed with magical, divine abilities, not to mention overentitling parents who encouraged their egotistical developments.

The timing was perfect . . . like all the planets aligning . . . this was the stuff myths, fables, legends, and national economies were based upon. We had a new crop of MedStuds and a fresh cadaver pulled straight from a sewage storm drain.

Vlaud had earlier determined it was death by drowning. Sadly, this individual appeared to be a homeless man who lived in the typically dry storm drains of the city. Flash rains had caught this poor soul entirely off guard . . . but the set of wind-up teeth with feet and little book of vulgar jokes found in his pockets told us that this guy probably appreciated going out with a postmortem bang.

The surgery students might as well have had little men in gaudy clothing running ahead with little gold trumpets heralding their arrival. What they weren't expecting was us; two large men, one who was VERY tall and VERY large, wearing dark grey scrubs with evil-looking black latex smocks over them *(these had to be purchased online from an S&M website)*. That, along with a half dozen "bad" – aka removed – overhead lights gave the morgue an appearance only found in horror movies. Vlaud, with his deep, guttural accent and baritone voice, only encouraged the sinister atmosphere.

*"Velcome 'udents. You have de honor of vitnessing a *real* autopsy. Not vone of those pandering, soft, peace'ully dead corpses. Our revered dead today drown in a dank sewer drain, crushed by a torrent of thousands of gallons of vater. I have taken measures to preserve the look of horror on his face . . . Follow me."*

It was apparent that over two-thirds of this group was wishing they were somewhere else, preferably where sun, fresh air, and alcohol was readily available. This also made it very clear who the "leaders" were; these individuals would receive some extra attention. The enthralled crowd of 18 students filed in after Vlaud. I, hiding a maniacal grin, filed in after them. The resounding heavy metallic sound of the doors being slammed shut made half of them jump and my emotionless apology didn't seem to settle any nerves . . . *perfect!*

Dr. Kreloshki turned down the evacuation vacuum a little on the room so the nauseating smell of cadaver was heavier then usual. Personally, I wanted to leave bubbling pots of liquid nitrogen on the floor for a nice covering of mist but agreed it would be too theatrical.

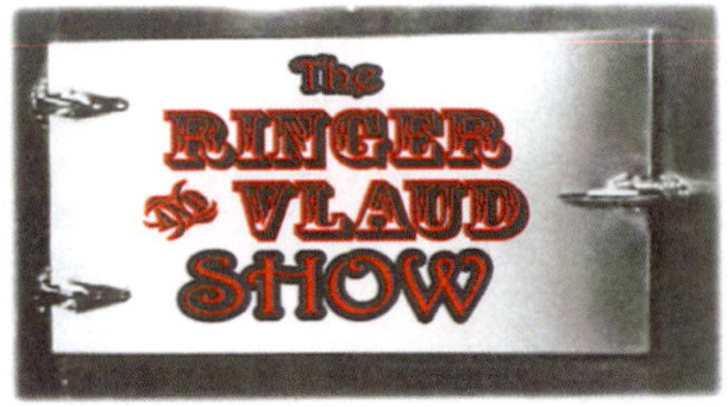


During a pause in the introductory monologue, I (still standing behind the med students) made a loud, and thoroughly unexpected announcement that if anyone felt sick, dizzy, or faint, they were to grab a partner and head out of the room to the morgue lounge. While everyone was staring at me, I got a thumbs up from Dr. Kreloshki as half the group had jumped excessively and now looked ready to change professions . . . probably to librarians.

- Two girls didn't make it beyond the chest saw and were taken out by two others **(14 left)**.
- After I loudly closed one of the freezer doors, another kid *(man?)* excused himself, thoroughly unnerved **(13 left)**.
- One girl ran out of the room when we pulled open the chest, one guy threw up in a trash can and left to clean up, another flat passed out at the smell of decay and was helped out by a second student **(9 left)**.
- Two excused themselves stating they had rounds to make *(bullsh*t!)* . . . just as we were looking for volunteers to help remove the organs **(7 left)**.

The two Ego Brothers (the leaders) were the best. Vlaud had picked them out at the beginning and the entire time they'd been making snide remarks like the egotistical, disrespectful asses they were. Dr. Kreloshki had given them front row seats for the abdomen inspection.

*"Have you two ever seen vhat the large bowel looks like up close?"*

*"Of course we have!"* answers Mr. Arrogant Ass #1.

*"Ah . . . but have you seen it corrupted by disease and decay!?"* With that, he slides his scalpel across the transverse bowel. With a sickening SLURKL sound, the contents of the bowel spill out and into the catch basin Vlaud placed under it. The smell made me retch from ten feet away. It was obviously far more enjoyable for those up close. Mr. AA#1 retched twice and threw up in his hands while Mr. AA#2 promptly passed out from the sight of it all and was dragged out by two other students **(2 left)**.

*"Dr. Kreloshki, this session has been most educational . . ."* Both Vlaud and I were instantly eyes-fixed on this cute, mousey little brunette 20-something woman, *". . . if you would not be offended, we would like your permission to step out to attend a cardiac bypass surgery."*

Vlaud looked absolutely floored, *"So you've known all this time?"*

The tiny med student smiled and said, *"My sister is a nurse in this hospital and had told me about the **RVS** adventures . . ."* she looked out the door, *". . . but more than that, I now know how to deal with those assholes. Fainting and throwing up on yourself isn't something you easily live down when your ego is a megolithic tower."*

Dr. Kreloshki just smiled at her and said, *"Vell now... I think I have a new friend today. You two keep this little melodrama our little secret yes?"* Silent nods, impish grins and gloved hands shook one another among the four of us.

***Damn this hospital is fun!*** +

# I Can't Believe It's Not Real Butter!

I did my residency training in pathology at a military medical center. For a while, the U.S. military had forces stationed in Haiti. Medical assets were deployed in support of the operation to provide care for sick or injured military personnel, as well as to perform humanitarian aid to the local people by providing them with modern medical care. Haiti is a desperately poor nation, and many of its citizens have never in their entire lives encountered modern medicine.

The deployed surgeons would send bizarre specimens to our pathology department in the United States. We saw mastectomy specimens that literally consisted more of tumor than normal breast parenchyma. We saw parasites that are almost unheard of in America.

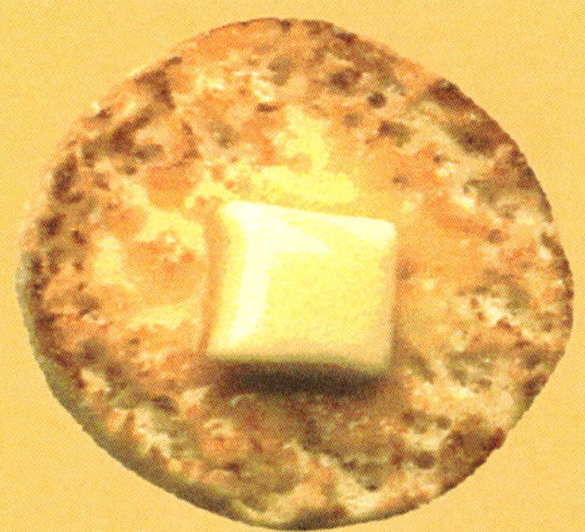

One day, I received a specimen labeled "breast cyst." The specimen had settled to the bottom of the transport container and formalin fixation had made it firm. It now bore the shape of the bottom of the container — a tan-white disc, three centimeters thick and ten centimeters in diameter. I bisected it to reveal that the specimen was filled with a semisolid bright yellow exudate. Given the shape of the specimen, after I bisected it, it looked exactly like a buttered English muffin. Microscopic examination revealed the lesion to be a lactating adenoma. The exudate was the result of breast milk which had been shaken. *It was actual butter!*

+

*EDITOR'S NOTE* - The authors recommend that the above exudate not be eaten.

# Medical Algorithm of Reality

## Risk Stratification for CHEST PAIN

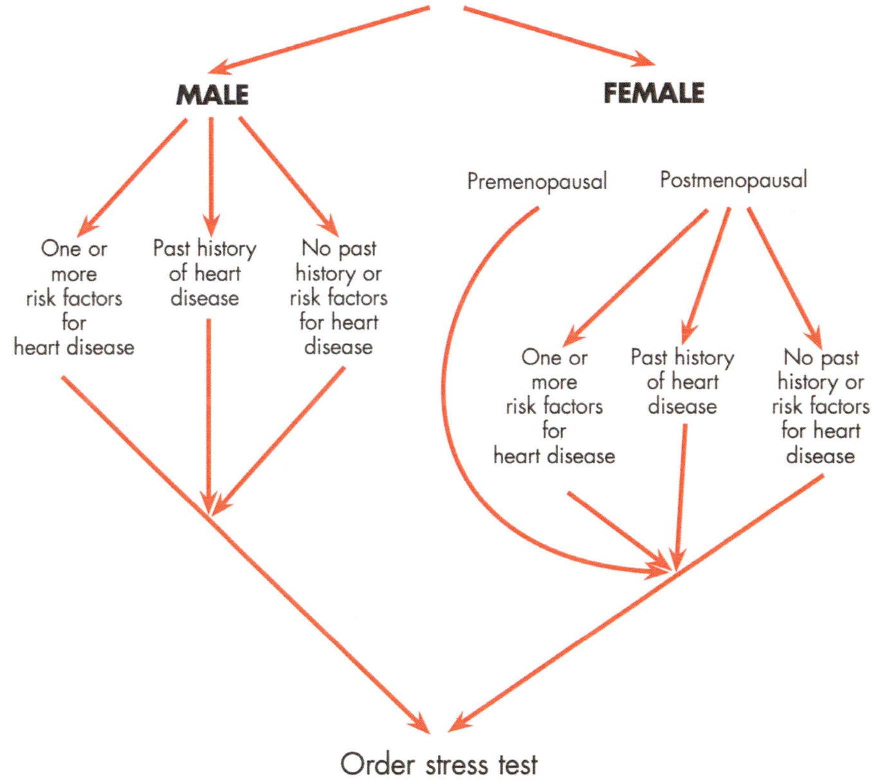

A drug rep left us a pan of fresh, warm cinnamon rolls in the break room yesterday. For the benefit of the member of our staff who was raised by wolves, and who ate the middle out of a roll, *Placebo Journal* presents:

# CINNAMON ROLL ETIQUETTE

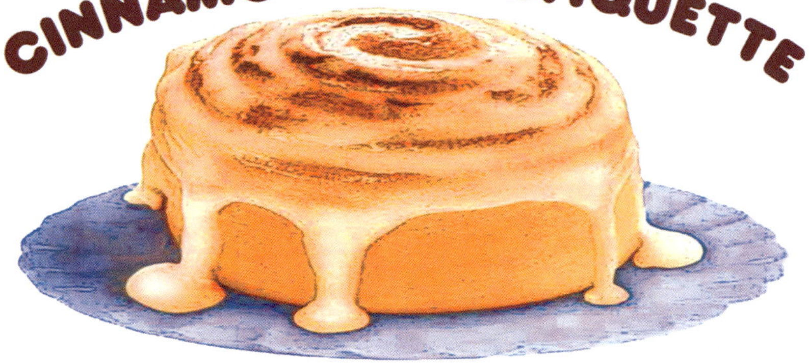

**PART ONE** (Cinnamon Roll Basics)

Cinnamon rolls are one of the culinary world's greatest paradoxes. They look delicious through and through, but often this appearance is misleading. The sad reality of the cinnamon roll world is that most cinnamon rolls actually are dry and crusty and less tasty on the outside 2/3 diameter of the roll, despite the tasty frosted appearance. We will refer to this outer dry area as *"The Wasteland."* Although most cinnamon rolls have *"The Wasteland"* on the outside, the majority have a moist and delicious center. This is the part of the cinnamon roll we will refer to as *"The Promised Land,"* or *TPL*.

The authors would like to point out that there are sometimes cinnamon rolls that are made to perfection and are tasty, moist, and delicious through and through. In essence, these rolls are all *TPL*, and are typically hyper-buttery and often have cinnamon-laden butter dripping down the edges, even when unheated. These are the cinnamon rolls dreams are made of, as well as heart attacks and strokes. Very few cinnamon rolls have such artery clogging perfection.

The responsibility of the cinnamon roll eater is to endure *"The Wasteland"* in utter and complete anticipation of *TPL*. Knowing that they will rarely find a rare perfect roll, the cinnamon roll eater will always enjoy *TPL* after eating *"The Wasteland"* and the gallon of milk it took to get it to go down. The guilt in knowing that *"The Wasteland"* is full of unenjoyed calories is completely erased by the deliciousness of *"The Promised Land."*

**PART ONE: SUBSECTION A**
(Wastefulness and Strict Diets)

The inconsiderate cinnamon roll eater will discard *"The Wasteland"* and enjoy only *TPL*. This is considered rude to the baker of the roll, and there is generally no excuse for such behavior. For the eater who is on a very strict diet, it is generally considered acceptable to skip to *TPL* but the eater must discard *"The Wasteland"* in a place where nobody will ever find it, such as a pop can, a toilet paper tube, or the desk drawer of a disliked coworker. Also note that the strict dieter has no business eating any cinnamon rolls in the first place, so if the dieter does eat a *TPL* while properly and discretely disposing *"The Wasteland,"* they should not be observed doing any of this. If a dieter is observed behaving in such a barely acceptable manner, they will be known as a "diet hypocrite" and should expect to be ignored by peers and anticipate social isolation for days to weeks. Such isolation can be cut short by the busted dieter if they bake a pan of cinnamon rolls and bring them to the office but don't eat any.

**PART TWO: THE WHOLE PAN PHENOMENON**

Occasionally, the reader will find himself in the coveted position of having an entire pan of cinnamon rolls at their disposal, rather than just one roll. The most common setting for this blissful encounter is at a social gathering or a break room at work.

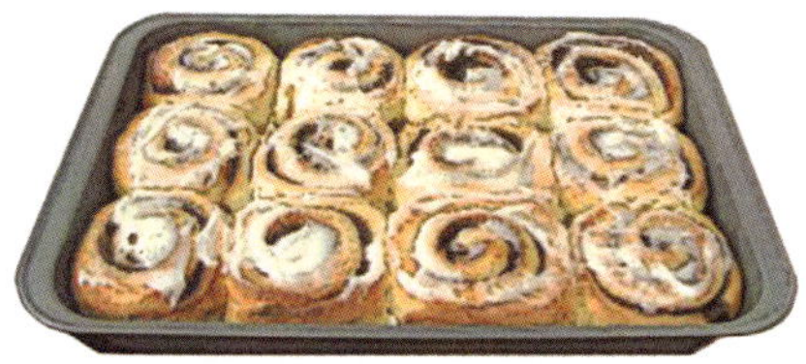

**PART TWO: SUBSECTION A**
(Roll Selection from a Pan)

The first point of etiquette at the pan encounter is the choice of roll. There are two kinds of rolls, those that are in the center of the pan (no borders with the edge of the pan, and thus less crust) and those that have one or two borders that were in such contact. In older more formal days, proper cinnamon roll etiquette dictated that the first eater to encounter the pan was to start in the upper left corner of the pan and no other roll was a polite choice. Subsequent eaters worked their way from left to right and down, as if reading a book, but more tasty.

More liberal thinking is the norm in the early 21st century, and as some eaters might enjoy a no-crust roll, any roll is fair game, as long as the roll can be removed without damaging the rolled structure of any adjoining rolls. If any roll is damaged while removing a center roll, the eater must refrain from removing the originally targeted roll, and instead remove the damaged roll and keep it for them self.

**PART TWO: SUBSECTION B**
(The Chief Rule of Cinnamon Roll Eating)

This point of etiquette was added in the 20th century after several children were found living outside a suburb of London in a forest, having been raised by wolves. Prior to that, no humans, even the most profoundly handicapped of the mentally handicapped, had ever lacked the common sense to violate the chief rule of cinnamon roll eating so no official etiquette rules to its effect were ever adopted. This rule was adopted after one of these feral children (who walked on all fours and cleaned himself with his tongue) was found eating a *TPL* after having cut it out of the center of a roll in a pan encounter. Without shame, he left *"The Wasteland"* for someone else to eat, but denied them the pleasure of *TPL*.

Obviously, the chief rule of cinnamon roll eating is that when an eater finds himself in a coveted pan encounter, the eater is to **NEVER**, under ANY CIRCUMSTANCES, **EVER** remove *TPL* from a roll and leave *"The Wasteland."*

But the biggest and most grievous error in etiquette that an eater could ever make, (and would subsequently rightfully cause all peers in his social group to assume that he was raised by wolves) would be to remove *TPL* from multiple rolls in a pan, leaving multiple *Wastelands* for their peers.

We hope that these have been useful guidelines for those of you walking around on all fours. ✚

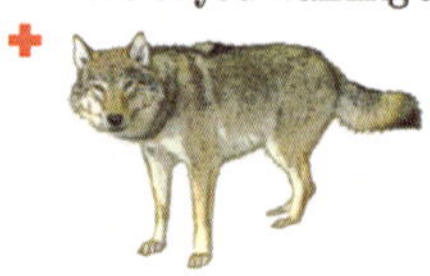

## PLACEBO JOURNAL

# TRUE STORIES OF MEDICINE

## EXPLOSION

In my former life as a surgical resident, *(liked the job, hated the hours, became a pathologist instead)* each resident did endoscopies one day a week. It is, of course, good medical practice to do a rectal exam prior to inserting the scope, and I did this while standing somewhat to the side of the frail elderly patient. Unfortunately, the two nurses assisting me were directly behind the patient because they could lean against the sink there. This was back in the era when nurses still wore white dresses, and many still wore nurse's caps. When I removed my finger, the patient had explosive diarrhea all over my two poor assistants. The nurses wore scrubs the rest of the day and probably the rest of their lives. ✚

## MORE TRUE STORIES

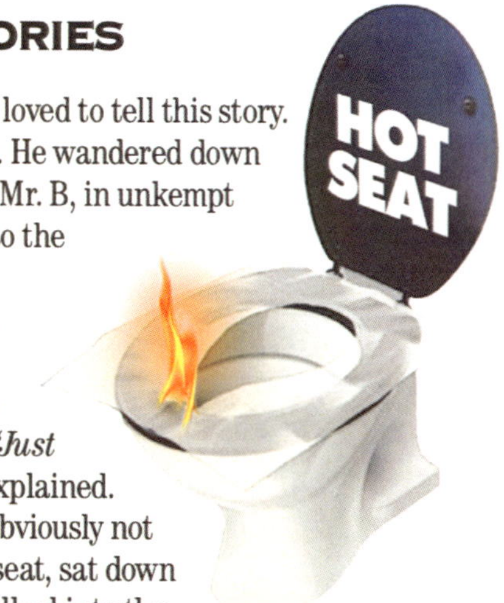


My late husband was a surgeon who loved to tell this story. He was on call and had a rare quiet night. He wandered down to the ED to visit with a couple residents. Mr. B, in unkempt clothes and a distinct body odor, came into the ED with his entire rear end and scrotum cherry red from burns. They asked how it happened.

He explained he went to a mall men's room and pulled out a paper toilet cover. *"Just wanted to have it clean, you know,"* he explained. Now this brought a smile as the guy was obviously not keen on hygiene. He put the cover on the seat, sat down and lit up a forbidden smoke. Someone walked into the men's room so to hide the evidence he tossed the cigarette in the toilet. But the little paper perforated center of the toilet cover was still intact. **It caught fire and flared up.** He flew off the john but it was stuck to his butt until he pulled it off. They treated him for second degree burns and sent him on his way. ✚

## A DIFFERENT ANIMAL ALTOGETHER

I had heart surgery (a valve replaced) and went to rehab on *Lovenox* shots twice a day. When I was released from rehab I went home with the *Lovenox* and instructions on taking it. My physician hubby was in Chicago teaching. Not to worry, I was well versed in giving injections and had no qualms about doing it myself. But my daughter, a vet tech for the Army, was visiting. That afternoon I showed her the meds and syringes. She said she would take over the *Lovenox* injections for the duration of her visit. She prepared the injection, popped it into my belly smoothly then smiled wickedly.

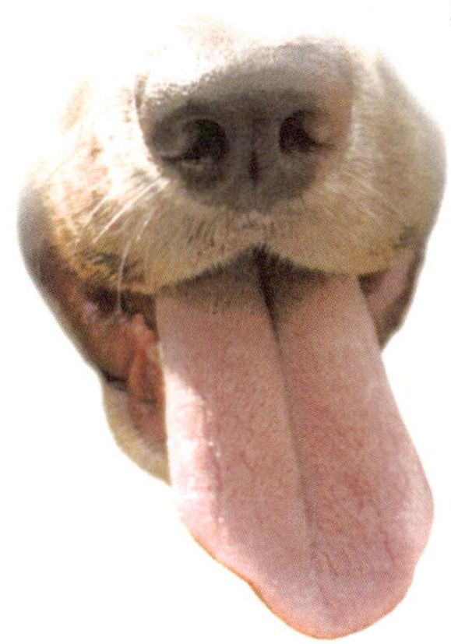

I asked, *"What's up?"*

She said, *"You are the first human I ever did that to. Most of my patients usually howl or lick my face."*

I declined to lick her face. ✚

# PHOTOCOPY THESE PAGES AND HAND OUT TO YOUR PATIENTS

# American Family Practitioner

## INFORMATION FROM YOUR FAMILY DOCTOR

## The Common Cold: What You Should Know

### What is a cold?

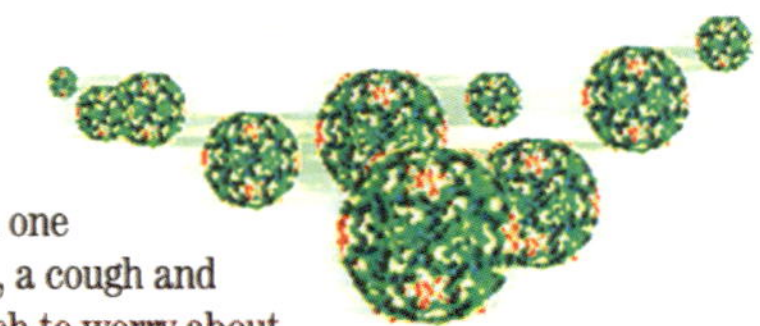

A cold is a virus. It is very common. In fact, most people are aware that there is not much we can do for it. It spreads from one person to another. You may get a runny nose, a cough and a sore throat. In any event, it really isn't much to worry about. This begs the question why you have shown up to our office today?

### What should I do if I have a cold?

First off, in the future, don't come in to see me. Second, don't call. You can try anything you want from over the counter at your local pharmacy. None of it will work, but it will buy time so that you forget about bothering our office.

### What is the difference between the flu and the cold?

There is tons of literature which describes the difference. All of it is bullsh%t. The bottom line is that the treatment is the same. Do nothing. Unless of course you are a wussy. Then I will be forced to give you a placebo disguised as an antibiotic or anti-viral medication.

### There must be something you can do to cure a cold.

Is there some type of disconnect here or are you just an idiot? I said there is nothing I can do. Suck it up.

### My Uncle says he rubs *Vicks Vapor Rub* on his feet and goes to bed with his socks on and he is better the next morning. Can I try that??

Dude, you can jam a pineapple up your ass for all I care. It ain't going to help, but as long as you don't bother me then I am fine with it.



**Please note:** The information presented is the best we could make up. Depending on our mood, this could always change. Some of this material is not suited for anyone.

### What about using *Zithromax*?

All right, now I am getting pissed off. *Zithromax* is an antibiotic. It won't help viruses. Get it. It is like spraying a bug killer on weeds.

### They say zinc works. What are your thoughts?

I am thinking that I would like to pummel you. Unless you want to go into the smelting business, you don't need zinc. If you continue to ask ridiculous questions I cannot be held accountable for my actions.

### When will my cold go away?

I'm serious. You need to stop.

### Do you think I should take some herbal remedies?

That's it . . .
I am going to kick your . . .

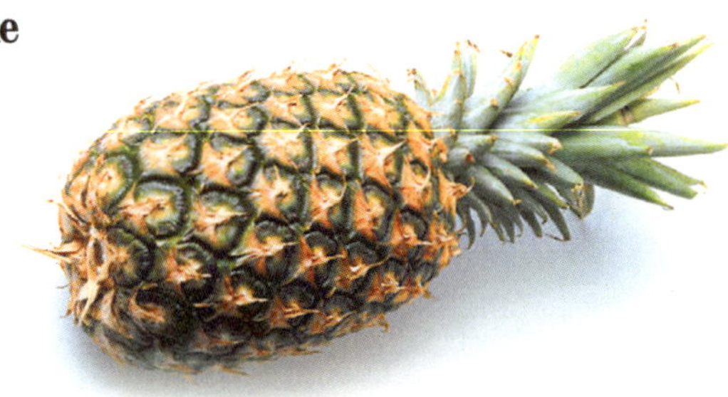

*This handout provides a general idea of this topic. Not everyone will like what they read. For those people, we recommend talking to your own family doctor.*

CORNELIUS PARODY MD AND ARISTOTLE JONES PHD

*Below is a case study which reveals a new but common syndrome plaguing many medical offices around the country. Drs. Parody and Jones use their unique style to address this disorder and give some recommendations for treatment. Please review carefully.*

# Disabilicus

**CC:** Chronic back pain

**HPI:** Jim is a 29 year-old white male who states he has had chronic back pain since he was 6 years of age. He feels that he has never had relief from this pain. Any type of physical work or job actually makes it worse. He has *"never been happy and has tried many different antidepressants but they have been no help. The only medication that did help was Ativan® or Valium® but his last doctor "shut me off. I hate that dick!"*

Jim is newly employed at a large textile mill. This was his twelfth job in the last three years. On the third day on the job, he states he stepped on a loose screw that was left on the floor. He claims to have heard an audible *"pop"* from his back, which made him fall to his knees. Jim's bosses made him go to the ER. All x-rays were negative and he was sent home on Darvocet® and *"lots of Valium"*.

Today Jim seems to be in agony after entering the room. This was a marked change from his laughing in the waiting room while speaking to his friends (something noticed by the receptionist). He describes his pain as a 20 on a 1 to 10 scale. It is diffusely located throughout his lower back and radiates into both legs, both testicles and his left forth toe. The pain never leaves and nothing has ever helped it.

**PMH:** Cellulitis secondary to infected scrotal ring

**SxHx:** none

**SH:** Never married. Two children but never sees them. Dropped out of high school after eleventh grade. Rides a motorcycle and snowmobile. Loves NASCAR racing. Goes to bed at 2:00 AM after playing Play Station® all night. Sleeps until noon. Drinks over two cases of beer a week. Smokes six to seven joints of marijuana a day. Smokes two and a half packs of cigarettes a day. Arrested on multiple occasions for driving under the influence, possession of a handgun, selling marijuana.

**FH:** Brother has bad depression and is on **disability**. Sister has chronic cystitis and is on **disability**. Father has been on **disability** since he was age 24 for alcoholism. Mother on **disability** for *"something to do with her ear"*.

**Meds:** none

**All:** NKDA

**Pertinent ROS:** Tired all the time, poor dentition, occasional sores on his penis, anal warts.

**PE:** **HT** 5'11", **WT** 138 pounds, **BP** 111/59, **HR** 79

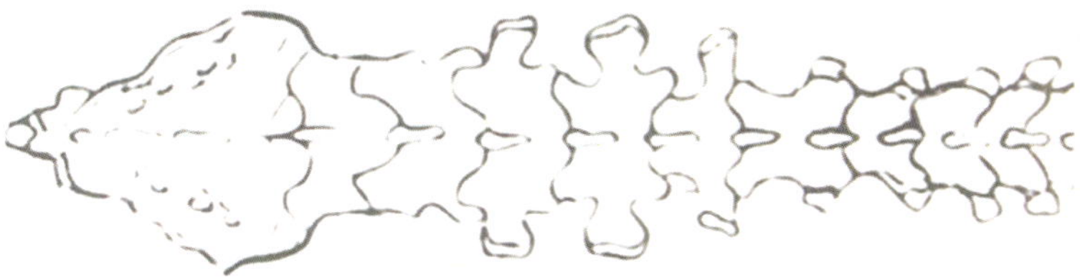





**Gen:** Poor hygiene, marijuana smell pervasive; Very relaxed but poor eye contact; limping while getting up, but left the office without a limp

**Neck** - supple
**Lungs** - occasional wheeze
**Cardiac** - mildly tachycardia
**Abd** - soft
**Ext** - no edema
**Back** - exaggerated pain with normal straight leg raises, easily distractible, muscle soft as fresh dough and without spasm
**Neuro** - normal sensation to light touch and pain, normal DTR

**Workup:** TSH normal. Sed rate normal. MRI, EMG ordered by an ER doctor was all within normal limits. Refuses any type of tox screen.

**Diagnosis:**

**Disabilicus**

**Discussion:** **Disabilicus** is a disease of increasing proportion as well as disturbing relevance. There is a good chance that many patients are diagnosed with other "diseases" or "syndromes" each year that are in fact true cases of **Disabilicus**. This is troubling as we are unable to truly estimate the exact amount of **Disabilicus** in the United States each year. We postulate it is in the range of 250,000 to 2,000,000.

**Disabilicus** is a strange disease that has been isolated to the short arm of Chromosome 7 or what we like to call the "Lazy" gene. Interestingly, the transmission is seemingly non-sex linked but is usually pervasive throughout a patient's family *(As we saw with our patient, Jim).*

All these patients have very similar attributes and should be easy to spot by a physician. Basically, they do not like to work. Ever. The cost of trying to prove or disprove their pain can be quite high. The authors feel it doesn't have to be so outrageous. Since there is no mystery to their case, the work-up should be very cut and dry.

In sum, with these types of patients, there is a lot less here than meets the eye.

**Treatment:** Treatment for **Disabilicus** is frustrating. Many patients will continue to somatisize new complaints or just fake them altogether. **It is not their fault.** Subconsciously, they just do not want to work. Their "Lazy" gene overrides any type of guilt they may have of sponging off their parents, friends and now the system. This does not make their care any less annoying. In fact, many physicians will use these patients as examples as to why they quit the profession.

The only success the physician can hope for is to get these patients out of their practice. Since these patients will never stop trying to get **disability** or worker's compensation, they will continually bother their practitioner until he or she succumbs to their efforts. Like the terminator, *"it's what he does. It's all he does!"* The fact that they have no job, your only chance is that their laziness will prevent them from following through on all the paperwork, doctor's visits, and phone calls that it takes to get to their goal. Unfortunately, in a strange ironic twist, patients with **Disabilicus** seem to be able to follow through on anything it takes to get **disability** and nothing else.

**Use This Knowledge Wisely.**

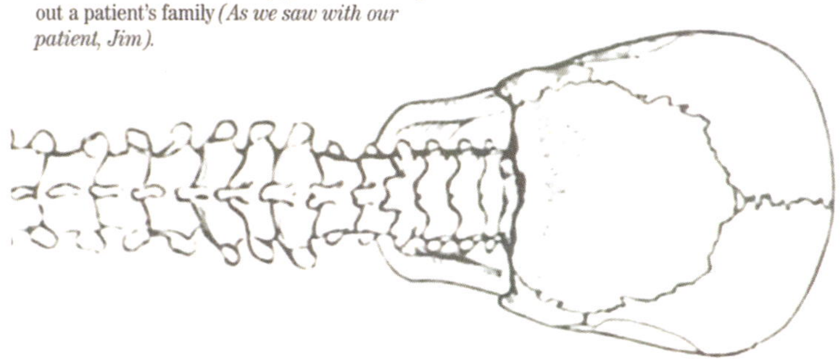

## MORE TRUE STORIES OF MEDICINE

# DON'T MUMBLE

Most of my patients in Internal (Eternal) Medicine are quite elderly and many are hard of hearing. I have tried to learn to enunciate clearly so miscommunications are minimal and instructions clearly understood.

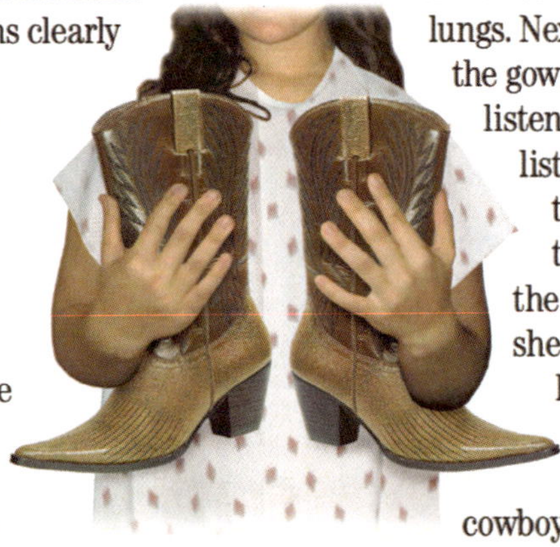

Once in awhile we do have the employed, well groomed, younger (under 80) patient who just needs a health maintenance visit. One attractive young lady in her mid 30s presented for a physical exam and was asked to put on the ubiquitous unflattering gown and have a seat on the exam table. As I entered the room I was relieved to be seeing someone who did not have seven or eight complicated medical issues.

After some small talk and history taking, I placed the stethoscope on her back to listen to her lungs. Next I placed it under the gown on her chest to listen to her heart. As I listened, I happened to glance down towards the end of the table and noticed she had removed all of her clothing except a fine pair of highly polished cowboy boots. I complimented her and said, ***"nice boots."***

She then turns, smiles and says: *"Oh you really think so? Thanks! My husband thinks they are too small."* +

# VIGOROUS TUG

It was the summer of 1980 and I was doing my pharmacy internship at *Upstate Medical Center* in Syracuse, NY. Every morning I would go up to the eighth floor which is a general medical unit and also a step down unit for the ICU at the end of the hall and I would check the med cart and refill the meds.

One morning I was at the nurses' station an one of the telemetry monitors suddenly showed Vfib. A nurse hit the code blue alarm and everyone went running. This included the three medical teams on the floor and the team in the ICU. The first nurse and physician burst into the semi-private room with many others close behind them. Fortunately, *or unfortunately*, the 18-year-old male patient who was alone in the room was not in Vfib but rather was exercising his forearm. +

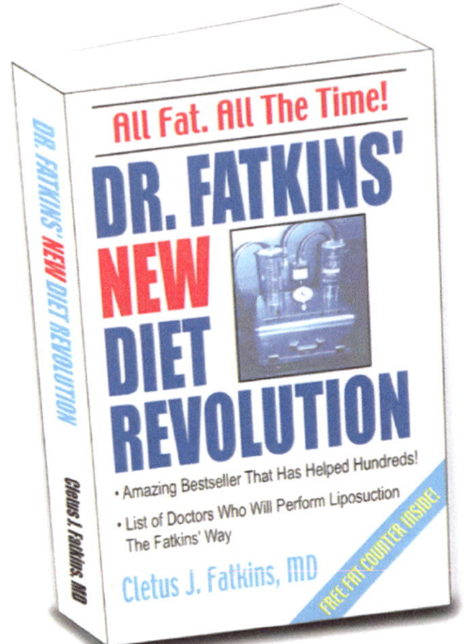


## NOW AVAILABLE FROM PLACEBO PUBLISHING!

**With the FATKINS Diet you can eat all the fat you want.**

**Nothing is out of bounds anymore. Deer fat, cow fat, and pig fat are just some of what you can have –**

## GUILT FREE.

**With the FATKINS Extreme Plan, Americans will even be able to feast on human fat.**

**Our liposuction recipes allow you to save your own adipose tissue for a tasty dinner treat.**

**Finally, your diet will be weight and calorie neutral**

## BECAUSE YOU ARE EATING YOURSELF!

The FATKINS Nutritional Approach rebalances your appetite and your body fat so that you improve your energy level and look great. Following this approach lays the groundwork for being thinner. It will, however, not improve your health.

The twelve-phase individualized eating plan allows you to knowledgeably select which foods to eat based on smell, appearance and animal from which the fat was removed. Selections will change in varying degrees depending on the species you choose starting from smaller animals (squirrels, rats, etc) and moving up to larger breeds (cows, moose, elephants, etc). In step twelve, participants finally hit the pinnacle of the FATKINS Plan and get to indulge on their own fat.

Recipes include:
Butter Nut Thigh Soup
"Indulgent" Cellulite Cream Pie
Fajita Fat with Peppers
Human Cheese Steak Surprise
Jamaican Jerk Fat (we are not able to list these ingredients as it may be too distasteful for some)

Customize the program to your own individual needs. You can even ask others to donate their body fat. *What could be better?*

**WARNING:** There is no actual science behind the FATKINS Diet. It may actually be a bad thing for you. Do not ask your doctor about the FATKINS Diet as he or she may laugh you out of the office.

*"After years of being on the road eating potato chips, I decided I needed a change. Now it's only pork rinds and meat grizzle for me!"*
David, reporter

*"My plastic surgeon gave me fourteen pounds of my own body fat back. I cook it in bacon grease and soy sauce and it is delicious!"*
Barbara, homemaker

*"I was obese with diabetes and heart disease. I couldn't fit into any of my clothes. Now I am thinner with diabetes and heart disease, but all my clothes fit great!"*
Randy, bus driver

**Dr. Cletus J. Fatkins** is a pioneer in barometric medicine and is the leading champion of the all-you-can eat fat approach to nutrition. He is an esteemed nutritionist who was never able to finish college. His degree is in results! Prior to creating this unique approach to diet, Dr. Fatkins received an internet diploma that has questionable legal ramifications. Thousands of people have heard him talk on informercials, which has only increased his credibility. Dr. Fatkins likes to play the flute, enjoys a faux tan, and even designs women's clothing.

# Feng Shui Tips For An Inner-City Medical Office

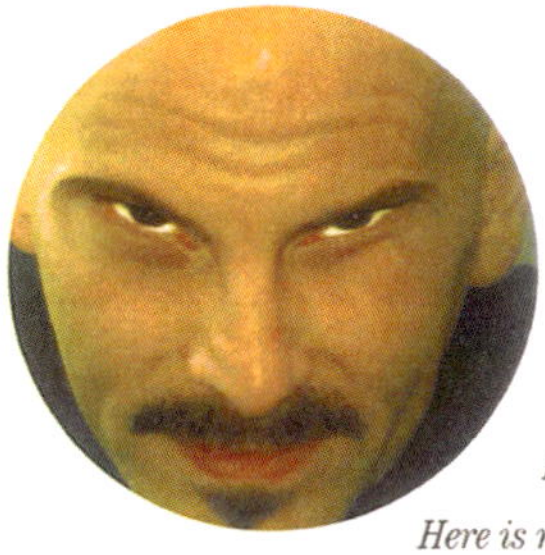

PRACTICE MANAGEMENT CORNER

Written by
Al Truistic B.S.

*Here is my expert advice to help improve your office environment. These Feng Shui recommendations will greatly transform your inner-city medical office into a more peaceful, roomy, and tranquil setting. The staff as well as other doctors in the practice will be amazed at the transformation. It will help you attain peace of mind, create more space and comfort and also allow you to become more productive! Most importantly, these tips will enable you live to practice another day. While I am no Feng Shui master, I did take a half-day community college course so I am pretty darn close. If you need more advice, I would need to analyze a specific problem for a proper diagnosis and then give you more tips that can be followed to keep your office in balance. My fee would be a bus ticket and possibly a warm meal.*

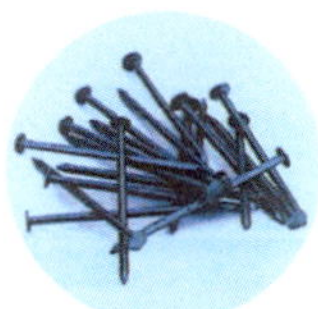

**1.** The arrangement of the waiting room chairs should be in a harmonious position so that chi is able to flow smoothly. Have a good amount of space between them so patients don't start fighting with each other. Nail all chairs to the floor to prevent them from being stolen or thrown at other patients.

**2.** You should not have any cactus or sharp-looking plants in your office as these plants have small sharp leaves and therefore cause "shar chi" in the office. It will also cut the sh*t out of little kids whose parents ignore your warnings and even encourage the little tots to play with them.

**3.** Use a metal wind chime made of six or seven metal rods about one foot long. The sound of metal is the best way to activate chi or disperse negative chi. Be sure it is not too accessible as patients will pocket it and possibly use it as a weapon or shim against you if you don't give them the narcotics they are craving.

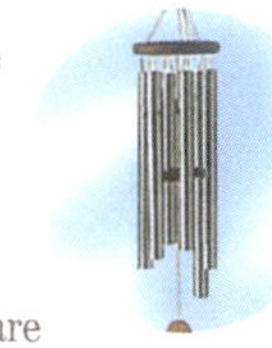

**4.** The chi from the main entrance of your office should not meet a wall inside the office. Instead use a metal detector, which will cause the chi to be more vibrant while also repelling those patients with semi-automatic weapons.

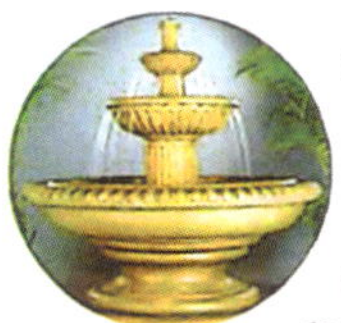

**5.** One may consider placing an indoor fountain in your waiting area to activate chi in order to bring a sense of calm to the patients. Be aware, however, that there is a good chance some of your patients will urinate in it.

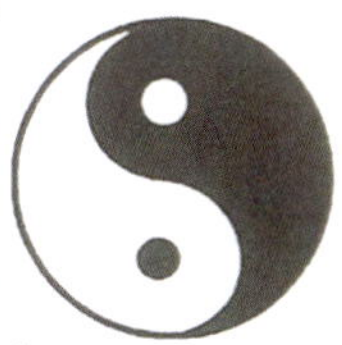

**6.** Have a good balance of yin and yang when decorating your medical office. Balance light and dark colors, soft and hard surfaces, insurance and Medicaid patients, fat and skinny nurses, and young and old doctors.

**7.** Keep your electrical cords to your office equipment well hidden. This will eliminate clutter and allow for the free flow of chi. It will also decrease the chance of some of the pediatric patients from chewing on them and the subsequent lawsuits that will follow.

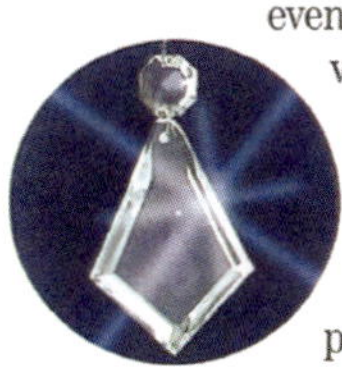

**8.** Try using a hanging crystal in your office entrance to enhance chi. To enhance the chi even more, purchase a video surveillance system to put inside the crystal. Actually this does nothing for the chi but will enable you to see which one of your staff is stealing all the petty cash.

**9.** When in an examination room, always sit with an open door behind your back to ensure that you have an easy exit from violent or threatening patients.

**10.** Chi should flow freely through your office, entering through the front door and exiting out the back. Clutter, sharp angles, nooks and crannies, and storage areas can slow down energy and make it harder for the police to find and arrest your most difficult patients.

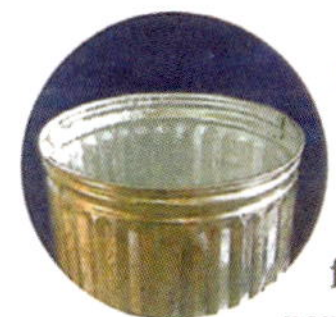

**11.** Do not have clutter in your personal office. Your desk must be kept tidy and clutter free. Since this is impossible for physicians to follow, just throw out all paperwork that cannot be quickly and mindlessly signed.

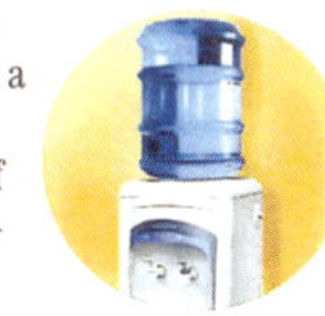

**12.** A powerful cure in Feng Shui is water. Water is able to transform the chi in your office to bring more balance and harmony. Have a water cooler for patients and liberally add samples of antidepressants and/or benzodiazepines.

**13.** Place a three-legged Toad God figure near your front office entrance to attract luck and wealth. Unfortunately, this will be stolen within one week.

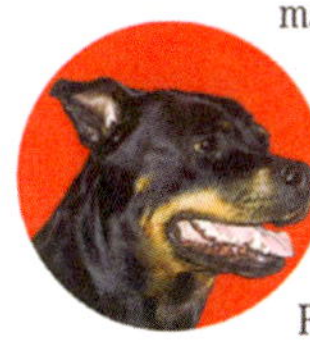

**14.** Try purchasing Fu Dog (male and female) figures and use them as protective animals when placed near the doorway of your office entrance to protect from evil influences. They are a symbol of valor and prosperity. These also will be stolen. Use live Rottweilers from there on out.

***AHHH . . . PEACE OF MIND***

**15.** If you have any negative energy directed at your front office door (vandalism), Ba Gua mirrors will help to disperse the negative energy. After this fails, hook up the surveillance video here as well.

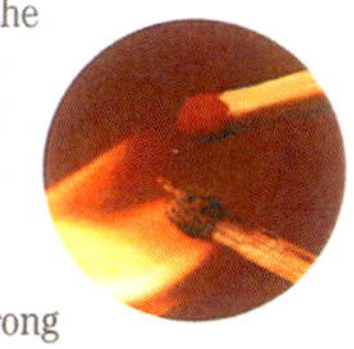

**16.** The bathroom is the most yin room in the office because of the presence of water. Yang elements, such as bright colors or candles may be added, but will do nothing without a really strong deodorant. At the very least, have the patients burn a match!

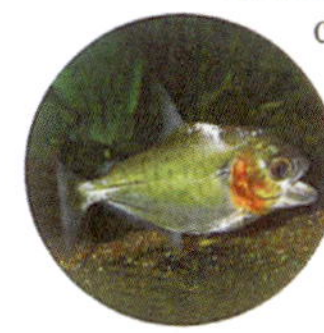

**17.** Place an aquarium in the east, north, or southeast of the office for calmness and tranquility. Use piranhas to balance the aesthetic chi with the chances of patients putting their hands in the tank and trying to steal the fish.

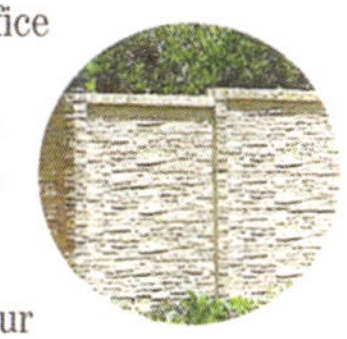

**18.** Use trees, shrubbery, and gardens outside the office to slow down or to screen out fast-moving or negative energy. When this fails, use concrete barricades.

**19.** Do not arrange your workspace so that you look straight out into a corridor or see the stairs, storage rooms, closets, elevators, escalators, or toilets. This improves your energy chi and decreases your chances of being shot.

**20.** Food represents wealth and therefore the office kitchen can generate general happiness. Three major elements need to be in balance:

a. Fire with its yang energy.
b. Water which is a yin force.
c. Drug lunches with its freebie chi and hot-looking reps. ✚

PJ PHARMACEUTICALS INTRODUCES

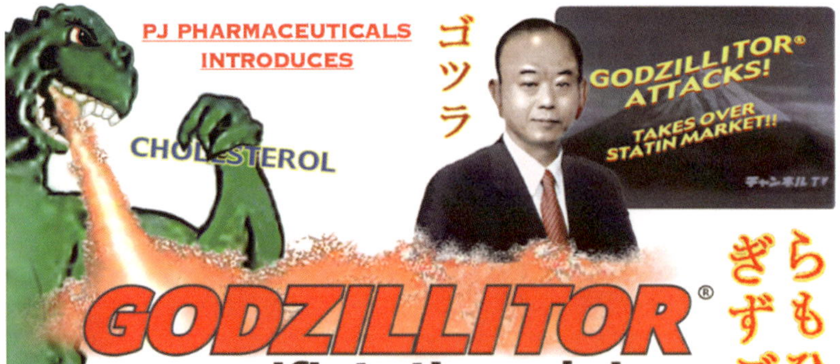
CHOLESTEROL
ゴッラ
GODZILLITOR® ATTACKS!
TAKES OVER STATIN MARKET!!

# GODZILLITOR®

## scifistatin calcium

らもひ
ぎずご

### "King of the Statins"

*Subtitles or not, GODZILLITOR®'s results will not be lost in translation.*

Finally, East truly meets West with GODZILLITOR®. Why do you think the Japanese have such little heart disease, anyway? You didn't think it was due to their diet, did you?

GODZILLITOR® is an invincible chemical creature created with incredible strength and efficacy. With its fiery statin blast, Godzillitor lowers any cholesterol in sight.

Did you know that a lot of people have high cholesterol? In fact, some people have such "fatty" blood that you can actually hear it move throughout their body.

*GODZILLITOR® is here to attack the problem.*

FACTS:

- Synthetically engineered and mutated by atomic radiation.
- The next and last step in statin evolution.
- Has a refreshing minty taste!

*GREAT FOR PATIENTS ON THE FATKINS 'DIET!*
(See advertisement on page 19).

Who needs all that cumbersome outcome data? Not PJ Pharmaceuticals. Sure, we don't have any lipid lowering studies, but our sales are through the roof and we have the best direct-to-consumer ads ever created!

GODZILLITOR is a prescription medication for use in obliterating any kind of cholesterol. In clinical studies, almost 40 percent of patients completed the regimen. The most common side effects are muscle pain, death, burtsing livers, constipation, weakness, stomach pain, nausea, chest pain, herpes, dengue fever, hemorrhoids, death, drooling, vaginal or penile discharge, rash, death, open sores, ear aches, sniffles and death.

After starting GODZILLITOR you should still follow a diet low in fat and cholesterol and exercise regularly. Since we all know that there is no way in hell that you will do that, just take GODZILLITOR and hope for the best.

Only your doctor can decide if GODZILLITOR is right for you. Be sure to tell your doctor if you:

- Have any money or insurance.
- Drink alcohol like a fish.
- Have a living will.
- Are very litigious.

COMING SOON:
Mothracol • Rodanitor • Megalonizol
from PJ PHARMACEUTICALS

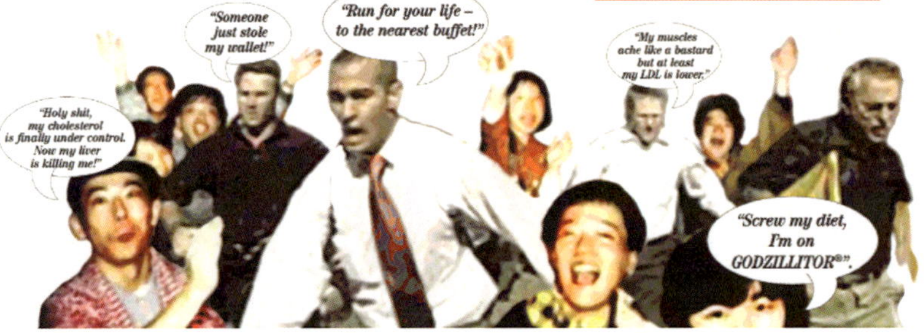
"Holy shit, my cholesterol is finally under control. Now my liver is killing me!"
"Someone just stole my wallet!"
"Run for your life – to the nearest buffet!"
"My muscles ache like a bastard but at least my LDL is lower."
"Screw my diet, I'm on GODZILLITOR®".

MEDICAL PRACTICE OF THE FUTURE

# IF HMO's HAD THEIR WAY. . .

***In the future, patient gowns will come complete with Easy-Access Openings so you can save time and see more patients.***

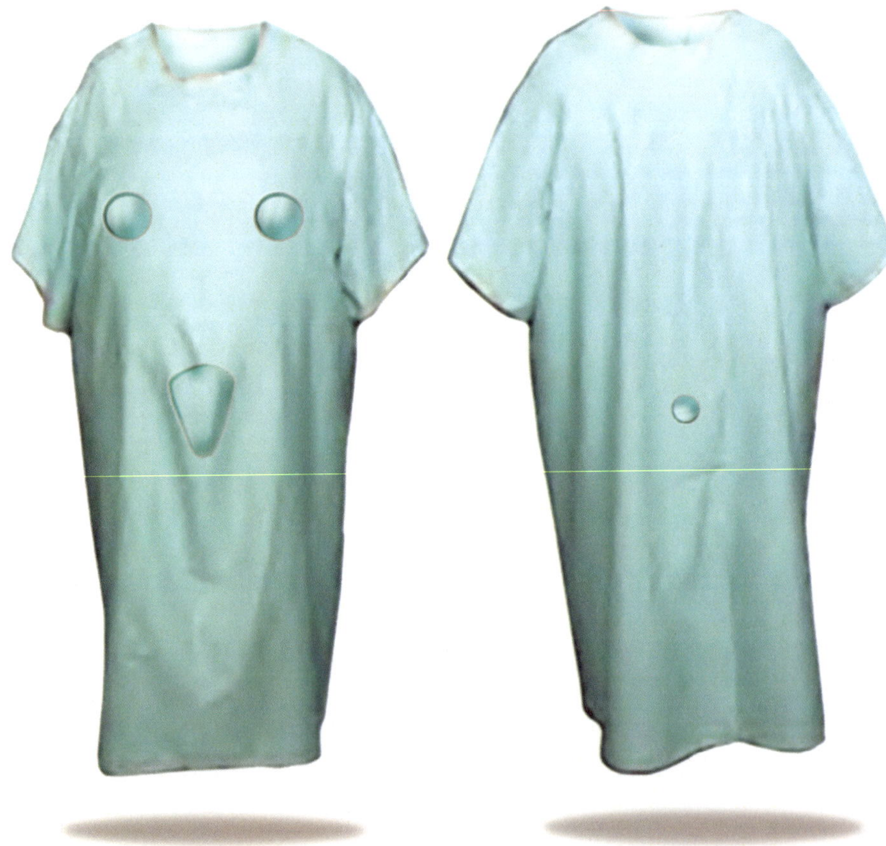

## ANOTHER TRUE STORY OF MEDICINE

# CAUGHT SWEARING

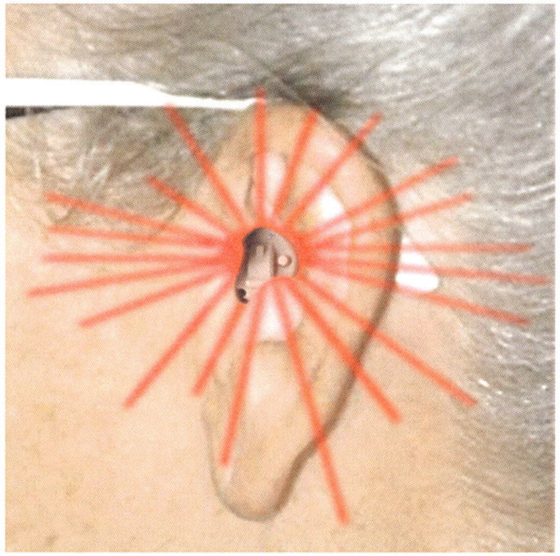

I work as a female internist in a large HMO and I have a panel of 50 to 90 year-olds, mostly women. They come in with long lists *(as always!)* of screening tests and printouts from the internet *(yes, even the 80-year-olds!)* One day, I had an 84-year-old patient who was extremely hard of hearing come in. She was wearing a hearing aid with a microphone. She had come in for a full physical, including Pap smear, despite the fact that I had told her repeatedly that, given her lifelong history of normal annual Pap smears, she really did not need them anymore.

As I saw her chart on my desk, I started cursing loudly to my medical assistant, ***"G*&@D*@*@, Mrs. Taylor! I F*@#&#^ TOLD her that she does not need Pap smears any more, there is no G*&@D*@*ed WAY I am going to be able to do a full physical with Pap smear and follow her congestive heart failure and everything in 20 minutes – it's going to take her that long to get up into the F*@#&#^ stirrups with her hip arthritis!"***

I ranted for a few more minutes before looking at my medical assistant, who was holding the patient's microphone in her hand, with the green light on *(signaling it was on!)*

I quaked as went into the patient's exam room, said, *"Hello, Mrs. Taylor! It is so good to see you!"* while pretending that nothing had happened.

At the end of the visit, Mrs. Taylor said to me, *"Can I say something?"*

*"Of course, Mrs. Taylor!"* I said, bracing for the worst. I could just imagine the complaint that she was about to file to the management. She leaned over to speak to me confidentially, *"You might want to talk to your assistant about her language. I'm afraid I heard her swearing about one of the patients."*

I promised her I would. +

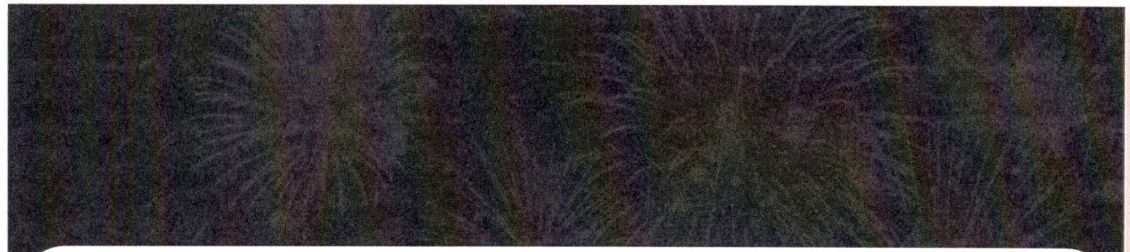

## THOSE DARN NARC SEEKERS

n the way the patient tells the story than from the story itself. *James B. Herrick*

### TRICK OR TREAT?

**Mr. Tricket presented to my Occupational Clinic for a Work Comp injury. Just out of my Family Practice residency, I was eager to impress my colleagues in the department. Unfortunately, I was also rather naive regarding "narc seekers". As I perused the intake form I noted that he was employed as a "Pyrotechnic Engineer" and his complaint was low back pain from lifting heavy fireworks. More curious about his career than the back pain, I saw him over about four months while he related wonderful stories about huge firework displays that he "engineered" for the City of Chicago's Fourth of July, etc. Also during that time, I wrote about 400 Vicodin® for him. Fortunately, one of my colleagues happened to see him when I was out of town, and pulled me aside to "enlighten me".**

**On the next visit, I confronted Mr. Tricket and never saw him again . . . *well not exactly.* About two years later I was walking by our reception area and recognized Mr. Tricket checking in to be seen for back pain. My receptionist stepped into my office concerned that the patient had no form of identification and refused to give a name, and thus could not be seen. I told her that we would make an exception since I couldn't wait to see him again. I reviewed his occupation which noted "Central Intelligence Agency". Upon entering the exam room I asked why he didn't have any ID.**

**He said, *"Well doc, you see I'm working undercover on special assignment with the CIA, and they don't give us anything, so if we're ever compromised they can deny ever knowing of us . . ."***

**I said, *"No credit cards, health insurance card, driver's license, nothing?"***

***"Nope"*, he responded.**

**I subsequently confronted him regarding his previous occupation, upon which he stood up and left without saying a word. *I wonder what he'll be next year?* +**

HiFI

# HIP FRACTURE INSTITUTE

*Because Sometimes Science is Painful!*

As a pharmaceutical company, you depend on good data. Elderly patients on a fixed income need free samples of drugs and some extra cash for the Early Bird Special.

***At the HIP FRACTURE INSTITUTE located in Key Biscayne, Florida, we can help you bring the two together in order to get the results you depend on.***

In today's expedient society, many drugs never get the rigorous testing they need. The osteoporosis literature, for example, is missing much of the data needed to prove which drugs are better. There are just not enough studies with the biphosphonates to see which one truly prevents fractures.

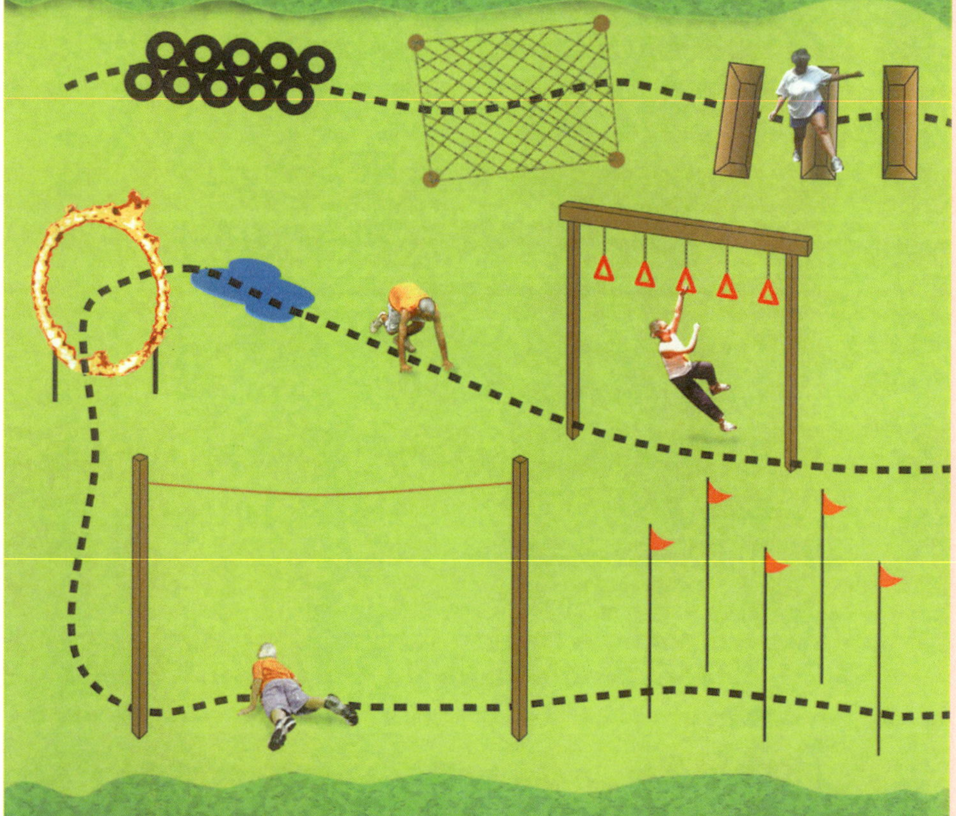

***Making Them Fall To Get The Data***

**Our specially designed obstacle course for the osteoporotic elderly is perfect to prove whether your product is worthy.**

## YOU GET THEM ON YOUR MEDS AND WE MAKE THEM FALL.

## *IT'S THAT SIMPLE!*

Each patient is given a free track suit, a free pair of walking shoes and an orientation to the course. After a brief radiological work-up, we let each patient loose on the course. We adhere to any methodological research standard you set in place and finish each patient's run through with another radiological view.

***Did your drug truly decrease the fracture rate? Now you can know for sure and get rid of all those hassles from the FDA!******

***The patients you send us will love it!***

The ones who survive will even receive their own **HiFI** T-shirts.

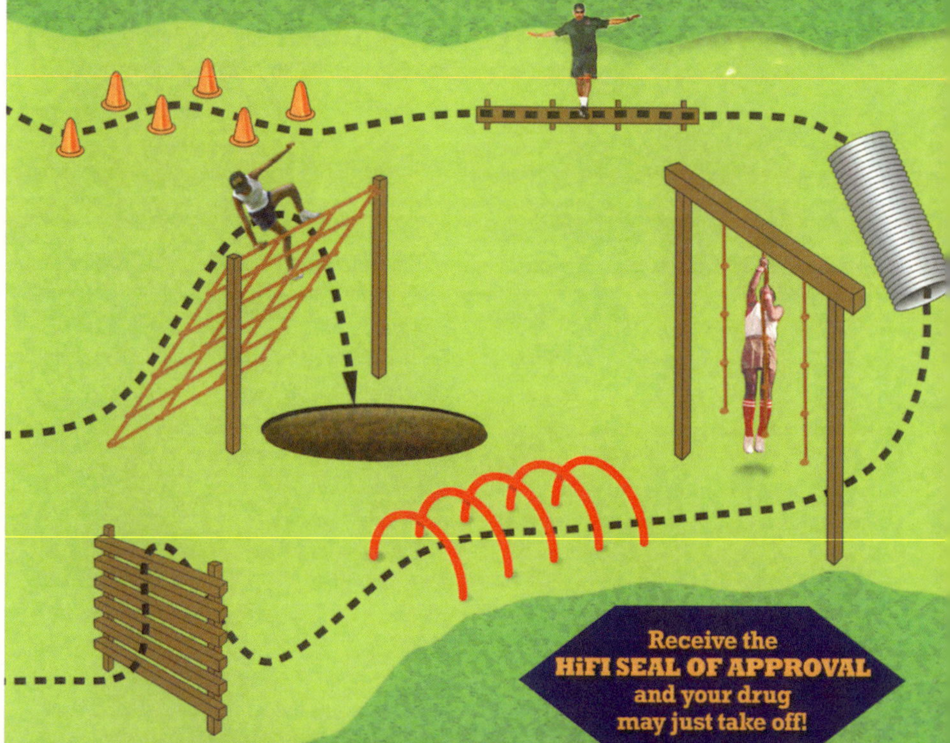

**Receive the HiFI SEAL OF APPROVAL and your drug may just take off!**

*HiFI is not approved, endorsed or condoned by the FDA. They hate us.

**CALL 1-555-FRACTURE TODAY**
**and let our research team make you billions.**

# iGOMER *The patient simulator of tomorrow*

*The newest innovation in medical education technology is finally here!* No industry involves more life and death decisions than healthcare. The problem is that most patient simulators are not realistic enough. The engineers at *PJ Technologies* have come up with one that may change medical education as we know it.

**iGOMER** is capable of exhibiting many of the same symptoms, communicable diseases, and pseudo-complaints you see in the ER. All of **iGOMER**'s reactions are wirelessly controlled by a computer and a barely awake instructor.

For more information on the **iGOMER** and how to purchase one for your hospital, call *PJ Technologies* at **207-555-GOMER** and see how you can train your staff in the most realistic fashion possible. +

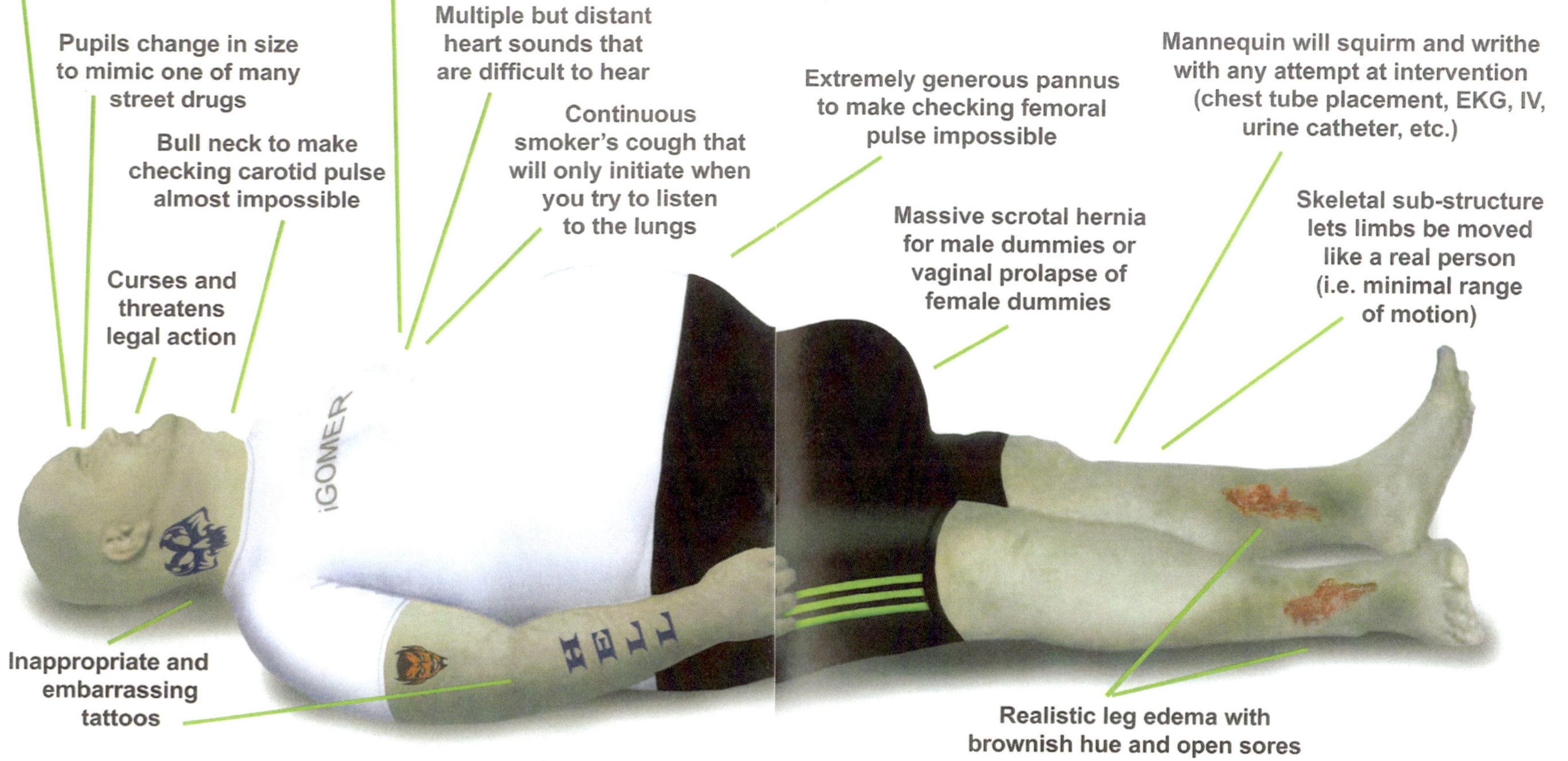

MORE TRUE STORIES OF MEDICINE

# JUST HUSKY

Although I am not a doctor, this is one of the most embarrassing moments I've had as a physician assistant. I had taken care of a pleasant 5 foot 7, 350+ pound lady who was very pleasant, just "husky." We'll call her "Frieda." She had been having vaginal discharge for a month or so. I had given her everything from an empiric standpoint I could think of as not to have to do an actual vaginal exam. I know, "Bad PA." You can "whip" me but wait until I finish this story!

Frieda had not had a Pap smear for some time, although I always grudgingly offered it to her at her yearly physical. With no luck from medications, she presented with the complaint and said, *"I can't stand it any longer. Let's just do what we have to do."*

I left the room to start slitting my wrists while my medical assistant got her double gowned and ready for the procedure. Little did I know it would be such an eventful exam.

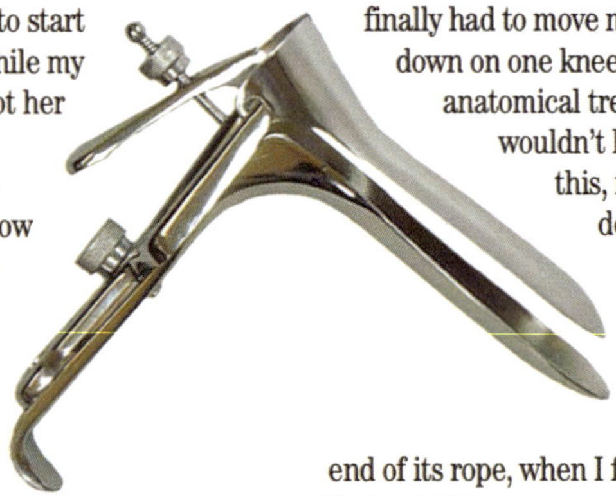

As you can imagine trying to manage even getting Frieda into the proper position was a task. When she was finally up in the stirrups, I inserted the largest speculum I had. Unfortunately, the deeper the speculum penetrated, the more adipose tissue obstructed my view. I searched for a couple of minutes with no success for "Cervical Gold." Frieda then magically remembered that her last physician told her that her uterus was extremely "tipped." Damn! As I was just about ready to give up after searching for what felt like a lifetime, my speculum crossed the posterior aspect of her cervix. *No freakin' kidding it was tipped. Climbing the face of Everest might have been easier!* I couldn't put any more torque on the speculum because the handle was hitting the table. We tried helping her scoot down a little more, which of course was a huge task (no pun intended.) I was bending over so far that I considered having my medical assistant start filling out a workman's comp. claim for a severe lumbar/ cervical strain. I finally had to move my stool and get down on one knee to visualize our anatomical treasure. I normally wouldn't have done all of this, nor should I have done it but that's why gynecology gets paid the big bucks.

My empathy was near the end of its rope, when I finally found the "jackpot." There was no turning back now. By the time I had the full cervix in view, I was on one knee and sweating profusely. As I started to obtain a sample, Frieda commented,

***"You don't think this infection could be caused from using sex toys do you?"***

By that time I was so exasperated that I just shook my head and started to laugh. Of course, she started to laugh which made the exam all the more challenging to complete. The more she laughed, the more the speculum moved in all directions. There was enough tissue crossing my view I could of sworn I saw a uvula in there! We finally accomplished the exam, which was in part due to the efforts of my trusty sidekick (medical assistant) lifting and contorting Frieda as if she was on a conquest to find a gem, like out of an *Indiana Jones* film.

As we finished with the exam and helped her sit up, I felt like I had just competed in the "World's Strongest Man Competition." I looked at my medical assistant who was red as a beet and was beginning to pass out. Frieda looked at me, laughed a little bit, and then said,

***"No really, could sex toys cause an infection like the one I have? I keep them extremely clean."***

At that point I just looked at Frieda and said, *"No, dear, you are fine as long as they are clean."* As my medical assistant and I walked out the door we made a commitment to each other that there would be no vaginal exams in our office on patients over 250 pounds. ✚

## STILL EATING

An interesting thing happened at the office last week. My patient, Mr. Jones, likes shiny beer cans (about 12 a day in fact). One day the glare from a can must have temporarily blinded him as he fell down the front steps of his home and suffered an intracerebral hemorrhage. He ended up on my service in an inpatient rehab hospital with a PEG tube sticking out of his abdomen primarily because his head injury made him forget how to eat.

On his first night here, **Mr. Jones gave the tube a yank and it broke in half.** He was found with the outside part clutched in his fist and a presumably larger piece still inside his stomach.

He was shipped back to the BIG hospital where he was made NPO (no food) and scheduled for an EGD the next morning. Mr. Jones was not amused and told his family that he was being tortured so they brought in an *Extra Value Meal* for him to eat. Well, the next morning he pooped out the wayward piece of tubing and felt great afterwards.

Not to be upstaged in this manner, the gastroenterologist scoped him anyway and pronounced his upper GI tract free of foreign bodies. Mr. Jones is now back in rehab sans PEG tube, free of obstruction and eating like crazy.

The moral of this story is, ***"Would you like fries with that EGD?"*** ✚

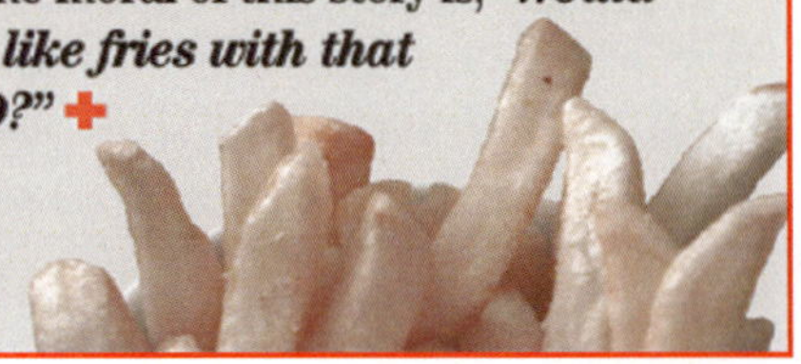

# NARCOTIC SEEKING DETECTION 101

***(In hindsight, of course!)***

*Three weeks ago a young male came to my office seeking narcotics and I prescribed them. In retrospect it is quite clear to me that I was fooled by a professional narcotic seeker. Here is my story with some educational commentary along the way.*

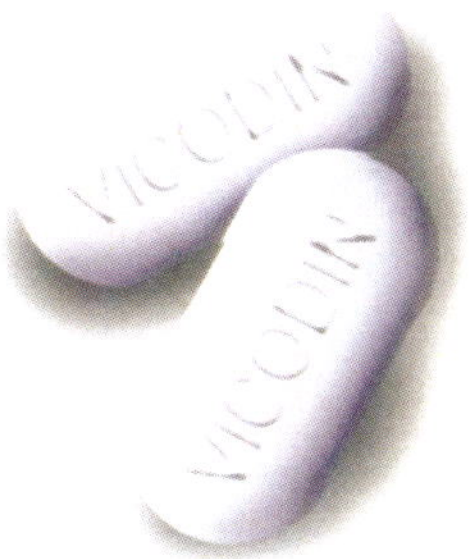


## THOSE DARN NARC SEEKERS

Jimmy was a 27-year-old male who presented with a sole history of asthma.

*Note: No history of back injury/surgery or need for narcotics for pain were discussed in the history.* **(Clue #1 and Lie #1)**

In the interview, Jimmy initially addressed his asthma by saying that he was on some sort of inhaler. He let me guess.

*"Advair?"*

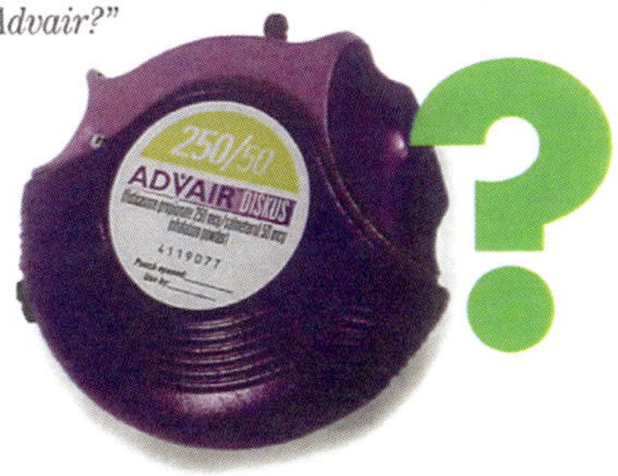


*"Good,"* he cooed. I felt smart. *This was going well!*

*Note: Jimmy was playing dumb and giving me kudos for being smart.* **(Clue #2)**

Next comes the *"Oh, by the way . . . can you cover me for my Vicodin? . . . I don't use it very often . . . just when it starts to get cold my back hurts."*

*"How come?"* I ask innocently *(with some trepidation).*

*"Oh, I had back surgery after a sky diving accident and several motor vehicle accidents."*

*Note: If some incident sounds too miraculous for the person to have survived, it probably isn't true.* **(Clue #3 and Big Lie #2)**

I asked, *"Who prescribed your last pain meds?"*

*"My PCP, Dr. Kendall, last fall. However, he is no longer in practice."*

*Note: If a doctor is out of practice it is darn near IMPOSSIBLE to get records to verify patients' stories and this is a great NARC SEEKER TRICK.* **(Clue #4 and Big Lie #3)**

At this point, I am getting uncomfortable with the direction we are going.

*Note: A sense of being uncomfortable and that you have a problem when discussing narcotic use with a new patient approaches PATHONOMONIC that you are dealing with narcotic seeking patients.* **(Clue #5)**

I ask questions about pain management concerning non-narcotic or NSAID use. Motrin doesn't work. OK, I'll prescribe a stronger medicine (I start writing an Rx for Naproxen). Jimmy says, almost spontaneously, *"Oh, yeah, and I'm allergic to Naproxen."*

*Note: Allergies to non-narcotics or classic selective direction by the patient is being performed. I am feeling hemmed into writing narcotics.* **(Clue #6)**

I pull my trump card, *"No, I will not prescribe narcotics for you. I will refer you to the local pain management clinic."*

Jimmy responds, *"Oh yeah, Dr. Sorenstam, he's OK, but he uses too much heavy narcotics!"*

I try my best to ignore this while filling out the referral *(I have found an out and am so happy with myself).* Jimmy is also helpful in this department too. He knows the pain management clinic's phone number BY HEART!!

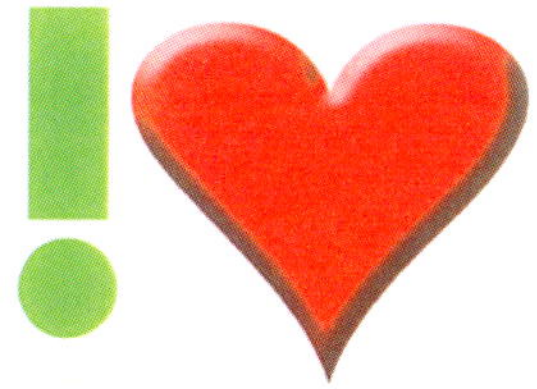

*Note: If your patient is seeking narcotics and knows the pain management clinic phone number by heart, then you pretty much don't need to go any further.* **(Clue #7)**

I step out of the room to go get a sample inhaler for Jimmy and return to give him the sample and the referral. Now Jimmy pulls out HIS trump card, *"What about pain meds until I get into pain management? . . . It takes two months to get in!" (Jimmy's demeanor was angry and intimidating at this point).*

I think to myself, *"He's right."* I start writing out a 30-day supply of Vicodin with a one month refill. The patient takes the Rx and leaves the exam room and walks out into the parking lot to his car without stopping at the desk to make his one-month asthma follow-up.

*Note: His closer was better than mine. There are two clues here. The first is the "No to Yes Phenomenon," in which the physician is skillfully moved from a No on prescribing narcotics to a Yes in prescribing narcotics. And this is another PATHONOMONIC clue for narcotic seeking patients.* **(Clue #8 and #9)**

The final **Clue #10** is that the patient's problem has now become the doctor's problem. I had allowed Jimmy to wear me down and paint me into a corner. Writing the Rx's at that time seemed like the only reasonable option.

Aftermath: Jimmy had a positive narcotic Rx from eight other doctors in town including a different pain management clinic than the one I referred him to. The local police had been looking for Jimmy and appreciated our sharing information about him. His home address was falsified too. A disgruntled family member snarled, *"He don't live here no more!!!"*

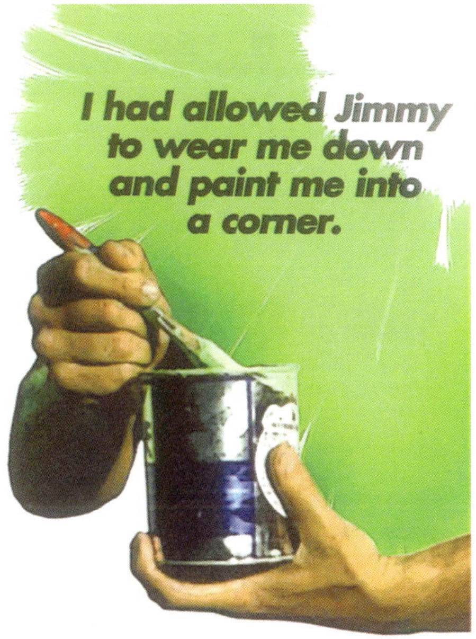


***What have I learned?*** Well, I have done a lot of research on narcotic diversion and I'm going to give my findings in a presentation to local residents. *Who knew that being a doctor means you need to figure out more clues than a police detective?* **Jimmy knew, that's who.** ✚

### MEDICAL STUDENT ADVICE 101

Second biggest lie to tell a patient?

***"I know what is causing your problem."***

First biggest lie to tell a patient?

***"I know how to fix it."***

# MEDICAL JOURNALS THAT NEVER MADE IT.

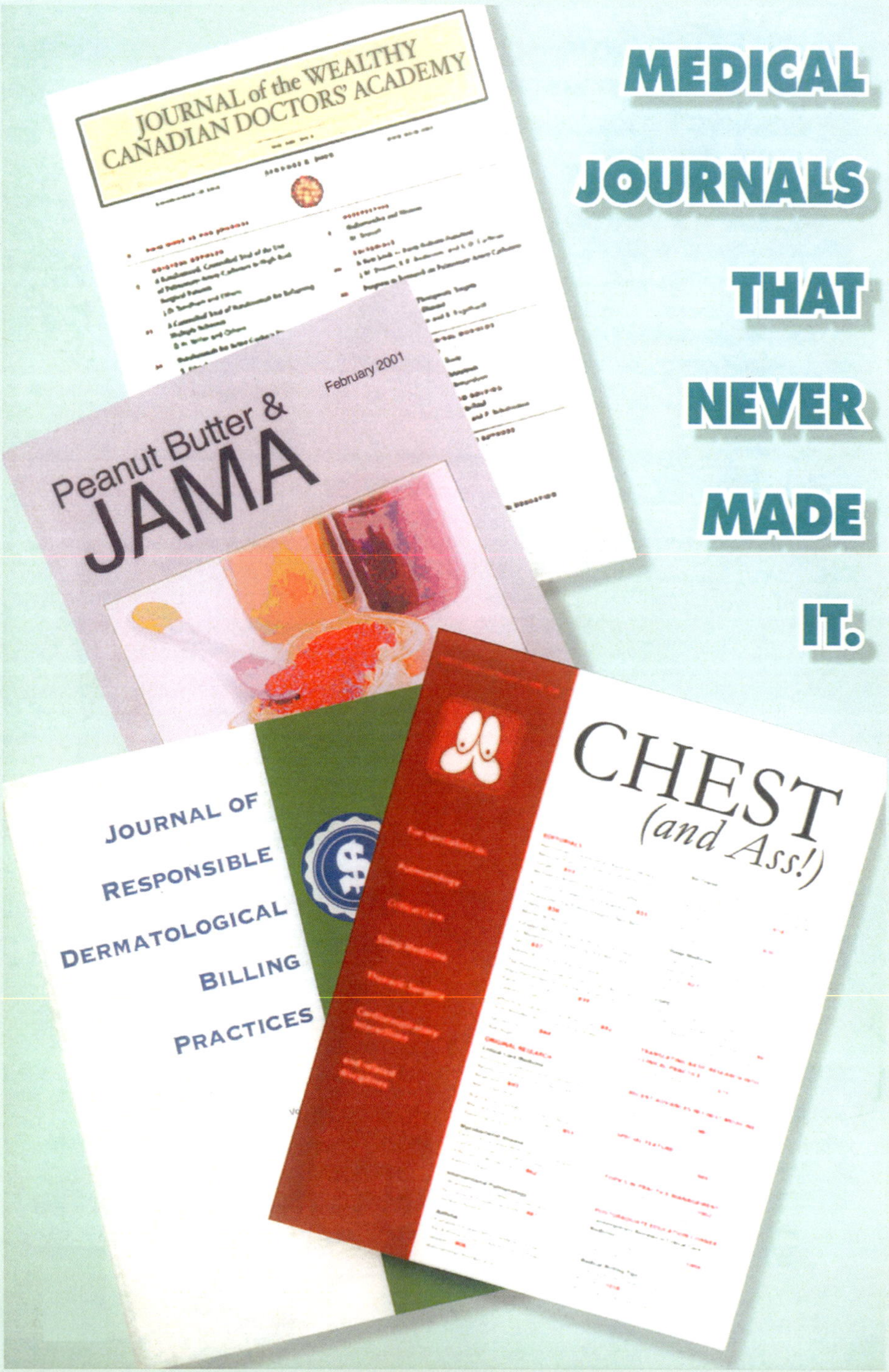


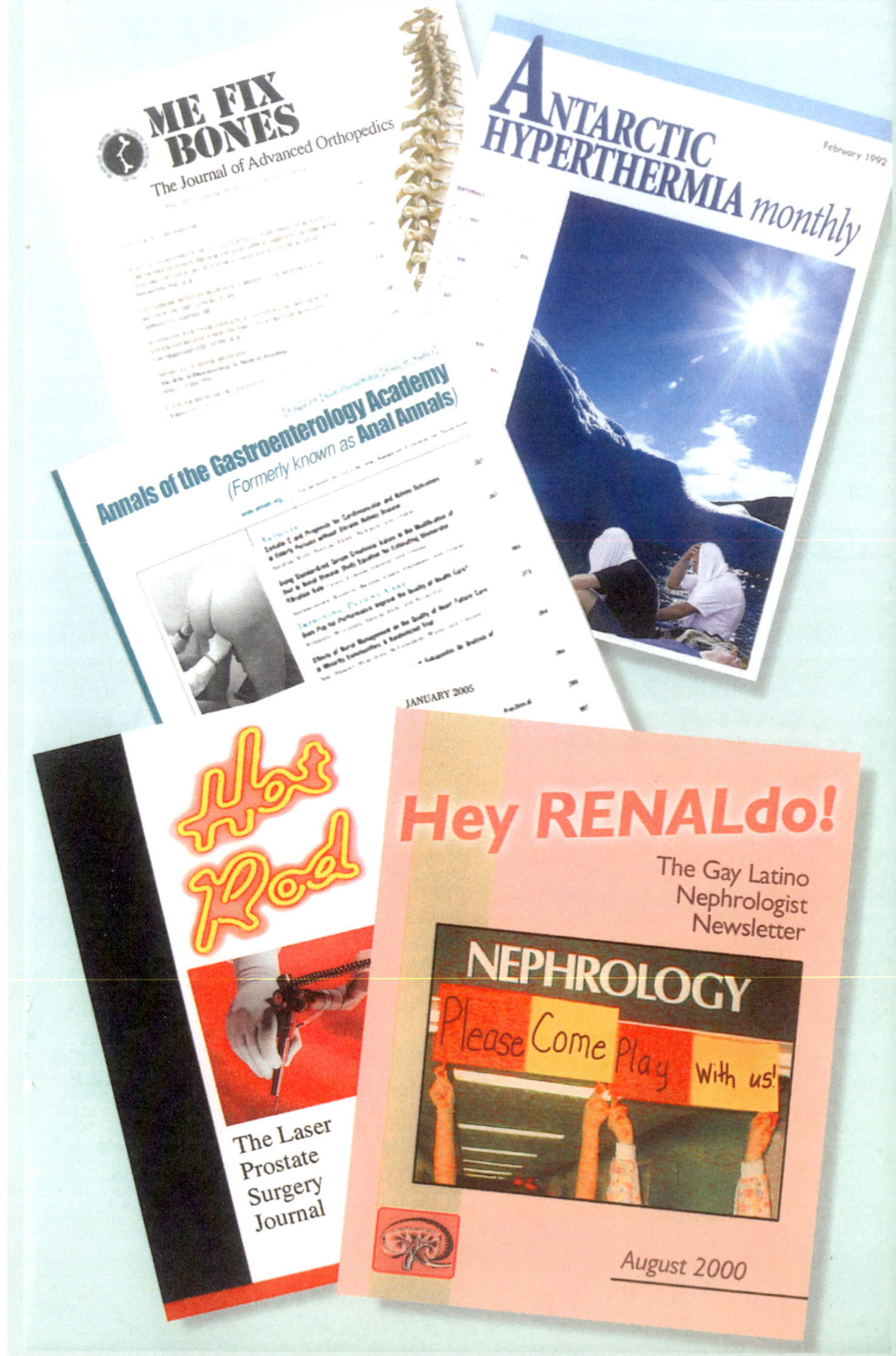

# MALINGERERS SAY THE DARNDEST THINGS!

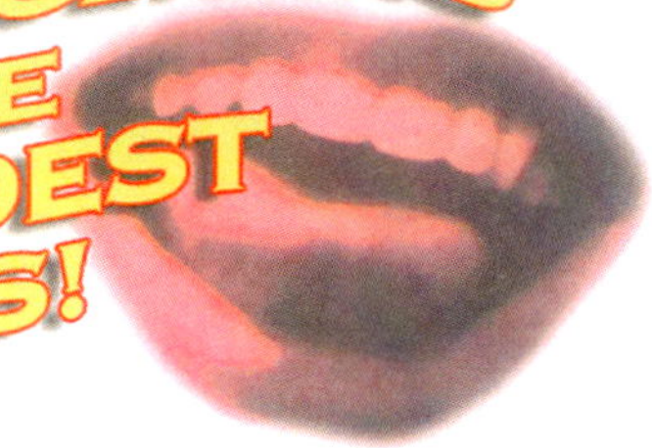

## Worker's Comp Claim Gone Wild

Mr. Q presented with back and foot pain which he felt was related to working at his job in delivery services for a local hospital. Sometimes the packages were heavy. Mr. Q was in his forties and he had worked there for ten years. He had gone to a different workers' comp doctor who wrote him light duty work.

***"But I'm in too much pain to do anything!"***

He had his wife drive him to the office. They were chatting, looking comfortable. He had been diagnosed with plantar fasciitis and mechanical back pain by the previous doc and had some mild heel spurs. X-ray of the back was negative. We discussed heel cups, home stretches, and physical therapy.

***"But I'm in too much pain for that."***

I told him that he needed to at least try and that the anti-inflammatories would help.

The next day he was back, this time with his son who drove him in. His son looked very young – maybe fifteen at the most. Both he and his dad were sitting comfortably, chatting on respective cell phones. Mr. Q had self-procured a cane . . . but he was walking without any real limp. Again I asked him to try light duty.

***"But I can barely walk! And I don't think I have heel spurs either."***

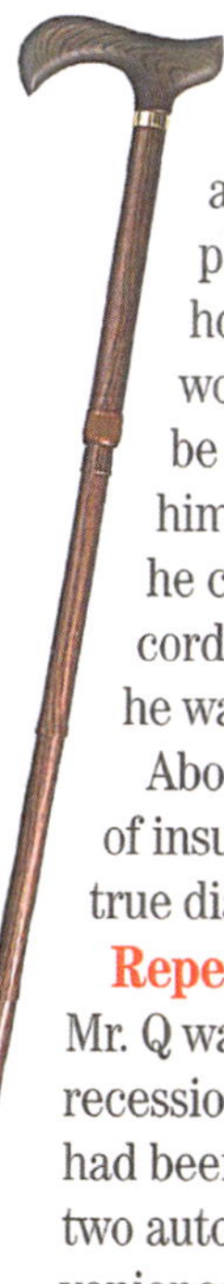

He argued extensively with the front desk and again I asked him to please try to walk for just two hours a day and to do light duty work. I advised him that I could be accused of fraud if I wrote him totally off work if it appears he can do something. He was cordial but really didn't seem like he was going to try my suggestions.

About a week later, with the help of insurance company video, the true diagnosis was made:

**Repetitive Shopping Disorder.** Mr. Q was on video, shopping like the recession had never happened. He had been at three hardware stores, two auto supply stores, and one convenience store. He had been in and out of the car for hours – and all this without the aid of a cane.

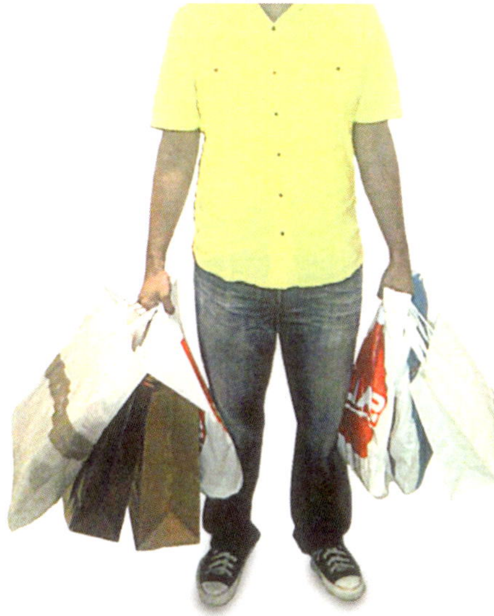

Also, the time he had come to my office with his son, Mr Q was on tape driving away from the appointment!! At the same time I was looking at the video, Mr. Q was calling our office saying he was completely bedridden and was in too much pain to come in for a follow-up visit later that day.

To spare Mr. Q pain, not to mention my staff and myself, we talked on the phone. *He didn't remember shopping!!* I asked that he follow up with his family doctor because, at this time, his workers' comp claim was very difficult to support. I told him he was on video, walking, driving, working on his car and looking really good. The following day, he called asking for the week off.

***Keep on shopping, dude!!*** ✚

**SUBMIT YOUR TRUE STORIES OF MEDICINE.**
**WWW.PLACEBOJOURNAL.COM**

## ANOTHER TRUE STORY OF MEDICINE

## THE FRENCH CONNECTION

A robust French Canadian lumberjack came to my office and was perturbed that appointments were running late. He was swearing in French, and apparently the language was very foul.

@!#*%!!

He obviously thought no other patients in my waiting room in a small Pennsylvania town understood French.

However, sitting across from him was Father Dooley whom I know was fluent in French, in addition to knowing the best swear words himself.

When Father Dooley arose to come in to the office, he said in French to the lumberjack, *"Your choice of words is superb."*

Finally, the lumberjack was visibly embarrassed and had met his match. ✚

## LAST CALL

Recently I was paged to the emergency department at 3 a.m. to stitch up another Jethro. This guy was totally hammered. The story was he was drinking peacefully with his honey when all of a sudden she up and smashed him in the head with a beer bottle.

*Damn!* Second time she's done that this month! Funny how these guys fall prey to so many unprovoked attacks. I've had several drinks with my wife over the years, and I honestly can't recall her ever bashing my head in with a beer bottle.

Anyway, I set up all of my suturing equipment, cleaned off his shard-filled forehead and was just about to start stitching when he announced, *"Hey! W-w-w-wait a minute!"*

*"Why?"*

*"I gotta take a leak."* He rolled off the stretcher, staggered to the adjoining bathroom and slammed the door shut.

Moments later, we were treated to the sound of a torrential stream of used beer. A minute later he was finished. Watching him navigate his way back to the stretcher brought to mind images of a sailor trying to walk across a ship's deck in the middle of a typhoon. He plopped back down on the gurney and promptly fell asleep. Within a minute he was snoring like a hippo.

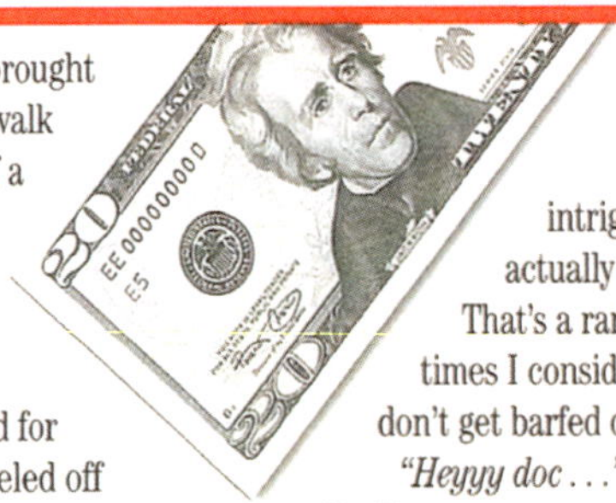

I quickly sewed him up (no need for local anesthetic this time, folks), peeled off my gloves and got up to make arrangements for him to be observed in the department for a few hours. I was halfway out the door when I heard a slurry, nearly unintelligible, *"Heyyy doc, hang on a shehcond . . . come ovah here . . ."*

I turned back, intrigued. Was this guy actually going to thank me? That's a rarity at 3 a.m. Most times I consider myself lucky if I don't get barfed on.

*"Heyyy doc . . ."*

*"Yes?"*

*"Can you lend me twenty bucks?"*

✚

## NO REHAB

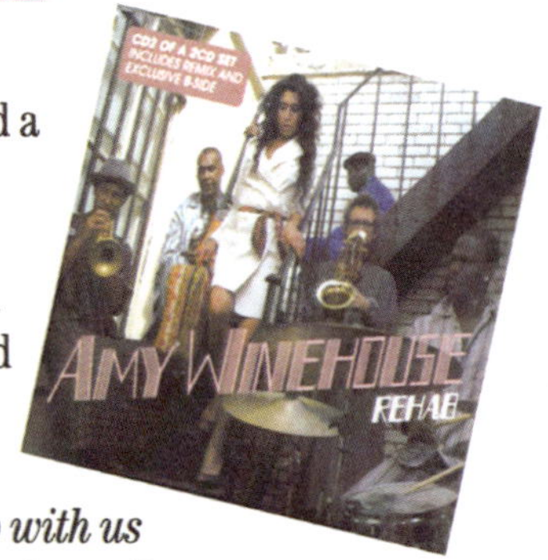


Mrs. L. was a lady in her sixties who had had a stroke and was being treated on my service. Her stroke had left her with left sided hemiplegia and at times some neglect. So I wasn't surprised when one morning she asked me if she would be allowed to go to work the next day. I assumed she was just unaware of her weakness. I gently said, *"No, Mrs. L. You aren't able to walk. You'll need to finish up with us and then you'll probably need to go to rehab to get better."*

Without missing a beat and with a totally deadpan face she sang, ***"You try to make me go to rehab, but I say No, No, No."***

Who knew a 61-year-old woman would listen to Amy Winehouse?! ✚

## HEARD IT ALL

Yesterday I got a request from a patient who I had treated several years ago for injuries sustained in an auto accident. Unfortunately, I have been the only person that would listen to all of her complaints, and believe me they are numerous. She asked me to write a letter to her insurance company so they would cover her health club dues **for LIFE**, a massage therapist **for LIFE**, and last and least we forget –**her dog.**

Her dog apparently has hip dysplasia and must get his exercise. Since my patient is so disabled, she has not been able to walk and exercise him.

She also wanted me to include a request to have them also pay for a Dog- Jog treadmill so he can get the exercise he needs that she can't give.

Talk about milking the insurance companies. *Now you've heard it all.* ✚

# How To Be A New Medicare Patient

● You must be accompanied by (1) a spouse, (2) one of your adult children, or (3) a friend who is at least as old as you are.

● After being roomed, go to the bathroom for half an hour and wait until concerned people start knocking on the door.

● When the doctor asks what your problem is ask, *"I only get to have one?"* Then pronounce your diagnosis and ask the doctor what can be done for that.

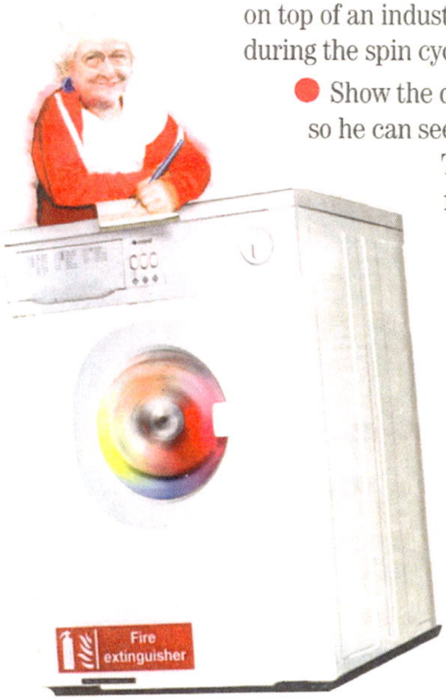


● Every third question, argue with the person who came with you. The doctor should feel like Bob Eubanks running the *Newlywed Game from Hell*, but with sick people. Example:

Doctor: *"Does it burn when you urinate?"*

YOU: *"No."*

Other person: *"Yes! You always complain about that."*

YOU: *"No I don't."*

Other person: *"Yes, you complained about it on the way over."*

YOU: *"That wasn't burning. I said it was like hot tingling,"* and so on.

● Bring a list of medications. It must have a at least 10 wrinkles or folds and be written in a light feathery script or faded pencil. It should always appear that you wrote it while riding on a roller coaster. If you have legible handwriting, re-write the list while actually riding on a roller coaster or write it on top of an industrial washing machine during the spin cycle.

● Show the doctor your pill bottle so he can see what you are taking. The bottle should be faded and completely impossible to read, except for the expiration date: June 8, 1978. If the label happens to be legible, point out to the doctor that those pills are not the ones that originally came in that bottle, as if the doctor had not already deduced that from the fact that there are ten different pills in it, as well as some *Smarties* and *M&M's*.

● As the doctor goes through the medication list, start looking at it too and point out the medications that you are no longer on. Then tell the doctor that there are some new medications that are not on the list and only identify them by their first letter and the color of the pill.

● You must list "sulfur" as an allergy but forget the reaction you had because you were so young at the time.

● When asked to open the top button on your shirt, completely disrobe before anyone can stop you. This is also acceptable behavior when the exam room door is wide open.

● No matter how loud the doctor talks, insist that you can't hear. Keep turning to the Other Person for translation, and turn up your hearing aid.

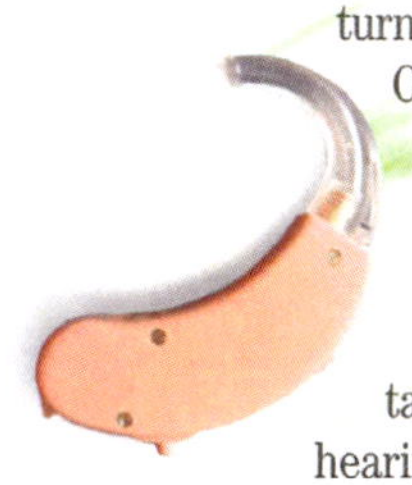

● When you take out your hearing aid for the ear examination, do NOT turn it down first. The resulting ear-splitting high-pitched feedback that you can't hear not only serves to sonically sterilize the room, but it also keeps dangerous rabies-infected bats at bay.

● If it is a pain complaint and you are a man, start your history with a military injury: *"I think my back is bad because of all the planes I jumped out of in Korea,"* or *"I have a retained arrowhead in my leg from the French & Indian War."*

● Ask a question early on. It doesn't matter what it's about. Every few minutes ask the question again like it's a new question (which it is for you).

● If you aren't sure about an answer in the ROS, discuss it with your Other Person for five minutes. You should do this at least once for each organ system.

● Forget half of the surgeries you had and then remember them one by one every two minutes while the doctor is asking questions about something else.

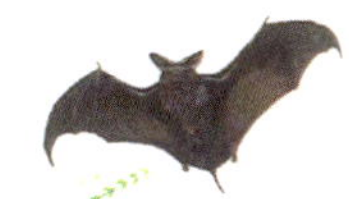

● During the physical exam, suddenly recall the name of one of your new medications. Do this for each anatomic system. Women should jump off the exam table while totally nude and start going through their purse because they just remembered they have the bottle.

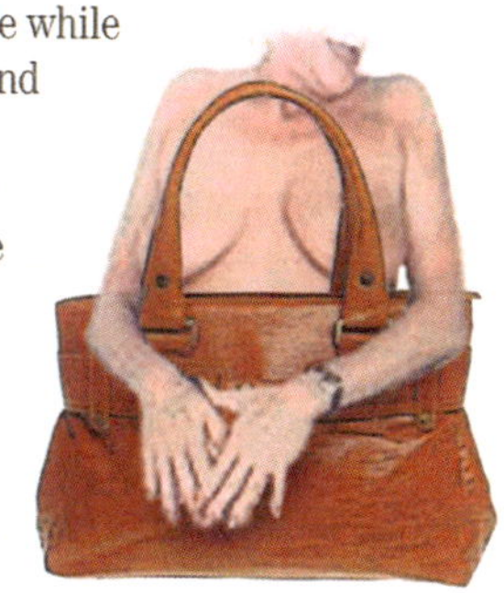

*and last . . .*

● If you are a post-meno-pausal woman over the age of 70, scold the doctor at the end of the visit because you weren't asked if you had osteoporosis.

## TRUE STORIES OF MEDICINE

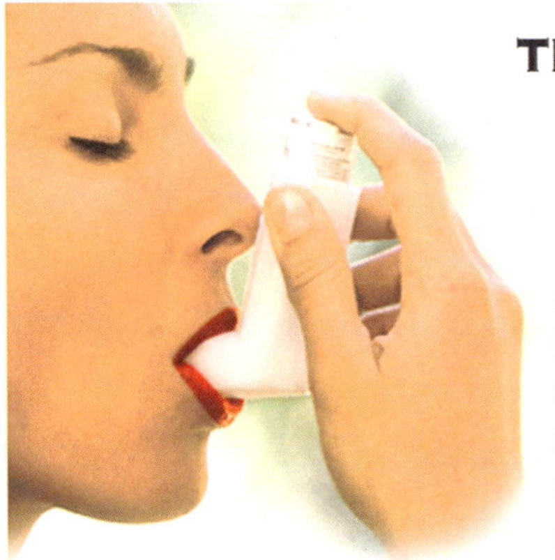

# SWALLOW

I had a 46-year-old female patient who came in with a nagging cough she had been having for a few weeks. My exam did not reveal anything serious and I thought a steroid inhaler would help her more than anything else. I gave her an *Asmanex* powder inhaler and instructed her on its usage.

***"Take a breath and blow out completely, then put the tip of the inhaler in your mouth and suck in deeply."***

She did fine, took the inhaler out of her mouth, revealing lipstick around the tip. She continued to hold it up and inquired, ***"Do I swallow now?"***

I couldn't contain myself, started laughing, and then she joined me, realizing what she had said. ✚

# WHERE, OH WHERE

About 30 years ago, in a small exam room, with the patient in her seventies, her daughter, my nurse and I in the room, I was doing a pelvic exam on a lady who had had a hysterectomy. The exam would have been much more easily accomplished if I had remembered the hysterectomy, but I did not.

After searching unsuccessfully for a cervix from which to obtain a Pap smear, I asked somewhat exasperatedly, *"What have you done with your cervix?"*

The lady's reply was immediate, *"Are you talking to me or your nurse?"*

My nurse had to leave the room. The daughter could not suppress her laughter. My red face was hidden by the drape sheet. ✚

# NOT POSSIBLE

I was seeing patients in a military acute care clinic and was presented a chart for a woman who had discharge from the navel. It took me several minutes to compose myself and try to determine if this was anatomically and physiologically possible after reading what the screening nurse wrote as the chief complaint:

***"pussy discharge from the belly button."*** ✚

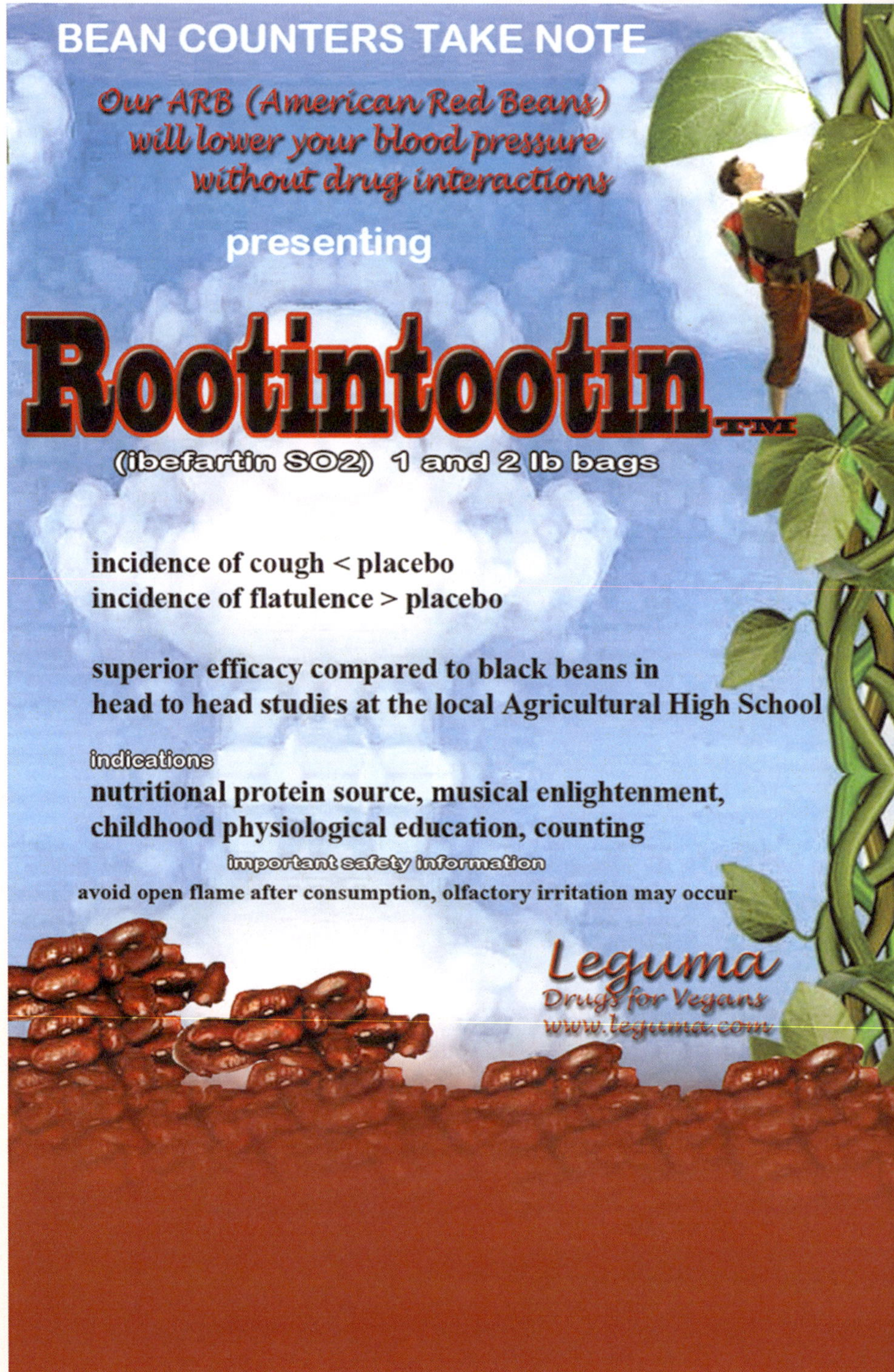
BEAN COUNTERS TAKE NOTE
Our ARB (American Red Beans) will lower your blood pressure without drug interactions
presenting
Rootintootin™
(ibefartin SO2) 1 and 2 lb bags
incidence of cough < placebo
incidence of flatulence > placebo
superior efficacy compared to black beans in head to head studies at the local Agricultural High School
indications
nutritional protein source, musical enlightenment, childhood physiological education, counting
important safety information
avoid open flame after consumption, olfactory irritation may occur
Leguma
Drugs for Vegans
www.leguma.com

## 3 NEW STORIES!

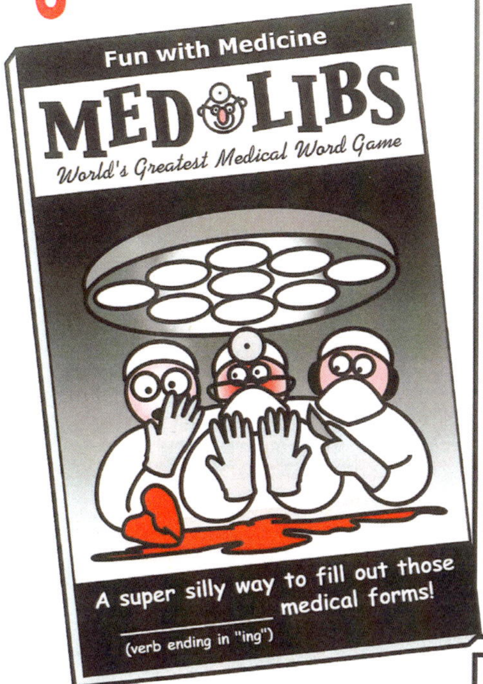


### MED-LIBS INSTRUCTIONS

Med-Libs is a game for physicians who basically are tired of all the damn paperwork in medicine.

**Directions:** The first part (this page) has blank spaces for words you use over and over again in your dictations. Do not look at the story (next page). Have your nurse or one of your physician partners ask you for a word for each of those blanks. *Be creative.*

**To Play:** When you are done, place the words in their matching blank spaces in the second part (story). Read aloud the crazy, ridiculous, outlandish dictation that you have just created. You will realize that it is basically the same as every other dictation you do. *It's great fun and depressingly revealing all at the same time!*

ONE MORE STORY ON PG.32

### A NEW OB PATIENT VISIT

(fill in the following)

FEMALE RELATIVE ____________

ADJECTIVE ____________

NUMBER ____________

NUMBER ____________

ANOTHER FEMALE RELATIVE ____________

NUMBER ____________

NEGATIVE ADJECTIVE ____________

BOGUS DISEASE ____________

A THIRD DIFFERENT FEMALE RELATIVE ____________

SLANG TERM FOR BREASTS ____________

A TYPE OF BABY FORMULA ____________

### A NURSE MESSAGE

(fill in the following)

A LAST NAME ____________

NARCOTIC MEDICINE ____________

ANIMAL ____________

TYPE OF CAR ____________

BODY PART ____________

NUMBER BETWEEN 11-100 ____________

BENZO ____________

ADVERB ____________

NSAID ____________

SYMPTOM ____________

DERMATOLOGIC LESION (PLURAL) ____________

## MED LIBS A NEW OB PATIENT VISIT

Doctor, I just wanted to let you know that I am certain that I will need a C-Section to deliver my baby. My ____________ (FEMALE RELATIVE) had one, so I know I will need one, too. My uterus is ____________ (ADJECTIVE) so that also means I will certainly need one. For the last ____________ (NUMBER) of my pregnancies I was in labor for an average of ____________ (NUMBER) hours. Also, my ____________ (ANOTHER FEMALE RELATIVE) had her baby early and although he had to stay in the NICU for a long time, he was fine. So I probably should have my baby ____________ (NUMBER) weeks early, too. Oh yeah, I will probably have to be excused from my ____________ (NEGATIVE ADJECTIVE) job, because I am sure I will have a problem with my ____________ (BOGUS DISEASE) soon. One more thing. I won't be able to breastfeed, because my ____________ (A THIRD DIFFERENT FEMALE RELATIVE) tried and her ____________ (SLANG TERM FOR BREASTS) wouldn't make any ____________ (TYPE OF BABY FORMULA).

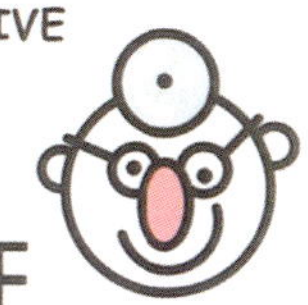

## MED LIBS A NURSE MESSAGE

Mr. ____________ (A LAST NAME) called, he needs an early refill on his ____________ (NARCOTIC MEDICINE). He knows the clinic policy of not refilling narcotic medications early, but his pet ____________ (ANIMAL) ate the prescription and then the pet was run over by a ____________ (TYPE OF CAR). He is having excruciating pain in his lower ____________ (BODY PART). On a scale of 1-10 he rates his pain as a ____________ (NUMBER BETWEEN 11-100). He also needs an early refill of his ____________ (BENZO). He was opening the bottle and the pills ____________ (ADVERB) fell into the toilet. As you know he cannot take ____________ (NSAID) instead, because he is allergic. He had a horrible ____________ (SYMPTOM) and ____________ (DERMATOLOGIC LESION (PLURAL)) all over his body the last time he took it.

Finally, the first female libido-enhancing medication is now available!

# Ladies, are you ready for *Modic*?

modic®

(Meloxicum) patch

**Female sexual dysfunction, like many other women's health problems, has long been neglected by the medical world. Finally, PJ Pharmaceuticals has created a medication that will finally make women happy.**

## Who knew that all they needed was a little Modic?

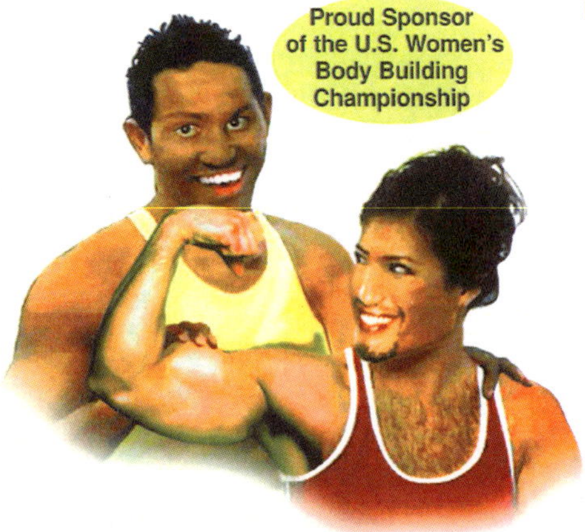


Do you have a decreased interest in sex, an absence of sexual fantasies or a grotesque and overweight husband?
**If you answered yes, then you need Modic.**

Missing some ovaries? No problem . . .
**How about some Modic?**

Feeling lonely? No problem , , ,
**How about some Modic?**

Hate your marriage? No problem . . .
**How about some Modic?**

PJ Pharmaceuticals is not afraid to ask the question . . .
**"Ladies, isn't it time you got some Modic?"**

**PJ PHARMACEUTICALS** *The Realistic Drug Company*

Modic is a testosterone-containing patch that artificially drives up your sexual desire. At least we think that is what is going on. In studies of women who had undergone ovary removal surgery or were menopausal, women taking a good amount of Modic for six months reported that they experienced an average of one additional episode of intercourse every four weeks compared with women given an inactive patch. Our own studies also show that by playing on women's insecurities about sex, we can make millions of dollars on those same women because they will subsequently seek prescriptions from their physicians. *Don't you think it's your turn to be experimented upon!*

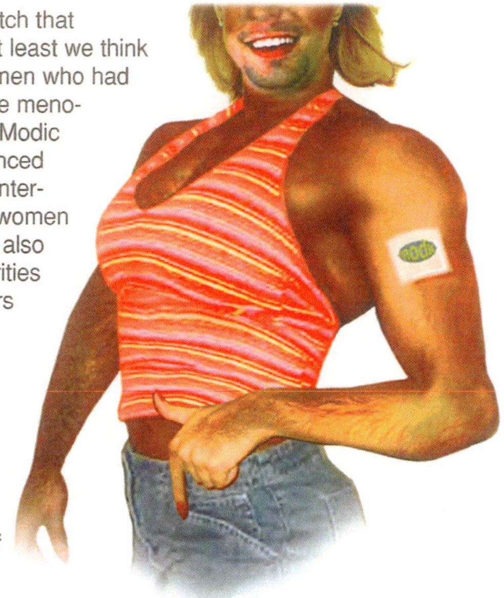

**We know that nothing will pique your sexual arousal more than Modic. Maybe you are suffering from a lack of Modic. Maybe you are just curious about trying Modic. You don't need any crazy blood tests of hormone levels or questionnaires about sexual satisfaction to determine that you just want Modic!**

**Ask your doctor now about whether you should get Modic You'll be glad you did.**

**FREE RAZOR**
**with each prescription refill!**

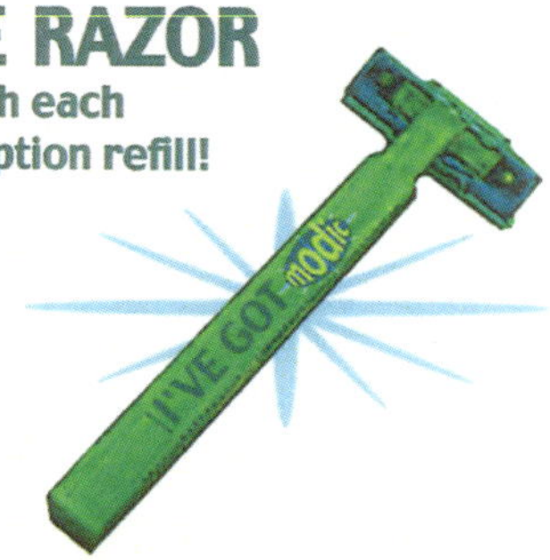


*"My doctor states that all I needed was Modic in order to feel better. He was right. I can't wait to go back to his office and get Modic directly from him!"*

JoAnne Moreno
5th Grade School Teacher

*"I love taking Modic! The only side effect that I felt was a very faint hairline. It's barely noticeable as it travels from my navel down to the tip of my newly formed penis."*

Breanne Lancaster
Exotic Dancer

modic®

(Meloxicum) patch

**SIDE EFFECTS – breast cancer, divorce, a whole smorgasbord of sexually transmitted diseases, unusually coarse hair growth in really weird places.** *© 2005*

## ONE MORE TRUE STORY OF MEDICINE

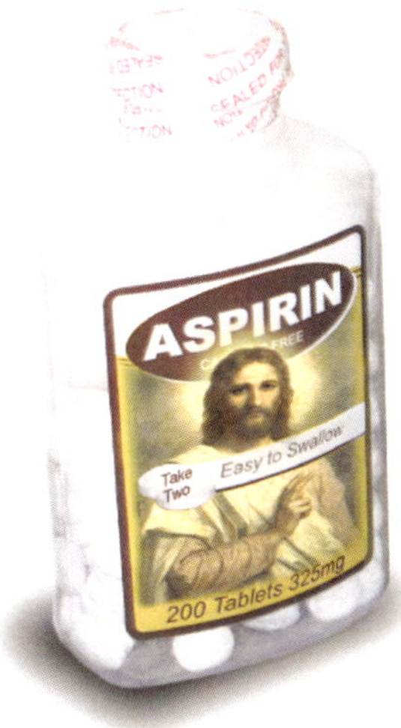

ASPIRIN
Take Two
Easy to Swallow
200 Tablets 325mg


# HEAVENLY TRIP

I'm a family physician by training, but I no longer do clinical medicine. Instead I am a revenue management consultant which involves extensive chart review. So far, this is the funniest history I've reviewed:

*"The patient is a little 81-year-old woman who took an unknown amount of aspirin and two bottles of diphenhydramine in an effort to see Jesus. Unfortunately, her trip was cancelled and she was brought to the emergency room for emergency treatment."* ✚

# Stupid Hospital Tricks

From a loyal reader:

*"This is a "GIFT" (I use the term LOOSELY) given to the ER and ICU nursing staff by our esteemed employer during Hospital Week.* **WOW.** *Words escape me. A pizza cutter . . . SERIOUSLY?!"* ✚

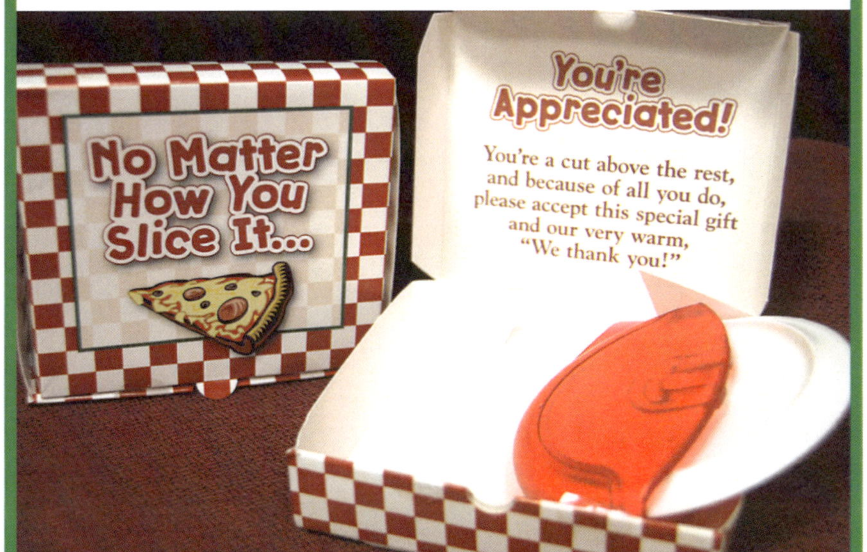

No Matter How You Slice It...
You're Appreciated!
You're a cut above the rest, and because of all you do, please accept this special gift and our very warm, "We thank you!"


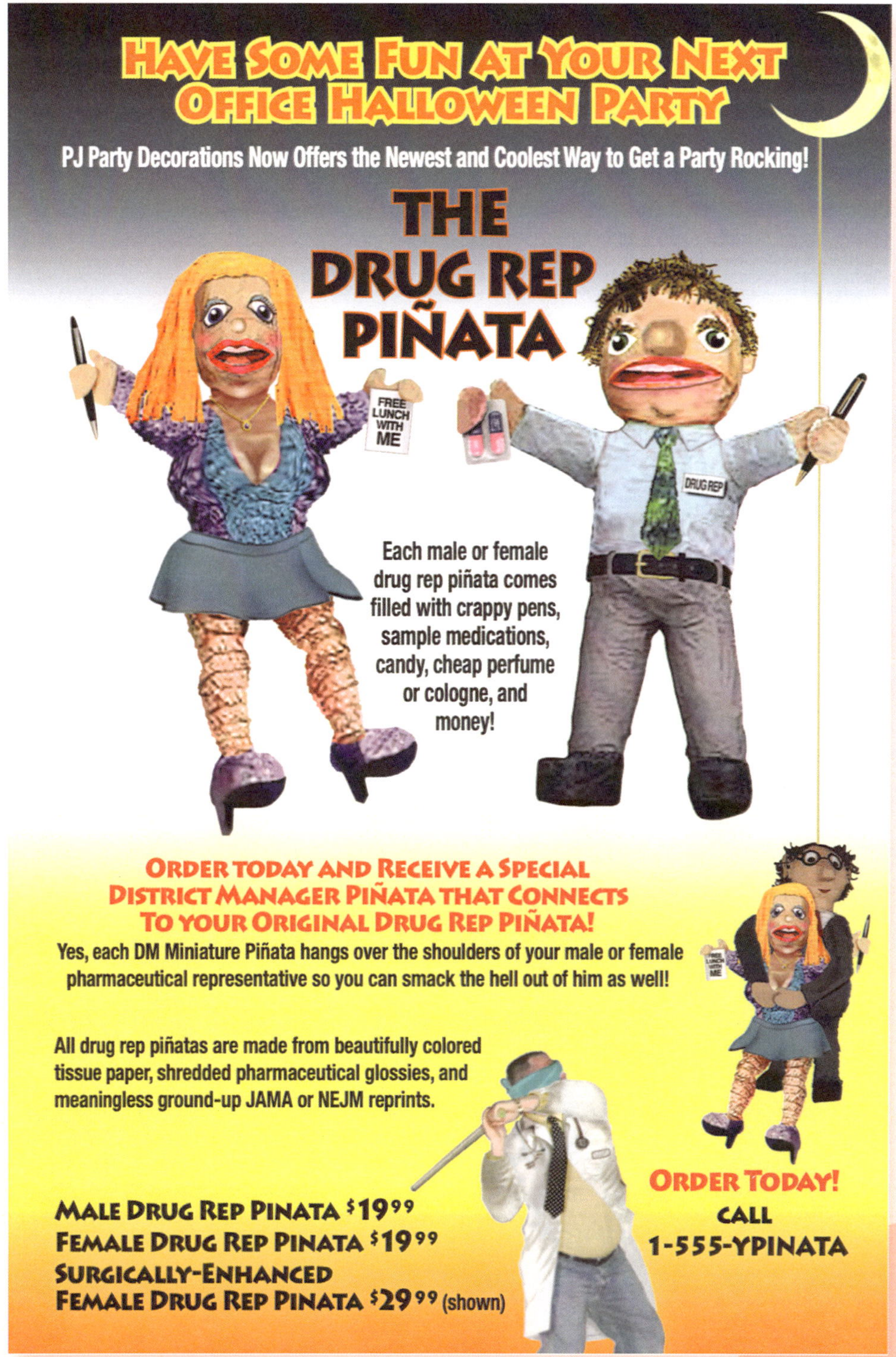

HAVE SOME FUN AT YOUR NEXT OFFICE HALLOWEEN PARTY
PJ Party Decorations Now Offers the Newest and Coolest Way to Get a Party Rocking!
THE DRUG REP PIÑATA
FREE LUNCH WITH ME
DRUG REP
Each male or female drug rep piñata comes filled with crappy pens, sample medications, candy, cheap perfume or cologne, and money!
ORDER TODAY AND RECEIVE A SPECIAL DISTRICT MANAGER PIÑATA THAT CONNECTS TO YOUR ORIGINAL DRUG REP PIÑATA!
Yes, each DM Miniature Piñata hangs over the shoulders of your male or female pharmaceutical representative so you can smack the hell out of him as well!
All drug rep piñatas are made from beautifully colored tissue paper, shredded pharmaceutical glossies, and meaningless ground-up JAMA or NEJM reprints.
MALE DRUG REP PINATA $19.99
FEMALE DRUG REP PINATA $19.99
SURGICALLY-ENHANCED FEMALE DRUG REP PINATA $29.99 (shown)
ORDER TODAY!
CALL
1-555-YPINATA

# Homemade Office Halloween Games

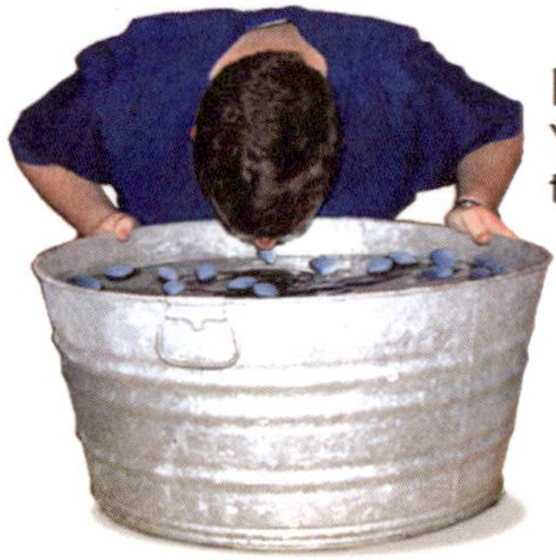

### Bobbing for Viagra
Your office staff and spouses will love dipping their snouts in the bucket with this one!

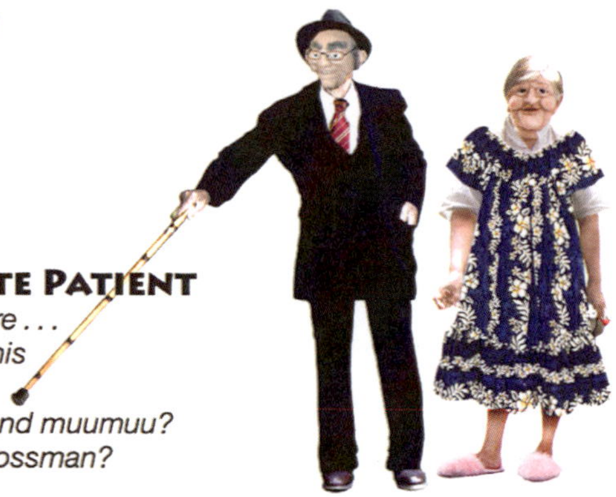

### Dress as Your Favorite Patient
This one is a blast! *Look over there . . . Is that Mr. Hendrickson swatting his cane at the receptionist? Is that Connie La Russo in her slippers and muumuu? What's that smell? Is that Mrs. Grossman?*

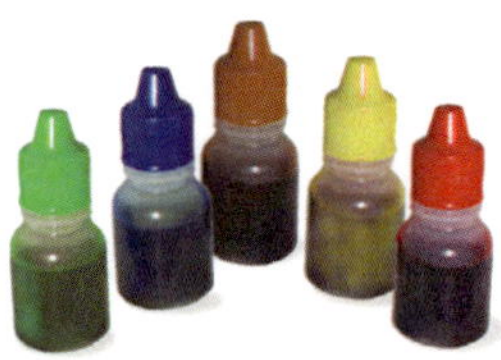

### Heme "Occult" Twister
Use some red, yellow and green food dye to stain some of your cards. Then collect all your month's sample cards that have been mailed in by patients. Intermix these blue-colored positive samples with the regular brown ones as well. Tape them all together and you're off! Create a spinning wheel and pray the arrow doesn't come up brown or blue for you!

**Truth or Scare** Sit around with your partners and staff and ask some medically-related questions. *"Doc, do you really know what the RDW on the CBC means?" "Mary, did you actually return Mrs. Griffin's call about her constipation or did you just write 'no answer'?" "Quick, where is the pharynx?"*

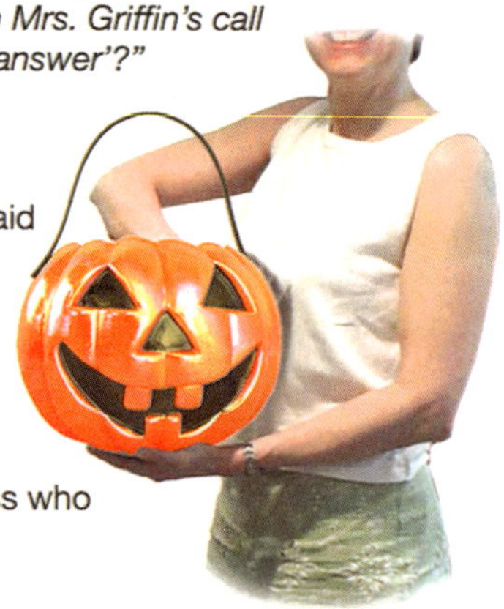

### Administration Pictionary
Write down the most asinine things that were said to you by your hospital administration over the past year. Divide into two teams and place the slips of paper into a plastic pumpkin. One player from the first team starts by picking a slip of paper from the pumpkin. Have each player read out loud the rubbish on the paper as their team tries to guess who said it! *It's hysterical fun!*

**Olden Days** Dress like it's the healthcare system of the1940's. *Make up some ground rules:* Nurses have to actually treat the doctors with respect. Smoking is encouraged and so is a little gin flask in your back pocket. Use only the four drugs that were available for all medical problems at that time.

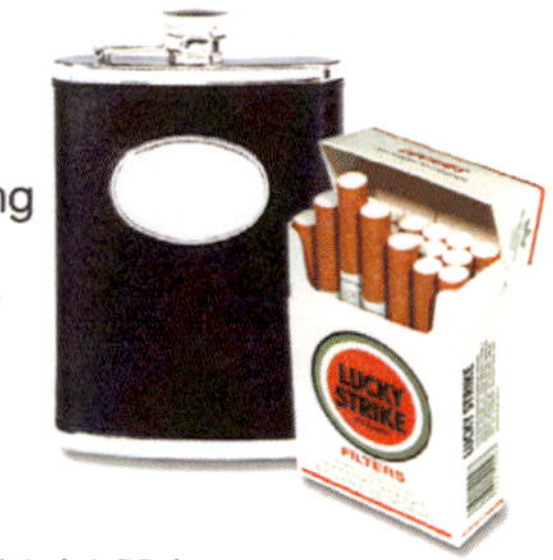

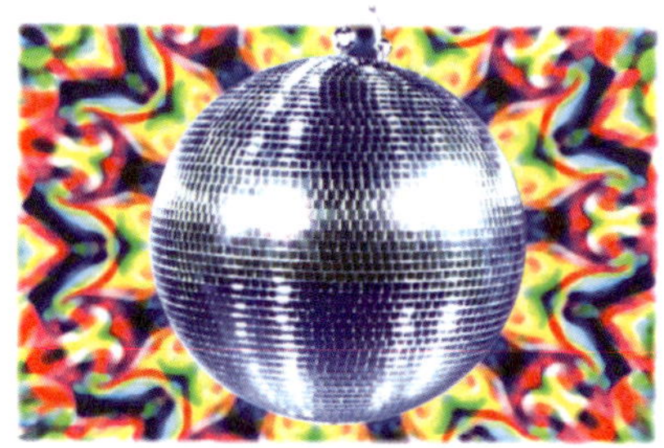

### Translymania
Have you and your staff swallow as many sample psychiatric medications they can find and then turn the lights out. Get a disco ball or strobe lights and play *The Doors* as loud as you can. See which one of you has a psychotic break first!

### Musical Flu Shots

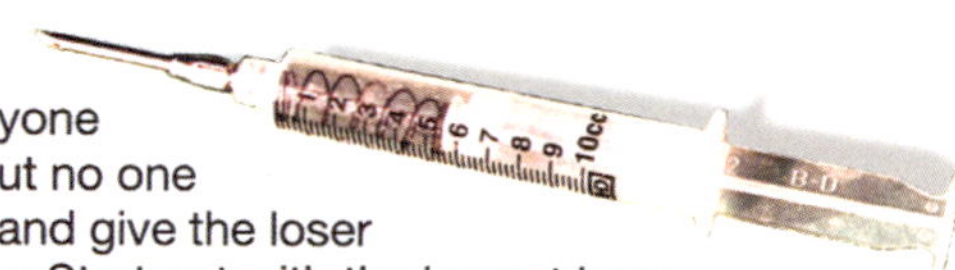

It's that time of year again. Everyone in your office needs a flu shot but no one wants one. Play musical chairs and give the loser his or her dose. *Here's the kicker:* Start out with the largest bore needles at first and work your way down to the normal size. You will never see your staff fight more then when they have to find their chairs!

**FrankenStain** Collect all the messes from the previous month – urine, stool, semen, blood, and who knows what else. Then, give out prizes for those of your staff that can guess the correct choice only by using their sense of smell. *A great time for all!*

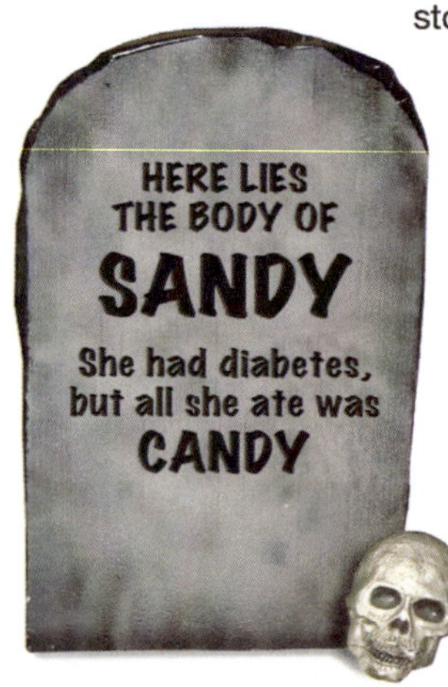
HERE LIES
THE BODY OF
SANDY
She had diabetes,
but all she ate was
CANDY

### Tombstone Mystery
Write an epitaph for the patients who you think will die in the near future and see who gets it right! A great way to decorate the office when you are done. *Warning:* some patients may find running into their own tombstone disturbing, so use first names only. +

**Happy Halloween**

## Grab your friends and get in the game!

# FANTASY Physician P4P

**By using Pay-For-Performance (P4P) scores that are published to the public, you can draft and play your own Fantasy Physician team.**

We all know how meaningless the report cards from managed healthcare companies are. ***That is until now!*** Create a private league and battle it out with your friends! Take on the world in a public medical league and show how your American team can kick the crap out of some socialized healthcare team!
Every day, statistics are downloaded into our database whereupon our propriety program analyzes such items as surgical outcomes, immunization records, HbA1C levels, and much, much, more!

**Tired of hearing how bad the healthcare system is?**
**Now you can use your opinion to make money.**
**With Fantasy Physician P4P, there are no more excuses.**

Become the coach and health care administrator. Run the team your way!

There is no more sitting on the sidelines reading about how this surgeon cut someone's wrong leg off or how that internist has committed fraud. Now it is your turn to pick the doctors that buff their charts to get good grades.

Search rosters from around the country and pick one hospital, one cardiovascular surgeon, one general surgeon, two family doctors, and two internists.

**P 4 P**

Get ready to experience the frenzied excitement as surgeons lose lives on the table and your score bottoms out. Watch as your family doctor attains a perfect score for treating asthmatics and her grades make your teams score soar! Discover how negative scoring (from post operative infections or worsening cholesterol levels) can lower your team score and put you at the bottom of the heap.

**Whether you're a grizzled gomer looking for a new challenge or a rookie hypochondriac who just hates doctors, Fantasy Physician P4P leagues are the place where patients of all levels can give their skills a true workout.**

Sure, Pay-For-Performance is an unethical way to practice medicine. Sure, grading doctors has never been proven to improve healthcare. *Who cares?* Especially when you can use this data to make cash and win with your league.

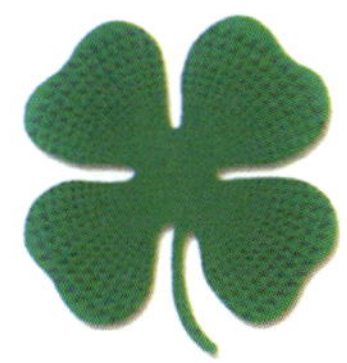

## Week One

Lucky Psychos

Red Hot Iguanas

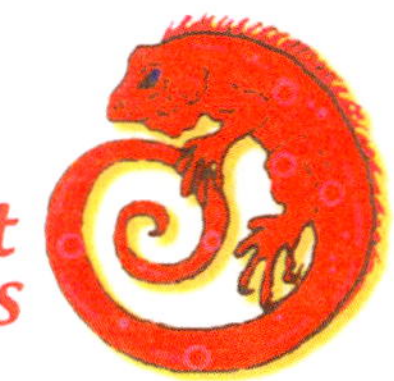

| Doctor | Grade | Doctor | Grade |
|---|---|---|---|
| Mercy Hospital (FL) | 68% | Parkview Hospital (NE) | 49% |
| Dr. P. Jones (CA) – cardiovascular surgeon | 74% | Dr. E. Ochi (AK) – cardiovascular surgeon | 86% |
| Dr. L. Smith (FL) – general surgeon | 67% | Dr. Q. Cronauer (KY) – general surgeon | 91% |
| Dr. R. Clark (HI) – family doctor | 98% | Dr. Z. Norman (OK)– family doctor | 94% |
| Dr. S. Martinez (NM) – family doctor | 81% | Dr. M. Howell (NH) – family doctor | 54% |
| Dr. RH Littman (MA) – internist | 34% | Dr. H. Speranza (NY) – internist | 90% |
| Dr. K. Hymon (GA) – internist | 89% | Dr. W. Morin (ME) – internist | 71% |
| TOTAL | 73% | TOTAL | 76% |

Fantasy Physician P4P is open to legal residents of the fifty (50) United States (excluding residents of Arizona, Iowa, Maryland, Montana, and Vermont since we don't like those states). Players must be eighteen (18) years of age or older or at least carry a firearm.

## A TRUE STORY OF MEDICINE

# THAT CAN'T BE!

It was a cold, snowy Friday night in late December of 1973. Patients occupied all seven ER rooms at a general hospital in Detroit. I was an emergency room technician working my way through *Wayne State University*. The event I'm about to tell you happened as I assisted Dr. Perkins and Nurse Crowley.

*"Dr. Perkins,"* said Nurse Crowley, holding a chart. *"I have a sixteen-year-old female patient in Room 3."*

*"What are her complaints?"*

*"Two day history of nausea, urinary frequency and low back pain."*

*"Any fever?"*

*"No."*

*"Did you get a urine?"*

*"Yes. It's normal."*

*"When was her last period?"*

*"Two weeks ago."*

Perkins introduced himself to the patient and her anxious parents. She was lying in bed holding her abdomen. A few minutes later, after examining her, he said, *"I need to do a pelvic exam. I feel something in her lower abdomen."*

The mother with tears cascading down her cheek, said, *"Is it a tumor, doctor?"*

*"Not sure,"* said Perkins, avoiding direct eye contact with the parents.

*"Oh, my God! Cancer runs in our family."* She reached over and grasped her daughter's hand.

Crowley and I took the patient into the GYN exam room. The parents waited in their daughter's room. I stood at the head of the exam table as Perkins completed the pelvic exam. He stepped back and removed his gloves. A solemn expression appeared. His shoulders slumped as he gazed down at the floor.

*"Do I have a tumor?"* asked the patient.

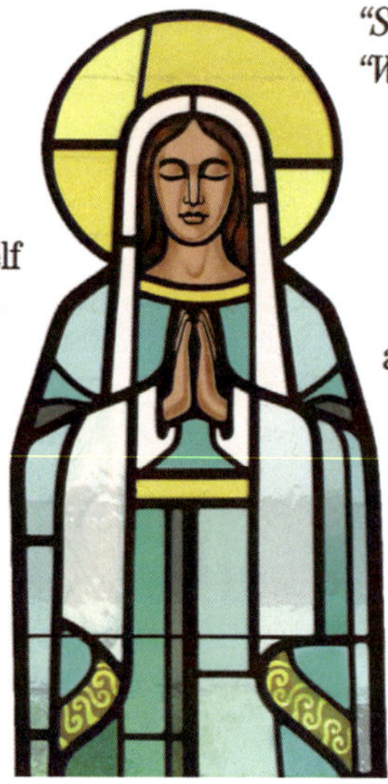

*"Sort of."*

*"What do you mean sort of?"*

*"You're pregnant."*

*"That can't be!"*

*"Why's that?"*

*"I'm a virgin."*

Perkins walked over to a small window at the far end of the room, peered upward into the night and said, *"It's another Immaculate Conception."*

Later, after a positive HCG, she admitted to having sexual activity to her parents. ✚

# MORE TRUE "PATIENTISMS"

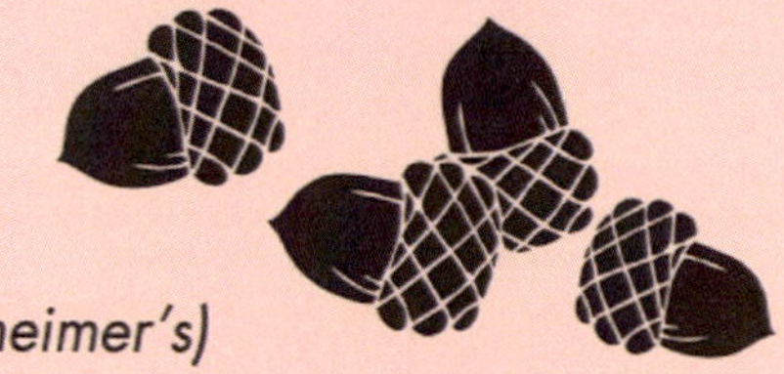

⑧ *"How bad is the pain on a scale of 1-10 with 10 being the worst ever?"*
**"10/10"**
*"The worst ever?"*
**"No."**

⑦ **"I have half-heimer's."** *(Alzheimer's)*

⑥ **"I took two *Immodium* before the *Eagles* game. I got stopped up for five days."**
*"Why did you take the Immodium? Did you have diarrhea?"*
**"No, I didn't want to go during the game."**

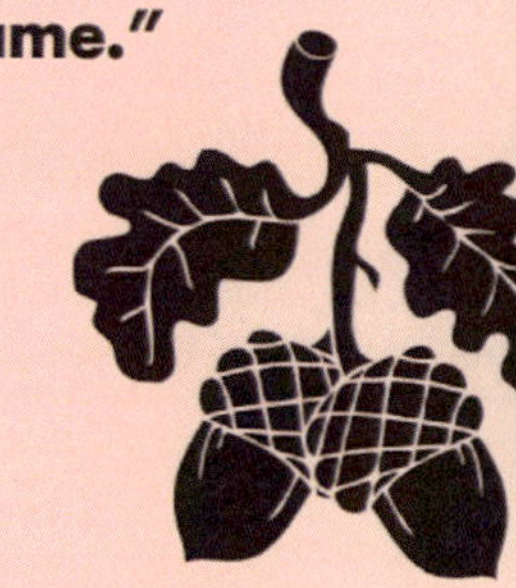

⑤ **"The twins are both five years old."**

④ *"When did you run out of the medication?"*
**"After I used it all."**

③ **"I'm here for ear pain."**
*"Which ear?"*
**"The left one. MY left one."**

② **"I've had no surgery, but I had my appendix removed in 1989."**

① **"I've been swimming a lot, in water."**

BELIEVE IT OR NOT.

# MY "REALISTIC WEEK" OF PAIN (PRACTICE)

## MONDAY

This weekend had been a full moon and I hadn't been on call, I thought with satisfaction. I was to pay for my smugness on Monday. My assistant said that two new patients had been added, one urgent from an FP I had a good relationship with (*I thought*), and one the new receptionist had double-booked *"because she was in so much pain."* New hires really screw with my schedule until they become hardened by the steady stream of narc addicts who will end up screaming at them, the most visible target before they are booted out the door.

The "urgent" patient had an impressive case of centripetal obesity that made my back hurt just to look at it. He regaled me with his 25 year history of back pain until I couldn't stand it anymore and I asked him what had changed that made his back pain urgent. He blinked in surprise and then announced, *"Well I HAD to be seen."*

I foresaw upcoming control issues so I had fun reading my narcotic contract to him line by line, outlining all HIS responsibilities. He wasn't taking it well and had had enough when I got to the part where he had to submit to random **urine toxicology screens** whenever I wanted them, not at his convenience. Problem solved.

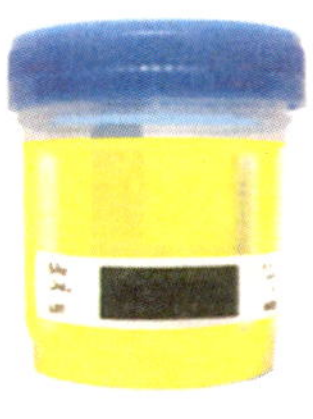

I watched second "urgent" patient waddle down the hallway to the exam room. Barely five foot tall, she weighed in at over 200 pounds. As I listened to her tale of woe of back pain that nothing had ever helped from three other pain doctors in town as well as a host of out-of- towners, I noticed a **urine drug screen** on the hospital browser. Quick as a wink, I opened it and noticed it was positive for cannaboids. She was astonished as I pounced on her about it, but she recovered enough to say that she HAD to smoke marijuana or she *"just couldn't eat for days."*

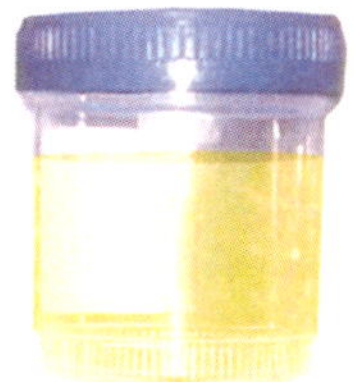

I saw her liver function profile and asked about drinking. Still unbalanced, she admitted to heavy drinking *"in the past"* but only had a few beers a day, wait, a month . . .

It was time for my ultimate weapon: the "holistic" approach to pain management: diet, exercise, and psychiatric consult. A face of blank incomprehension met mine. She started to explain how it was *"impossible"* for her to do *"any kind of exercise"* and that her only problem was back pain.

I gave her my sad little smile and gave her the final kicker – until she admitted she had a problem, no one could help her and if she changed her mind she could always contact us when she truly wanted help.

As she left the exam room, I heard her tell my assistant in wonder, *"That's the first time a doctor has every told me I had a problem."*

## TUESDAY

Since I am the only pain doctor to take the crappy military insurance, I get a mixed bag of patients, both good and bad. There are the hard working military men who just want to get better, the foreign wives driven to every psychosomatic complaint by living isolated in a foreign country, and the malingerers looking to comp out of the military (*they aren't as amusing as Corporal Klinger in* M-A-S-H).

## WEDNESDAY

Day off. My usual bank branch is closed for repairs, so I go downtown to another branch. There, on drug dealer alley, is a well known patient of mine I have been unable to bust up until now. Note to self: **time for urine toxicology screening!**

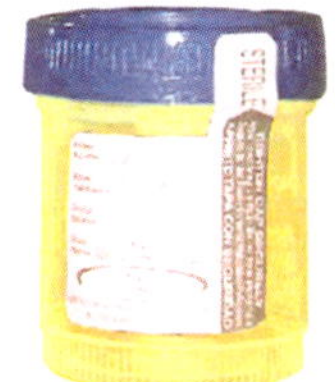

## THURSDAY

The patient from drug dealer alley comes in for his appointment. I knew the ante was going to be upped because he comes in bundled up with hat and scarf (it was 68 degrees outside) and looking miserable. I fire the opening salvo, *"I saw you on X street."* Shock, confusion, then a struggle to recover crossed his face. He mumbled a denial, but I was not to be deterred. I pressed my advantage and ordered a **urine tox screen**, confident that it's abnormalities would free me (*he refused it, so I was free anyway*).

It's good to be the queen.

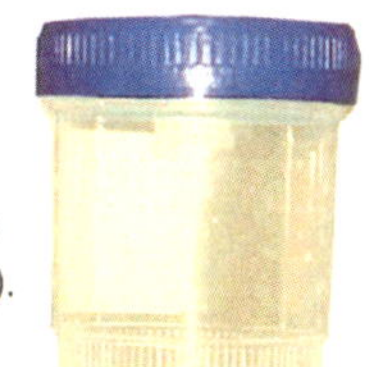

## FRIDAY

My assistant warns me that a husband and wife team is double booked. The referral is from the FP I've learned to wary of. I walk in to find the pathetic duo with all sorts of medical devices. It only gets worse as they launch into their stories of chronic back pain, failed multiple interventions and how a high dose of Oxycontin *"only takes the edge off."* Of course, they only want *"something"* for the pain.

I ask about their last prescriptions and they get evasive. I wrangle the name of the pharmacy from them and my assistant shoots out the door to call. They have enough for two more weeks so I order antidepressants and a recheck in two weeks to buy time.

As soon as they leave, I start calling the other pain docs in town. I hit paydirt with the second one I called. The receptionist politely asks which patient I am inquiring about and when I tell her, she exclaims, ***"Oh THEM! I'll interrupt the doctor for you!"***

**Time for more urine tox screens!**

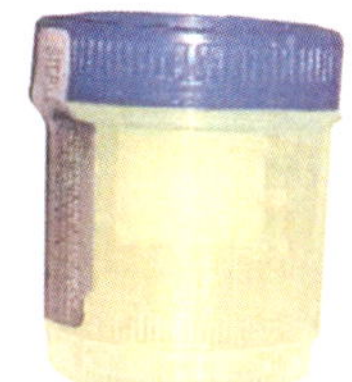

Friday night call. You know it's going no-where good when it starts with a message from my partner's patient: *"You've probably never had a call like this one . . ."*

I'm tempted to say, *"Oh yes I have,"* but call the patient back anyway. I wisely hold my tongue as the woman explains that she called the police on her husband who was taken away and that he wouldn't be in for his Monday appointment, but out of the goodness of her heart, she would still pick up his narcotic prescriptions. I assure her I will give my partner a message first thing Monday morning, although I doubt it is the one she is expecting . . . ✚

**SEND US YOUR "REALISTIC WEEK" OF MEDICINE.**

**IF WE PUBLISH IT, YOU GET A FREE ONE-YEAR SUBSCRIPTION!**

*11th Annual*

# NORTH AMERICAN PHYSIATRY CONFERENCE

Where: Sarasota, Florida When: September 10-11, 2009

**Sponsored by: PJ PHARMACEUTICALS**
Makers of *Oxycotton Candy* and *Cameloft*

## Audience

This conference is designed to aid physiatrists in evaluating and managing common problems in the field as well as to see some of the new and exciting trends in the specialty.

***Earn 15 hours of CMME***

## THURSDAY SEPTEMBER 10

7:00-8:00 a.m. Registration

8: 00 a.m. Welcome and Introductions

8:30-9:15 a.m. Specialty Introspection: *What The Hell Do Physiatrists Do Anyway?*

9:15-10:00 a.m. Plenary Session: *If Indeed We Actually Do Something, Does Anyone Ever Get Better?*

Refreshment Break

10:30-11:15 a.m. The Evolution of Creating A Special Spine Rehab Program: *How To Coax PCPs Into Sending Referrals for Epidural Injections On Their Patients Without Them Really Knowing*

11:30-12:15 p.m. Proper Fitting of Fuzzy Tennis Balls on the Four-Point Walker: *Are Generic Tennis Balls As Good As Proprietary Brands?*

LUNCH

1:30-2:15 p.m. Evidence Based Medicine and Stroke Rehabilitation: *Why The Two Will Never Meet*

2:30-3:15 p.m. Understanding the Side Effects of *Prednisone, Lyrica & Neurontin:* How To Turf Them Back To Their PCPs!

3:30-4:15 p.m. Bowel Programs: *Exciting New Trends That Will Blow Your Mind*

4:30-5:15 p.m. Physical Therapists: *Nemeses or Possible Gold Mines?*

Adjourn

6:00 p.m. Dinner and Music Provided by the Musical Group

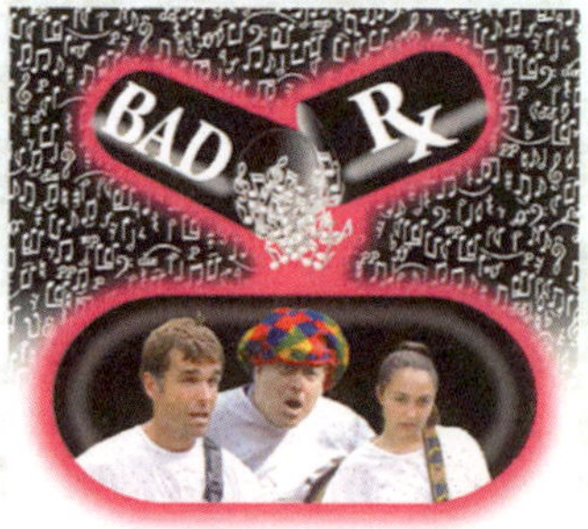
BAD
Rx

## FRIDAY SEPTEMBER 11

8:00 - 9:00 a.m. *Handle Long Meetings As Part of a 'Treatment Team' Without Wanting to Blow Your Own Brains Out*

9:15-10:00 a.m. Sexual Healing: *A New Focus of Rehabilitation* with Special Guest and Adult Film Star ***Conny Lingus*** (attendance limited due to high demand)

Refreshment Break

10:30-11:15 a.m. Finger Tingling, Headache, and Constant Hand Prutitis: *How To Obtain EMGs and Nerve Conduction Studies on EVERYBODY*

11:30-12:15 p.m. *Why P, M and R Should Stand for Planning My Retirement*

LUNCH

1:30-2:15 p.m. *New Product Information:* "PT in a Box" (comes with an exercise book, hot and cold packs, and a TENS unit)

2:30-3:15 p.m. *Clinical Pearls for Explaining the Difference Between Physiatry and Psychiatry When You Are at A Cocktail Party*

3:30-4:15 p.m. *How to Become a "Legit Front" for Widespread Narcotics Distribution*

4:30-5:15 p.m. Robotics in Rehabilitation: *How To Work Even Less & Make Even More*

**Special Closing Session**
(Dinner will be provided)
The Ethics of PMR:
*If an Epidural Injection Makes a Sound, Does it Matter If No One Really Hears The Patient Scream?*

Adjourn

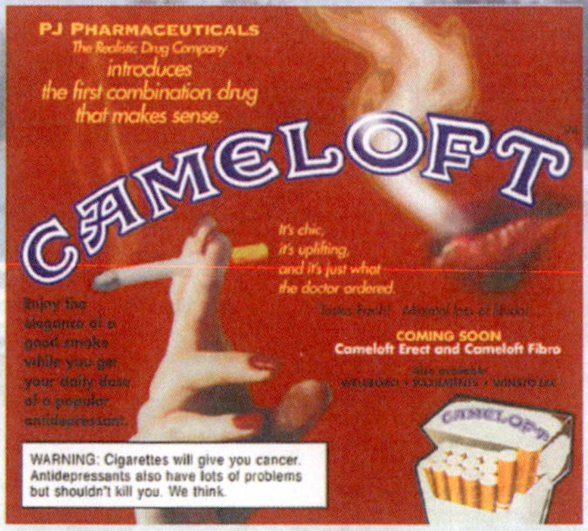


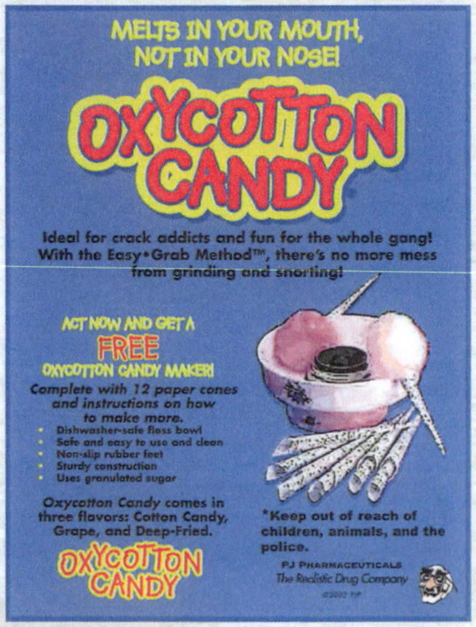
MELTS IN YOUR MOUTH,
NOT IN YOUR NOSE!
OXYCOTTON CANDY
Ideal for crack addicts and fun for the whole gang! With the Easy•Grab Method™, there's no more mess from grinding and snorting!
ACT NOW AND GET A
FREE
OXYCOTTON CANDY MAKER!
Complete with 12 paper cones and instructions on how to make more.
Dishwasher-safe floss bowl
Safe and easy to use and clean
Non-slip rubber feet
Sturdy construction
Uses granulated sugar
Oxycotton Candy comes in three flavors: Cotton Candy, Grape, and Deep-Fried.
OXYCOTTON CANDY
*Keep out of reach of children, animals, and the police.
PJ PHARMACEUTICALS
The Realistic Drug Company

***Proudly Sposored By***

## A TRUE STORY OF MEDICINE

# I LOVE ME SOME RESIDENTS

Back in the mid 90's, I was finishing my residency in Boston at St. E's in internal medicine. Little did I know, one day in medicine clinic would be like no other. I was an attractive 20-something woman who was married, but still enjoyed special attention from patients, staff, and my colleagues. *However, sometimes the attention is unwanted.*

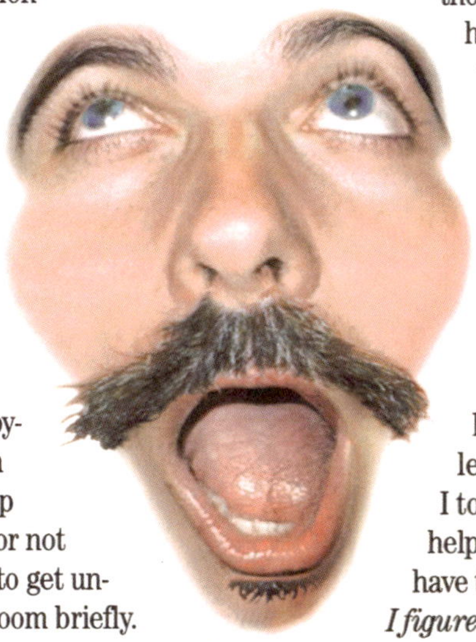

Mr. So & So was my first patient of the day, and he was in for a physical. I entered the exam room, and saw a creepy-looking short guy, with his mustache taking up too much of his face (or not enough). I asked him to get undressed, and left the room briefly. When I returned, the creepy guy was on the table and too "ready." I told him I would look at him from his head to his toes. My eyes and hands worked on him thoroughly, in the same fashion as I have examined hundreds of others.

When I got "down" to his scrotum he leaned back a little, let me palpate his junk, and without me asking if he wanted a happy ending, ***SPLOOGED*** all over my hands. *THANK GOD I was wearing gloves!* Sensing his embarrassment, I replied, *"Oh, that happens sometimes"* . . . . . . . . . (NOT!).

That was the finale to the physical, and I ran out of the room after I handed him some tissues. My preceptor thought the whole thing was hilarious. I told him that the experience was not what I considered the appropriate "doctor-patient relationship."

A few weeks later, I got a call from Mr. So & So, requesting another "clinic date." He said he was having some kind of problem with his netherparts. I told him that I could not help him, and that he would have to see another resident. *I figured that I did not get paid enough in residency, and certainly not enough for that kind of service!*

I still have not heard of any other doctor with the same experience, so I must be special. *In fact, some people who know the story wondered if they should make a physical appointment with me, too!*

I guess in these times of change in medicine, anything is possible! ✚

***Calling all physicians! Your prayers are answered. Finally there's a book that gives you the secrets to happiness on the job.***

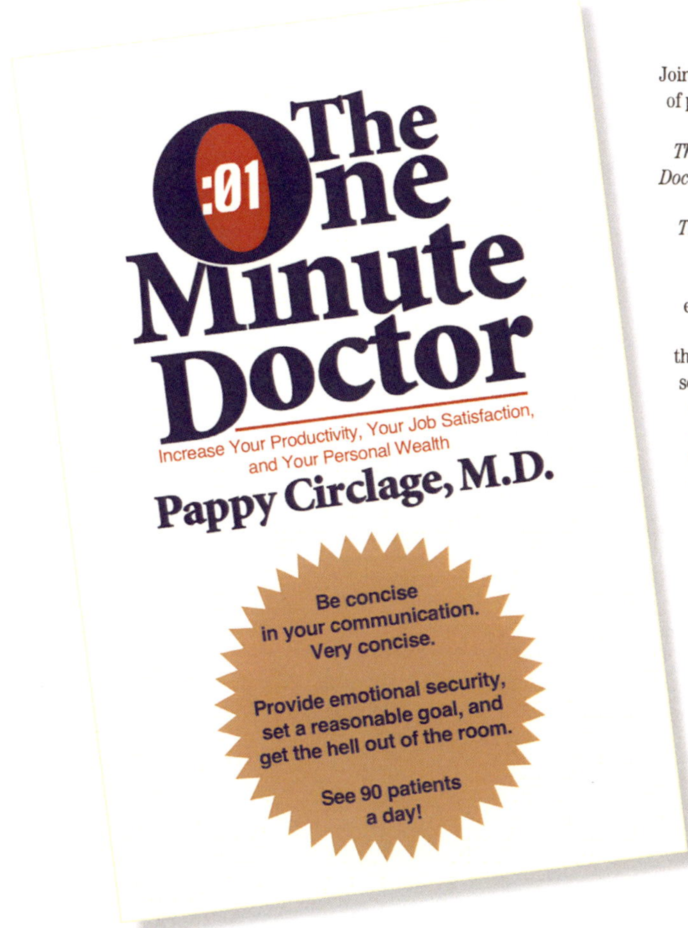


Join the thousands of physicians who have read *The One Minute Doctor*'s techniques.

*The One Minute Doctor* is a concise, easily read story that reveals three very practical secrets: create the illusion that you are there longer than you are, cut the patient off as quick as you can, and give them anything they want as long as they leave.

*Sponsored by more than two dozen managed care companies!*

**What others are saying about *The One Minute Doctor*:**

*"Though totally inappropriate, the lessons provided are profound, overly simplified, and tremendously reckless – but they work!"* **Jackie Ray Couglin, M.D.**

*"People who feel good about themselves will be better patients. So tell them anything they want to hear and give them some type of narcotic."* **Sebastion Flunhouser, DO**

**Coming soon: *The One Minute Lawsuit***

# A LANDMARK CASE STUDY

## Pinball Pain Syndrome with an Introduction of the Deep Purple Test

BY CORNELIUS PARODY, MD & ARISTOTLE JONES, PHD

*Below is a case study which reveals a common, but fascinating syndrome. Pinball Pain Syndrome is seemingly pandemic. Drs. Parody and Jones use their unique skills to address this disorder and give some recommendations to distinguish it from fibromyalgia. Lastly, a new diagnostic maneuver called the Deep Purple Test is introduced.*

### Chief Complaint:

*"I have low back pain radiating into the abdomen, up into the thoracic area, progressing up to my neck to the base of the skull and then down my left arm."*

### History of Present Illness:

Mrs. Feinman is a 63-year-old, white female presenting with complaints of abdominal pain radiating up into the interscapular area, then to the occiput, where it hangs a sharp left turn down the arm. She reports the onset of pain 50 years ago when she "broke her tailbone" after falling out of a tree. The pain has been gradually increasing in intensity until this morning at 3 a.m., when it became unbearable and she found the office number from the Yellow Pages.
She reports sensory loss in the eyebrows, fingernails, and behind her knees. She feels generally weak, and her legs "give out" suddenly although she denies any motor deficits. She reports dizziness and problems with her balance, which she thinks is due to sinus problems causing inner ear problems. After intensive research on the Internet, she is fairly convinced that she has both fibromyalgia (based on "hurting all over") and intermittent claudication. She does not actually have any pain with ambulation, but she likes how it sounds when she tells people she has "intermittent claudication."

### Past Medical History:

Migraine headaches since age two, irritable bowel syndrome and chronic fatigue syndrome.

### Past Medical History:

Laparoscopy x7 for pelvic pain, TAH/BSO (hysterectomy), laparoscopy x7 for pelvic adhesions secondary to surgeries above, exploratory laparotomy for small bowel obstruction x 7 secondary to all above.

### Social History:

Widowed times four, has been on SSDI for chronic headaches since age 46, smokes two packs a day, abstains from alcohol because both parents were alcoholics.

### Family History:

Unknown; *"I won't speak to them anymore."*

### Medications:

Xanax 0.5 mg tid, Vicodin 5/500 tid, Soma tid, Ambien 10 mg qhs, black cohosh, ginseng, Metabovegetan 99+, gingko biloba, Flintstones vitamins.

### Allergies:

All "cyclines", Thorazine, Prolixin, Haldol, lithium, Lactated Ringer's.

### Review of Systems:

Data entry form that she filled it has one line drawn from the top of the page to the bottom which denotes everything is positive (even penile discharge).

### Physical Exam:

Vital Signs: Weight 97 lbs., Pulse 134, BP 110/60

General: Very tan white female; thin and in no acute distress. Designer clothing with extensive makeup. Small lap dog named Chinchee.

Neck – no thyromegaly

CV – RRR no murmur

Lungs – clear with mild expiratory wheeze

Abdomen – thin; lots of surgical scars; diffuse pain throughout with no rebound or Murphy sign

Skin – tanned and smoked like leather, no rash or dysplastic lesions

Back – no spasm; soft

Musculoskeletal – tenderness with palpation of all body parts, including hair and even some items of her clothing.

Neuro – grossly intact, negative straight leg raises, normal reflexes

### Diagnostic Workup:

MRI reports from other practitioners were reviewed. These included studies of the neck, lumbar spine, and an MRA of the brain. All were negative. Plain films of the knees, lumbar spine and chest were also found to be normal. Also negative were abdominal and pelvic CT scans, extensive blood work, tea leaf readings, horoscope analyses, and three past life readings.

### Impression:

Possible Pinball Pain Syndrome

### Deep Purple Test:

Drs. Parody and Jones employed their new diagnostic procedure to elucidate the patient's true problem. By having the physician touch the patient firmly with his or her thumb, they were able to bring about a certain sound from the subject. Specifically, the sound was *"Oww!"* With proper training, the clinicians were able to rhythmically able to press enough areas to make the sounds as follows:

*"Oww, Oww, Oww . . . Oww, Oww, a-Oww . . . Oww, Oww, Oww . . . Oww, Owwwww!"*

With the right cadence and pitch, Drs. Parody and Jones were successful in reproducing the song *"Smoke On The Water"* by the rock group *Deep Purple*.

### Discussion:

Pinball Pain Syndrome is an interesting variant of a more generalized disorder, specifically fibromyalgia. Just as absurd, this disorder also possesses the usual complaints of fatigue, dizziness, weakness, and total body pain. Eerily similar to the "magic bullet" in the Kennedy assassination, it also has a very discrete pain complaint that radiates along non-anatomic pathways.

Pinball Pain Syndrome is often associated with the Tar-Baby Syndrome (also called Whack-A-Mole Pain), wherein successful treatment of any given pain complaint spawns two or more new complaints. It is called Pinball Pain Syndrome because it bounces all around. Etiology of this disease process is unknown, but it is postulated that there may be supratentorial "flippers" that keep the pain in play even if the physicians manage to fix something. The conclusions may seem fuzzy and devoid of logic, but it does allow the physicians to have fun at work.

### Treatment:

None. The authors recommend some basic steps to fix the problem. At the very least, cancelling the Yellow Pages ad would be a step in the right direction. One could also drop the patient's insurance plan immediately, but this may be sound better than it really is. Like the line in the movie *Last of the Mohicans*, patients always believe, *"I will find you."* Medication is truly useless and could change the Deep Purple Test in a way that would make the song unrecognizable or worse yet, sound something like a Barry Mannilow diddy. Billing the patient or insurance company for the Deep Purple Test is difficult but one can try using the code for prolotherapy since no one really knows what that is either.

### Conclusion:

The authors believe that Pinball Pain Syndrome is probably the same as fibromyalgia, but feel calling it something else would be the only way they could get published. It is also much more enjoyable. ✚

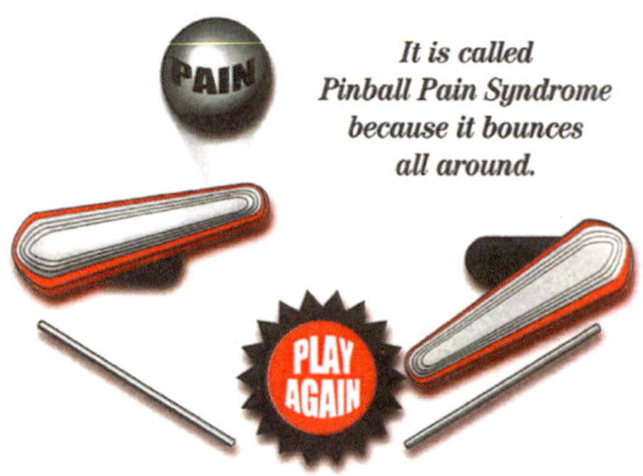


***It is called Pinball Pain Syndrome because it bounces all around.***

PHOTOCOPY THESE PAGES AND HAND OUT TO YOUR PATIENTS

# American Family Practitioner

## INFORMATION FROM YOUR FAMILY DOCTOR

## What Can You Do for Premenstrual Syndrome (PMS)?

**Please note:** The information presented is the best we could make up. Depending on our mood, this could always change. Some of this material is not suited for anyone.

### What are the symptoms of Premenstrual Syndrome?

Premenstrual Syndrome (called PMS for short) has many symptoms. The symptoms can occur a week or so before the menstrual period starts. They can continue for a week or so after the menstrual period ends. They can also occur throughout the whole month. Basically, you can have PMS whenever you feel like it.

The main symptoms of PMS are feeling irritable, anxious, short-tempered, and angry. In short, you are a raging bitch. Things on your body may swell, you may crave weird foods, and you may beat the crap out of your husband (especially if he mentions the swelling thing). This is normal and natural.

### How common is PMS?

Does it matter? The fact that you are cursed with PMS while your husband doesn't even know how lucky he has it is the main point here. Thank God for prostatitis.

### What causes PMS?

Contrary to a popular rumor, PMS is not another name for Mad Cow Disease. In fact, whoever originated that nasty joke will be found and dealt with accordingly. The causes of PMS aren't actually known, though most women believe that male scientists have known for years but have conspired together not to let the truth leak out. It is possible that your brain chemistry changes are occurring in order to make up for being the smarter gender. That is our story and we are sticking to it. Does anyone have a problem with that?

### How will my doctor find out if I have PMS?

You will tell your doctor you have PMS. End of story. If your doctor is female, she will understand. If your doctor is male, then make him understand . . . or pay.

Using a diary is a great way to get in touch with how you are feeling. We recommend photocopying a picture of your husband's face. Shrink it down and make enough of them for every day of the year. In your *Kathy* calendar, glue in all the pictures and then start doodling on them depending on how you feel. For example, putting scissors through his head is a catchy image to show you (and him) that you need to be left alone. At the end of the month, bring the calendar in with you to your doctor's office and see how quickly he or she gives you any prescription you want.

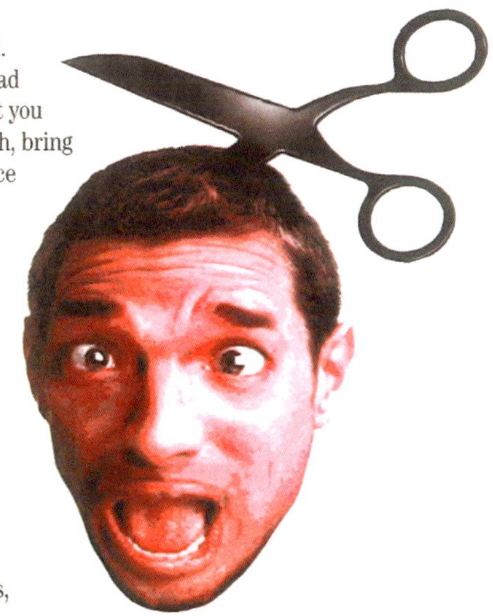

### Are there any treatments for PMS?

Yes. PMS can be treated. A combination of treatments usually helps the most. Your doctor may suggest using less caffeine, salt and sugar. He or she is wrong. Eat whatever or whenever you want. Take as much ibuprofen as needed so that you can fight the urge to tie a fishing line around your husband's testicles and play "start the lawn mower!" If all else fails, and you have already had kids, then send your uterus packing.

### The Bottom Line

With PMS, you make the rules. PMS can stand for either **Pissy Mood Syndrome** or **Potential Murder Suspect** depending on who pushes your buttons. The choice is theirs. These rules can change at any time depending on whether you want them to or not. Your husband can agree to this by ducking, groveling or feeding you tons of chocolate, or he can get the f*ck out! Of course, he must make that choice after he removes the scissors from his head.

*This handout provides a general idea of this topic. Not everyone will like what they read. For those people, we recommend talking to your own family doctor.*

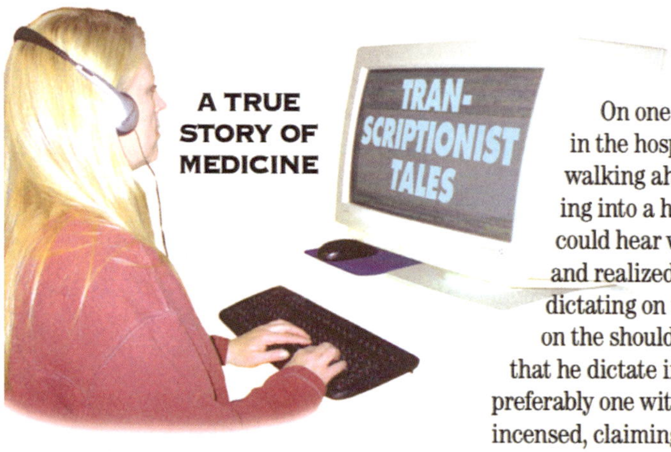


On one visit to see a friend in the hospital there was a man walking ahead of me speaking into a handheld recorder. I could hear what was being said and realized it was a physician dictating on the go. I tapped him on the shoulder and suggested that he dictate in an enclosed space, preferably one with a door. He became incensed, claiming no one had any idea what he was saying. I pulled him aside and repeated the patient's name, his diagnosis, and some of the medication he was on. *The doctor's mouth fell open.* I have no idea why he would think in this day and age of everyone talking on cell phones where everyone can easily hear all that is being said that no one would be paying attention.

At one of the hospitals I worked at as a medical transcriptionist, we had assigned areas during tornados and storms. When the warning bells went off medical personnel was told to go to their assigned area. Mine was post-surgical care. We all wheeled patients resting on their beds into the hallways and lined them up. Often after surgery one of the requirements before a patient can go home is that they pass gas. As the employees were sitting on the floor waiting for the storm to abate, one patient after another passed gas. The pitches were different and it almost sounded like music when you combined them. We were trying not to breathe, let alone laugh, until one of the patients looked at the patient across from her and said, *"I knew you was the long-winded one with all that talking in there."*

We couldn't contain our laughter and it all ended well. They all felt better and were laughing also as we took them back to post-surgical care. We were really happy we could change hallways.

During one dictation a physician was quietly dictating a history and physical, apparently while still in the patient's room. In the background I could hear the patient complaining about "foreign doctors." She kept screaming at him, *"I can't understand you. You can go back where you came from. I want an American doctor."*

He stopped dictating and I could hear him say to her, *"Ma'am, I'm from New York."*

While typing for a hospital in California apparently this physician was very, very tired. He received a cell phone call while he was dictating and I could hear him ordering a new *Lexus*. When he continued dictating he stated, *"The interior is blue."* As he was not a surgeon, I was not sure whether he was still talking about the car or the patient, so I flagged it just in case.

One of my favorite physicians was behind in his dictation. We had been warned by our supervisor that there would be extra dictation on the system and it would come up with a different code. He was scheduled to take his wife to Hawaii and the hospital had just informed him they would not release his check until all of his over 100 charts were dictated. He had three days to complete his dictation or he would not get paid. I was working the midnight shift and I seem to have gotten most of his dictation to transcribe. He must have waited until his wife was asleep. I listened as he whispered into the recorder and I tried to decipher his long-distance dictation. When he came back he personally brought me several fresh pineapples and a lei. He was a very thoughtful man and a thorough physician.

I typed for a physician who loved a play on words, as do I. He would always tell me a joke somewhere during the dictation and he always threw in a word that was close, but not correct to see if I was on my toes. I enjoyed his dictation immensely. He was dictating about a patient's foot, but said "helix" which is part of the ear. Hallux is part of the foot. He always knew exactly which patient he put the trick word with and as soon as I would bring him the dictation to sign he would go directly to that patient's dictation and check to see if I caught it.

I will never forget one patient who came in with her husband. She had poison ivy on a particular area of her upper body. As the physician dictated he noted her husband was also diagnosed with poison ivy and was the primary cause of his wife's discomfort. It was a joy to work for that physician. And he truly cared about his patients. He went above and beyond for them.

With voice recognition now I am thankful that the charts are edited. I typed a chart recently where we had to insert a line toward the bottom just above the signature line if a PA-C was the dictator. It should have read, *"This patient's chart was dictated by Jane Doe, PA-C for Dr. John Smith."* The dictator sneezed and coughed while dictating that particular line and Voice Recognition typed it out as, *"This patient was killed by Jane Doe, PA-C for killing Dr. John Smith."*

While that might have been the sentiment of the PA-C, I was pretty sure they didn't want it in black and white.

In transcribing, one letter can make a huge difference in the meaning of the sentence, i. e., *"The patient was now taking oxygen,"* to *"The patient was not taking oxygen."*

At one point I was working in a physician's office and I doubled as a transcriptionist and office assistant. On filling out the required form at my physician's office for my annual physical, in the box where it asked for my occupation I put *"office ass."* I had forgotten to put the "t" for asst. *They brought this to my attention after laughing about it for awhile.* ✚

Believe It Or Not.

# MY 'REALISTIC WEEK' IN PRACTICE

## I'M JUST SPREADING IT AROUND. AND AROUND.

### MONDAY

Let's hear it for the demented. They can drive you nuts but at least they aren't malicious about it. In fact, depending on your perspective, they can make your day. Take Theresa, for example. She has the disease bad. I have seen her decline over the years very rapidly. She now lives in a home for others with Alzheimer's disease and comes in every six months or so. She is in her late eighties and it seems her brain damage has left her a little less inhibited. Actually, she usually tries to hit on me with every visit and uses very inappropriate comments to boot. *Not a bad way to boost your ego on a tough Monday afternoon!* Usually it is something strange like, *"Close your eyes and I will give you a big surprise"*. No, I never close my eyes and there are never any surprises.

***"Boy, is this doctor handsome!"***

is her favorite line today. Being polite, I would then say, *"Thank you"*. Since she forgot she said it two minutes earlier, this interaction would repeat itself over and over. *Can you blame me for going into the room eight or nine times this afternoon?* Hey, it was tough day and I needed something positive; even if it was from a demented elderly female who has an inhibition problem.

Went to ER after work to admit a patient. As I was finishing up I could see the lowlife enter the area. No it wasn't a patient. **It was the ER doc you love to hate.** The one who never wants to do a full work-up. The one who thinks everything is an admission. **The one who is a complete moron.** I saw him scanning with his eyes just looking for someone to dump his work on. I knew he hadn't even really examined the patient in Bed 2. I slowly slinked my way past most of the nurses and was on my way out when I heard him questioning me, *"Are you covering for Dr. Smith?"* **Son of a bitch!** He got me again. It was going to be a long night.

### TUESDAY

After a long night on call, I physically got the sh*t kicked out of me by a four year old. By this age you would think Gina would be used to seeing doctors. No. She wasn't even sick. It was a "well child visit" that went awry as soon as she hit the hallway going towards the exam room. That is when I first saw her. Like an old western, our eyes met as we crossed paths and she stared me down with a scowl on her face.

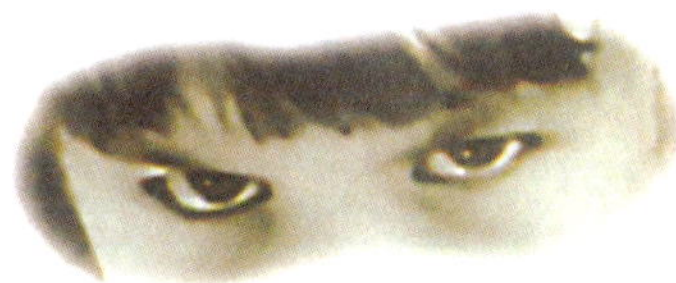

She was like a little Clint Eastwood and I knew this was going to be bad. The first part of the interview was going fine but she would growl every now and then. Each time we locked eyes she would squint and try to intimidate me. **It worked.** As the actual examine started, a slow crescendo of screaming and absolute terror began occurring. By the time I asked the Mom to remove her pants (the child's pants, not hers), Gina was ready for the big showdown. This little Tasmanian Devil wriggled and squirmed and screamed to her heart's delight. I went over to help Mom when Gina decided her feet should do the rest of her talking. **She kicked me about 12 times over the next three seconds.** It happened so fast that Bruce Lee would have been proud. That is when I removed myself from the room for a little quiet time. I returned, better composed, and went over some simple "anticipatory guidance" or instructions for parents and left the room with a smile. The exam was over for me, but not for Gina. My medical assistants were coming in with three immunizations to give her a taste of my little revenge.

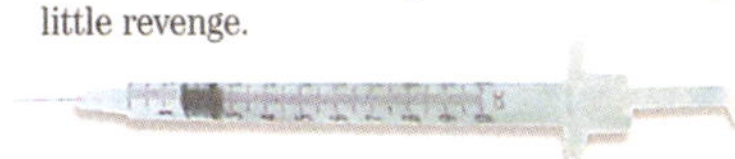

### WEDNESDAY

As my children get older I start to get melancholic more and more. It used to be that my day off was a way to have some peace and quiet. What broke the silence were my boys begging for my time and attention. I actually used to fight it. Now they want to spend time with their friends and it is me begging for the their time and attention. Today we went to the movies together. **I was happy.** They were tolerant. *Life is weird.*

### THURSDAY

Paper work kills me. I can't really "read" it all even though I know that if I sign it I am liable for it. *Doesn't matter.* The more I actually make myself read, the more I want to vomit.

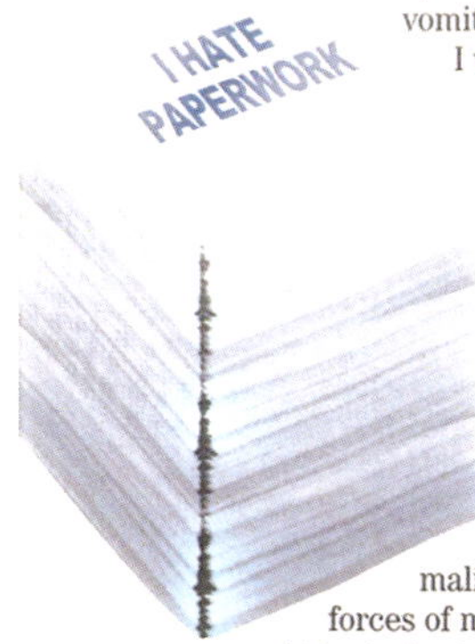


I was blowing through about three reams of absolute crap when I saw the note about George. *Ah, George.* He could never get better. He was on worker's compensation and they were investigating him for malingering. The two forces of me trying to heal him, and him trying to get his compensation check were the perfect example of the metaphorical rock and hard place. I sent him to every specialist in the world. His last stop over the past year and a half was with the chronic pain specialists. To be honest, their notes showed they were on the ball. These notes were the few I truly read because I enjoyed their description of George's **MOCUS.** Every letter started off detailing how George was doing worse, and ended with how George received a new injection, a new medicine, or a new therapy session and should progress well. **So naïve.** ***So humorous.*** Of course, George never did progress, but these pain specialists were eternal optimists nonetheless. Got to give them credit for that. **Today's note was the nugget I was waiting for.** The worker's compensation case with George was settled and they stated he entered the pain clinic with a shimmy in his step and a smile on his face. Now his pain was minimal, his energy was high and his future was bright. ***God bless modern medicine.***

### FRIDAY

Kelly is her mid-twenties and called yesterday at 4:30 pm. She wanted to be seen for back pain and headaches. We were able to finagle the schedule and see her the next day (today) at 8:45 am. We don't get a thank you. Today comes and there is no Kelly to be seen. At 9:05 am, Kelly calls the office and says *"I still have back pain and headaches. What am I supposed to do?"* My receptionist thought maybe she was hallucinating. **Didn't she have this same conversation at the end of the day yesterday?**

*"Kelly"*, my receptionist said, *"You were put in for this morning and missed your appointment which was twenty minutes ago"*.

Kelly responded in an indignant manner, *"Yeah, so, I overslept"*. Looking at her chart, I saw that she was my partner's patient and had missed three appointments in the last three months. I left him a note stating that she can get her back pain and headaches cared for by someone else in the future. She is never to be placed in my schedule again.

**Another "feel-good" case.**

Spent the rest of the day fending off latecomers who want to get in for minor issues before the weekend. As I was covering for three other doctors off for the day, my staff and I had to use all our powers to triage. Patients are getting good, however, in their anti-triage skills. Like Superman's Kryptonite, these special people can always say the right trigger complaints that get them right in. Things like "chest pain" when all they have is a simple rib strain or "shortness of breath" when all they have is a simple cold really burns my ass. Melanie was one of those who had the latter symptom and fought me hard when I refused to give her an antibiotic for her virus. I could have succumbed, but I was determined to do right by science. **I also wanted to give Melanie a dig back for weaseling her way in.** The exam ended poorly and the rest of my day had a black cloud over it. Sometimes these fights aren't worth it – even if you spread antibiotic resistance. ✚

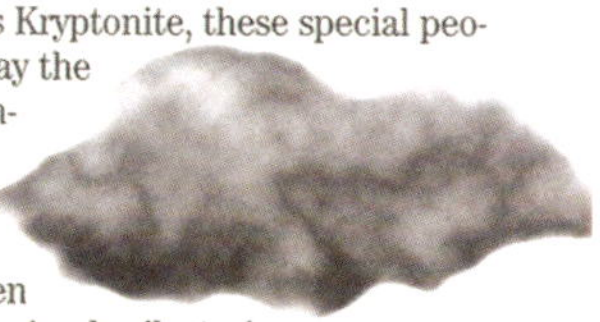

*Don't you hate it when a dermatologist gets paid $400 to freeze off a wart while you net $12 after spending an hour preventing death in an 80-year-old by managing a delicate balance of 25 medications and 12 chronic diseases?*

*Does the lack of reimbursement for cognitive skill and time investment (i.e. actually caring for patients) have you down?*

*Well buck up, little campers!*

The *Placebo Journal* Continuing Meaningless Medical Education Conference Series continues this winter with . . .

# Rejuvenescence!

*This important field of cosmesis is characterized by three important steps that those other "doctors" have known for years!*

**Participants will be able to employ the three steps and their varying applications:**

**STEP ONE:** Inject anything into any part of any patient for any reason, or shoot a laser at anyone for any reason.

**STEP TWO:** Bill with procedure code.

**STEP THREE:** Cash Check.

**Let our Aesthetic Medicine Professionals Show You *The Future of Medicine!***

This enlightening and "rejuvenating" conference will be held at the beautiful Wannabuyalexus Resort in Hawaii on Dec 19 - 20th. Classes are held from 9:00 to 9:15 a.m. on each day of the conference.

# Rejuvenescence!

**is a multi-level marketing franchise system proven to extract large amounts of cash from all ages, all skin types, and all types of rich patients.**

**Here is what past graduates have had to say about the conference:**

*"Before Rejuvenescence, my clinic barely broke even. I was often on call for their emergencies, and I often was late getting home to my family. I even had to drive a mid-size domestic sedan! Now, while those patients are either dead or seeing some other sucker, I inject wrinkles and zits, and I drive a Beamer! Did I mention I don't take any call anymore?"*

– Larry O'Brien DO

*"I don't even remember what congestive heart failure is. Now when I see an EKG, I think about injections that could smooth out that jagged line! Thank you for the amazing life-changing conference!"*

– Sasha Weinstein MD

*"Thanks to your conference, I learned that a patient's respect doesn't pay the bills. I got rich, divorced, landed an amazing trophy wife, and got good at golf! Thanks Rejuvenescence!"*

– Jack Winkle MD

**Rejuvenate Your Medical Career with Rejuvenescence!**

Call 1-555-REJUVENATE and reserve your spot today.

Only $1999 if you mention the code words: *"VANCE SENT ME."*

# A TRUE STORY
of all the weird, good, and bad things that happened in the Fall of my
# THIRD YEAR OF RESIDENCY.

### LATE AUGUST 2006:

**Sunday:** My wife and I noticed the smell of a dead rotting animal in our backyard. We figured a cat or rabbit or squirrel had died under our deck and we made plans to dismantle parts of the deck later that week to get it out.

**Monday:** A bat flew out of our furnace room and scared the crap out of us while we were watching a movie. We later found, caught, and released it.

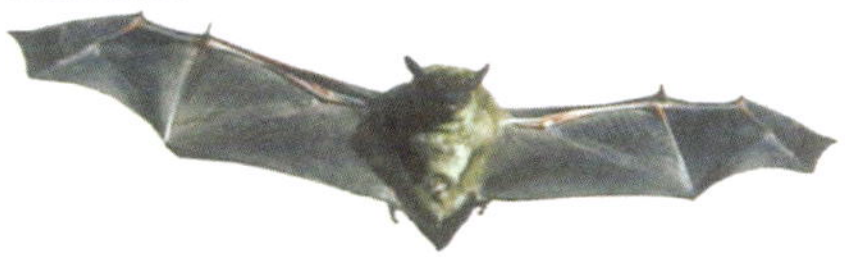

**Monday night, 11:30 p.m:** The sister of my depressed neighbor rang our doorbell asking if we had seen her sister. It seemed the neighbor had sent her 8-year-old son's Social Security cards to her brother in Colorado along with a note that said, *"I'm sorry."* I hazard a guess that the smell in our back yard was something bigger than a cat.

**Tuesday:** Her family managed to open her garage. She apparently had used a hefty dose of *Carbon Monesta* and took a really, really, really long nap lying down in the back seat. Based on all the evidence, she'd been dead for a week, lying in the 100+ degree heat and 90% humidity. *(All the upholsterers in the world couldn't de-violate this car.)* Our county coroner usually took a resident with him on coroner calls. Since I was right next door, guess what. *Yup.* It was horrible. I didn't puke but had to work really work not to.

**Wednesday:** The corpse was unidentifiable, and she'd had a bunch of oral surgery due to tongue/mouth cancer from smoking so they couldn't ID her with dental records. The cops called the coroner, who was just starting a 12-hour ER shift and asked him to go biopsy an internal organ for DNA identification. He couldn't get out of the ER so he called me, another resident, and another attending, and gave us the job. We went to the funeral home where she was in a cooler awaiting cremation *(the maggots are really thriving in there)* and using tin shears we got from the attending's garage and a disposable scalpel, we performed the thoracotomy and took a generous piece of her left ventricle. It was highly denatured but still had some mild resemblance to muscle and at least wasn't being eaten by worms. The cop was satisfied, thus ending the dead neighbor part of the story, except to say that I can get you a great deal on a slightly used *Buick*.

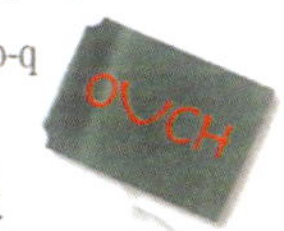


**Thursday:** I noticed a big sub-q zit on my scrotum. I though it was poppable so I cranked on it. *I'm a doctor for crying out loud.* I knew better than this. Many readers already know where this story is going. So all the squeezing I could muster caused only pain, and I was denied the highly satisfying reward of expression of anything but foul language.

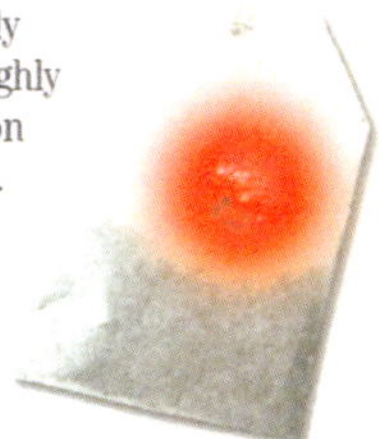

**Friday:** That little zit had turned into a sizable abscess so big it looked like a third nut. And it hurt. *Bad.* Something akin to keeping a big binder clip on there all day *(I would imagine.)* I now feared for the life of my coin purse and I called a friend who called me in some antibiotics and reminded me to sit in a tub of hot water several times a day.

**Saturday:** Pain. Hot Water. Pain. Repeat.

**Sunday:** Repeat of Saturday.

**Monday:** I worked all day long in clinic. I had never been so efficient. Something about a scrotum of fire will markedly increase your productivity.

**Tuesday:** I knew I was leaving for vacation in four days, and I also knew that something must be done about my teabag so I called a urology attending who got me in first thing in the morning. He thought there was some fluctuance there, so now . . .

*continued on next page*

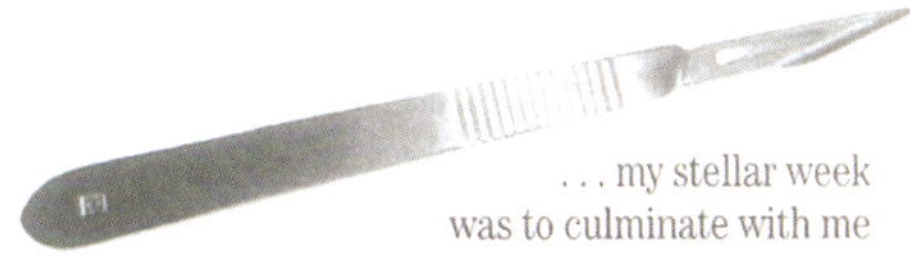

. . . my stellar week was to culminate with me watching him fillet my beanbag. If there is one place in the UNIVERSE I did not want to see a scalpel, it would be there. For whatever reason, all the lidocaine did not work. The English language has no words to describe what I experienced next so let's just skip to me leaving the clinic. I left in PAIN, with a nice 1/4" string of gauze hanging out of my balls, which actually looked kind of funny, like I had a intrascrotal tampon in place. *I guess I sort of did.* Hopefully not the kind that caused toxic shock.

**Wednesday:** Back to urology – packing comes out, more goes in, no anesthesia. If we ever get pregnant, I'm liable to be less sympathetic to the *"you don't know how this feels"* routine, because at least my wife can get an epidural. Preliminary report said staph. Antibiotics are changed *"just in case."*

**Thursday:** Same routine, except that this time an 18-gauge needle went into the incision and then superiorly into a very tender inflamed and very indurated area that he still suspected septated abscess in. *No anesthetic.* Lab comes back MRSA. Another antibiotic change. Knowing I was leaving for vacation, he taught my wife how to pack the wound and supervised her first attempt. She said she was sorry as the pain tore up my scroat thru the cord and then into my abdomen. I wanted to believe her, but inside I knew I should have done the dishes last week.

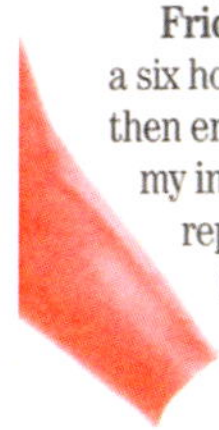

**Friday:** We drove three hours followed by a six hour plane flight the next morning, and then enjoyed a seven-day Alaskan cruise with my in-laws. For the first several days, my wife repeated the packing change. Although going on vacation in this situation was about the same on the fun scale as a week at work while getting kicked repeatedly in the nuts, at least it would be cooler there, and I was going to have nut pain anyway.

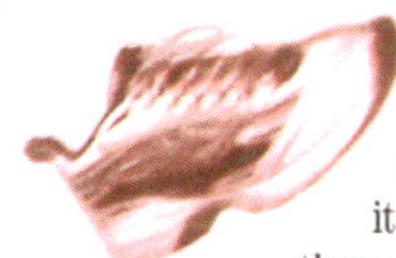

All the deck chairs on the cruise liner must be for decoration, because apparently the proper way to "cruise" was not to pig out on desserts and kick back with a book and a nice hot water bottle in your lap, but instead, to get off the boat and walk around tourist traps until you found the perfect collector's thimble or collect a cumulative total of 10,000 dirty looks from townies who both love and hate you. Other than walking five miles a day with my teeth gnashing and a pound of gauze stuffed into my underwear, going through a daily procedure that felt much like what I would imagine disemboweling to feel like, not getting to enjoy the 20 hot tubs on board or experience any marital bliss in the cabin for fear of my balls falling out of their protective case, I guess I couldn't complain about the cruise – at least I wasn't on call or *actually* getting disemboweled.

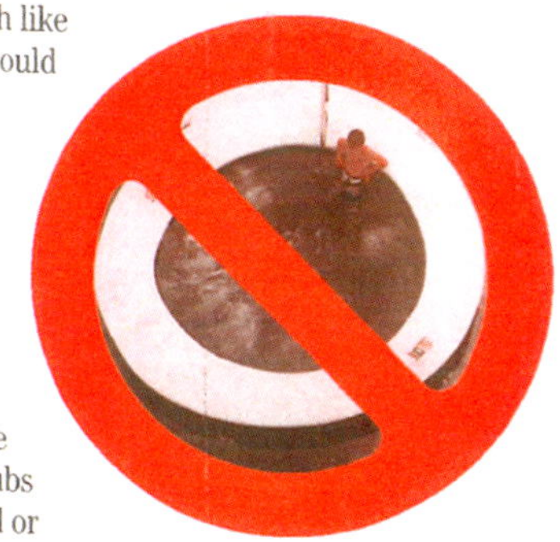

I got back home and the next day my wife told me we were going to have our first baby. *We were elated.* To top that off, after a couple of weeks of work I got to leave to receive an award that ultimately gave me a bunch of money and a free trip to the AAFP Scientific Assembly in DC.

We got to see lots of sights and met lots of people and walked until our feet were numb. By this point, the walking wasn't bothering me too much, at least not the first five miles or so. The problem there, was that we walked no less than 30 miles in two and a half days, and each night I was left with some good reminders of why not to try to pop zits below the waist.

### MID-OCTOBER 2006

Anyway, I was enjoying the turn around. Good stuff was happening to me again. So I got back from DC and rejoined the OB rotation and delivered babies for *(count 'em)* five whole days, when over the weekend the pendulum started to swing.

We went out of town to see some family and I started having some pretty serious abdominal pain. I made it back home Sunday night and couldn't sleep due to the pain. Luckily for me, I still had my denial, my pride, and a bottle of hydrocodone – all three leftovers from the nasty gonad incident from which I obviously learned nothing.

I was able to get to sleep with the help of the Vitamin L (or V, depending on which name brand you prefer when referring to hydrocodone). I woke up four hours later, pain worse than before and did the smart thing. I re-dosed the hydrocodone and went back to happy dreamland.

I woke up four hours later on Monday morning, and to my surprise, I was in terrible abdominal pain which until now I had refused to admit was at McBurney's point. (I had previously insisted that this "abdominal situation" was serious constipatory retaliation of cheesy corn dip. Friday night at a party, I encountered a huge bowl of very tasty cheese-corn-jalepeno dip that challenged me to a duel. I gladly accepted, and triumphantly threw down the entire insane amount and half a sack of tortilla chips. I spent the weekend convincing myself my symptoms were the last fighting efforts of defeated corn dip.)

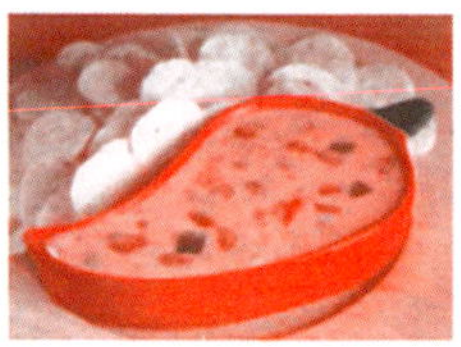

OK, back to waking up in pain: Pretty sure what was up, I called in sick and my boss ordered me some lab work and a CT scan, and of course I had a huge inflamed appendix. Now that I think about it, it probably was retaliation of the corn dip because, man, I ate a LOT of it.

That afternoon, I got to have my belly hair trimmed and a bunch of nurses I know got to administer some midazolam in pre-op and found out all the stuff they ever wanted to know about me. Did I mention that as part of the H&P I got to tell them that I was a probable MRSA carrier, and that I just got over a bad nutsack infection?

I then went through a very successful laparoscopic appendectomy in the afternoon and even got to come home that night to my newly made friend, hydrocodone. I spent the next day *(our wedding anniversary)* in bed. Not a lot of marital celebration went on, if you know what I mean.

A few days went by, and I was back to work. My life was now back to normal: incising scrotal abscesses, performing abdominal surgery, and prescribing narcotics to idiots who tried to pop scrotal folliculitis and ignored acute abdominal pain. ✚

MY APPENDECTOMY

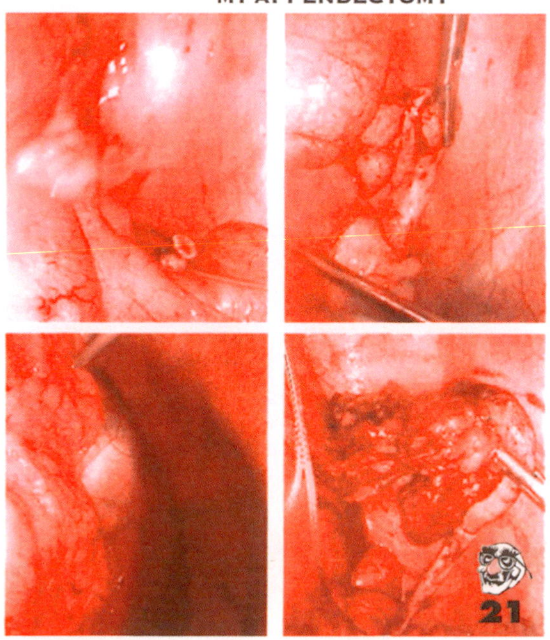


# X-Ray Files

## YIKES!

***Is this a CT of an alien's head?***
*(No, the patient moved during scanning.)*

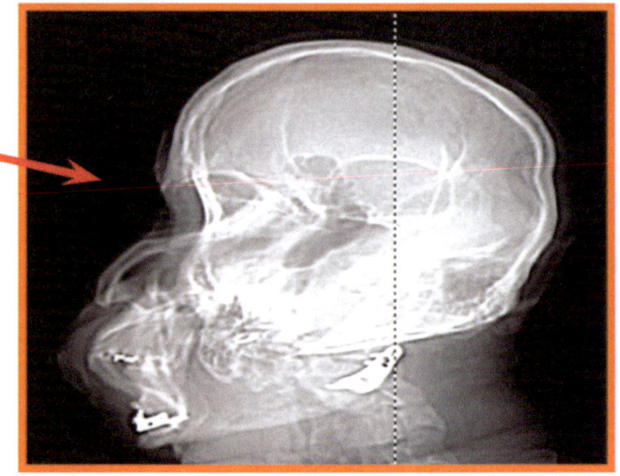

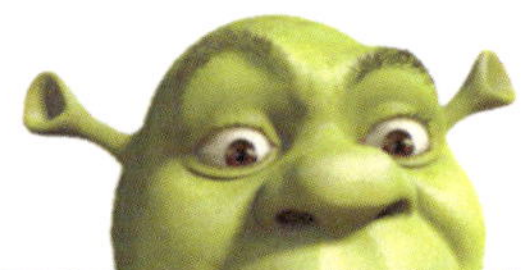

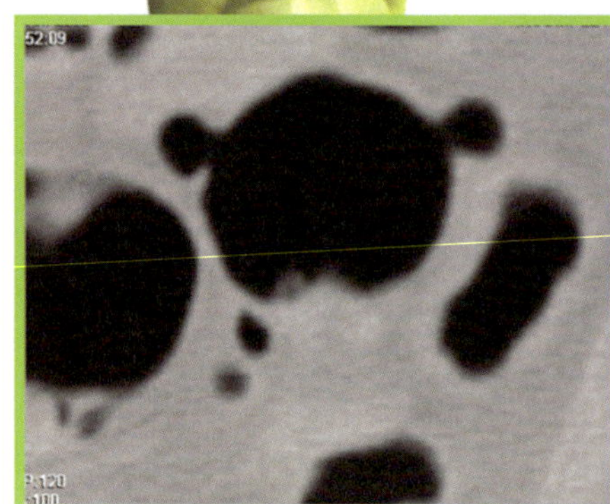


*Looks like Shrek® on a virtual colonoscopy.*

*Here's the Pac Man ghost on a CT of the abdomen.*

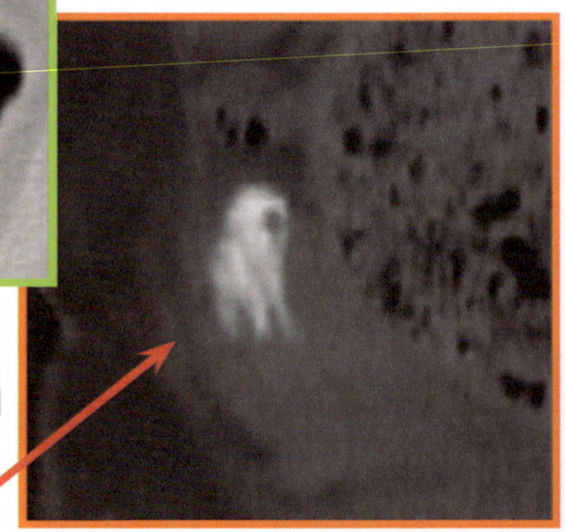

# BELIEVE IT, OR NOT. MY “REALISTIC” WEEK IN *“part-time”* PRACTICE.

## MONDAY

Take oldest child to school. First-grade teacher chirps happily about the class party tomorrow for *(fill in the blank for the holiday of the month.)* Groan and ask if I am required to attend. Shock teacher and earn looks of disapproval from the stay-at-home moms. Babysitter calls and says her child has fever so can’t come to watch my pre-schooler and toddler. Have choice of cancelling a full day of patients *(riot will ensue)*, finding another babysitter *(impossible)*, or swallowing pride and asking evil mother-in-law (MIL) for help *(odynophagia)*. Choose odynophagia.

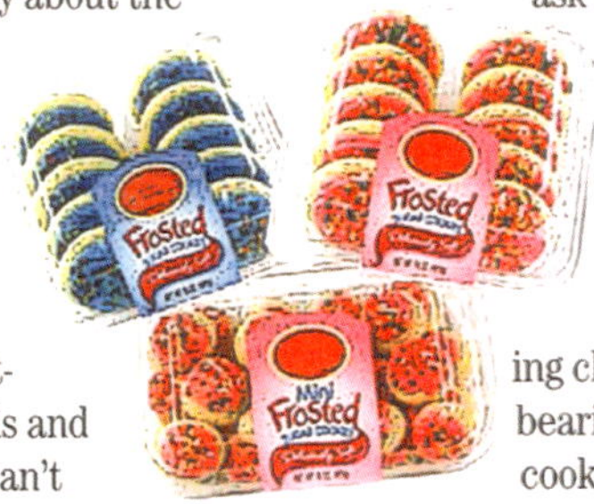


Arrive at combination Neurology/PM&R practice to have my neurologist boss call me “lazy” because I work “part-time” (due to my three children and anesthesiologist husband) – this from the man who has a stay-at-home wife to raise his three children. *Refrain from pointing out that not only am I doing his job, I am also doing his wife’s.*

Schedule is full of chronic back pain patients. The neurologist prescribed *Percocet* and now, tired of their demands, he has decided they need “rehab,” aka “dump the drug seekers.”

Stay until 6 p.m. wrangling with the narc seekers while boss went home at 4:30 p.m.

*SARCASM:*

## TUESDAY

My “day off.” Also,“party day.” Had to ask evil MIL to watch other two children so I can attend party *(more odynophagia)*. At party, children are dressed in appropriately themed and matching clothing with mothers bearing hand-made themed cookies and goodie bags. My child is in T-shirt and jeans. I hand over the store-bought cookies and spend rest of party right next to my child to avoid stay-at-home mothers’ scorn.

Evil MIL calls to inform me that 20-month-old has a fever and MUST go to the doctor. *I know it’s viral. You know it’s viral. I know the pediatrician won’t give antibiotics. You know the pediatrician won’t give antibiotics.* Evil MIL from era when every child who had a sniffle was given amoxicillin and INSISTS. She is also from the era when her child was prescribed phenobarbital AND donnatol for colic, *so there you go.* Call and wheedle the pediatrician’s receptionist for an appointment tomorrow morning *(my “morning off”)*, not above using my “doctor” title.

## WEDNESDAY

Drag my evil MIL to the pediatrician’s office with me so SHE can hear the pediatrician say no to antibiotics and why. She puts up a good fight but the pediatrician wins. It is a pyrrhic victory as now I must listen to evil MIL expound about how all her children got antibiotics and ask what is wrong with medicine today. It is my “half day” of clinic which officially starts at 1 p.m. but I allow my medical assistant to schedule urgent patients from noon to one. I am clever enough to schedule my half day in the afternoon rather than the morning, as all my other “part-time” doctor friends report their “half days” now run 8 a.m. to 2 p.m. instead of til noon.

## THURSDAY

Another full day which is packed through lunch. My wonderful medical assistant who must also endure taunts of being “lazy” *(since her doctor is “part-time”)* apologizes profusely.

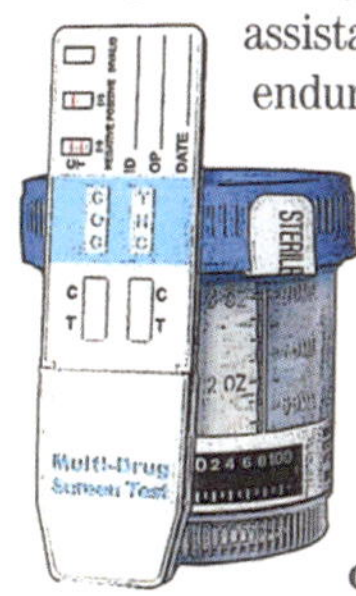


Halfway through the day, we decide on a new office policy: **All patients, whether 18 or 80, requesting pain medications must be drug tested prior to script being written.**

While I see patients during lunch, MA calls all the afternoon patients to inform them of the new policy. *My schedule miraculously clears* and I spend the afternoon with several sweet elderly patients with either neuropathic pain or shingles.

## FRIDAY

My other “day off.” It is filled doing laundry, grocery shopping, prepping for a meal, and taking care of children with residual illnesses. First-grader comes home with notice of another holiday party in two weeks and a blank to fill in what I want to bring. Shred notice into little tiny pieces.

On call tonight. Somehow it was decided that it was “fair” that I take full-time call even though I am officially “part time.” ER call at 11 p.m. from a patient complaining of a T4 sensory level. Perk up as this might be a real emergency. He is a patient of my PMR colleague who has a second office much further south. Refer the patient to the southern hospital where I don’t have privileges, explaining this is a real emergency and can’t be handled over the phone. Patient resists, so suggest the other southern hospital. He admits he has been to both southern ER’s and was D/C’d from both. Seems he thought the best treatment for his T4 sensory level was *Percocet*. Gleefully advise him to go to northern hospital where it just so happens my neurology boss is on call. He should reach the ER at midnight if his wife drives quickly, which will put the call through to my boss around 2 a.m. I sleep easy for the rest of the night. ✚

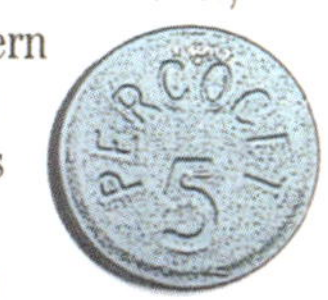


**SUBMIT YOUR “REALISTIC” WEEK**
**WWW.PLACEBOJOURNAL.COM**

# New and Useless Patient Self-Reporting Scales on the Horizon for the Joint Commission

**GOAL:** *To measure more and more in order to justify our existence.*

**OBJECTIVE:**
Use subjective evidence as much as possible
Validate vague complaints
Hinder clinical practice
Waste precious time
Confuse clinical acumen
Justify patient advocacy groups

## POOR SELF-IMAGE SCALE:

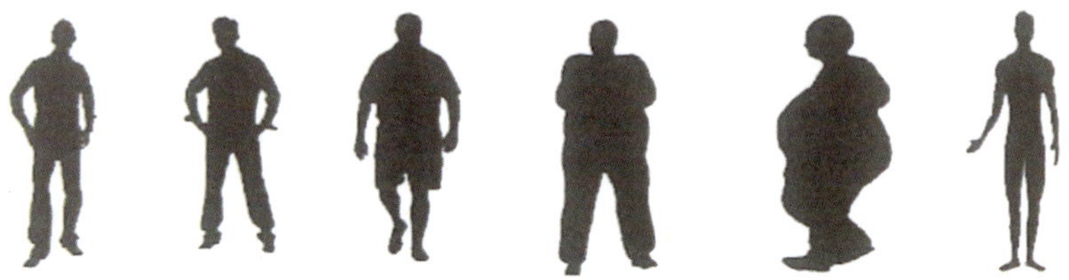

| *"I feel fine about myself."* | *"I wish I were thinner."* | *"I could stand to lose a few pounds."* | *"I could knock this weight off in a weekend."* | *"I'm just big boned."* | *"I'm too fat!"* |
|---|---|---|---|---|---|
| 0 POINTS | 1 POINT | 2 POINTS | 3 POINTS | 4 POINTS | 5 POINTS |

## *How hyperactive do you feel today?* SCALE:

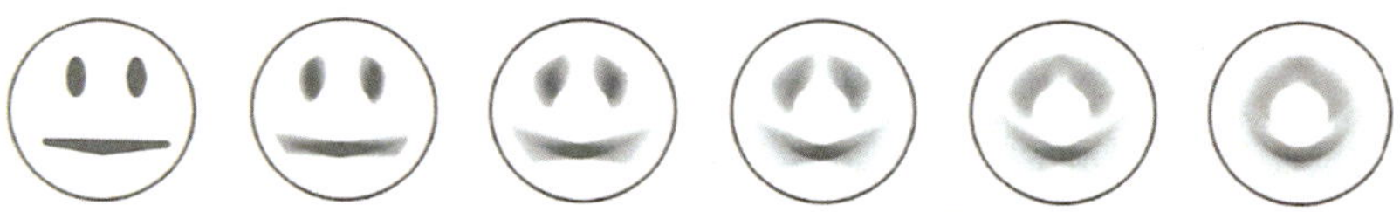

0 POINTS | 1 POINT | 2 POINTS | 3 POINTS | 4 POINTS | 5 POINTS

## *How tired are you today?* CHRONIC FATIGUE SCALE

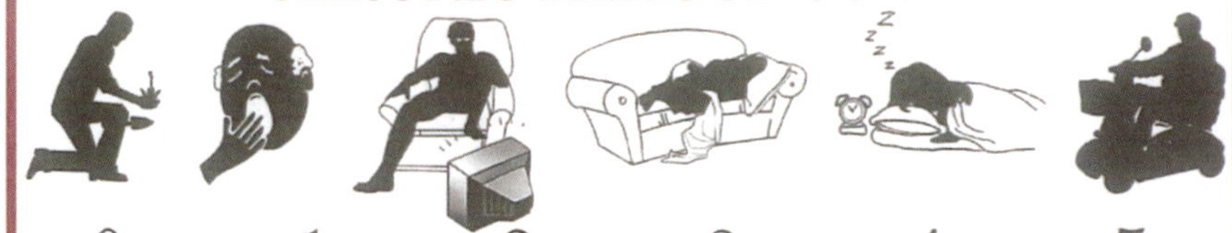

0 POINTS | 1 POINT | 2 POINTS | 3 POINTS | 4 POINTS | 5 POINTS

## VISUAL SEXUAL DYSFUNCTION SCALE:

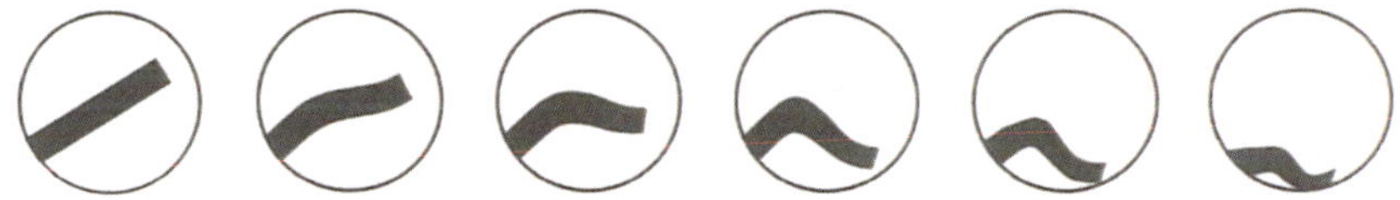

0 POINTS | 1 POINT | 2 POINTS | 3 POINTS | 4 POINTS | 5 POINTS

## *"How many narcotics do you want today?"* SCALE:

0 POINTS | 1 POINT | 2 POINTS | 3 POINTS | 4 POINTS | 5 POINTS

### *How much do you hurt today?* FIBROMYALGIA SCALE:

*"Ow!"* = 0 points
*"Oww!!"* = 1 point
*"Owww!!"* = 2 points
*"Owwww!!!"* = 3 points
*"Owwwww!!!"* = 4 points
*"Owwwwwwwww!!!!"* = 5 points

### *How normal is your stool today?* REGULARITY SCALE:

*Floop!* = 0 points
Chocolate Syrup = 1 point
Pudding = 2 points
Loaf of bread = 3 points
A bunch of rocks = 4 points
Bowling ball = 5 points

ANOTHER TRUE STORY OF MEDICINE

# BEHIND THE SCENES: THE INFAMOUS RECTAL FOREIGN BODY

Over the years in our practice, we general surgeons all encounter the famed "rectal foreign body" at some point along the way. Generally speaking, these stories are humorous by their very nature and many readers out there may have thought they had heard it all when it comes to this scenario. Still, we **relish** retelling the story to rustle up a few chuckles in our otherwise stressful and soul-killing field.

Last week, I had a reasonably quiet call day, and thought I was getting away with a good night's sleep when I received the dreaded 5:30 a.m. phone call from the ER.

*"Hi, are you on call for general surgery?"*

*"Ummm hummm,"* I mumble into my pillow.

*"Well, we've got a guy down here we need your help with. He's a 66-year-old man who was trying to have an orgasm and, er, one thing led to another and he ended up with a* **mustard** *jar wedged in his rectum. We can't get it out."*

*"Rough luck,"* I muttered, hoping this was a dream.

*"We've gotten all his labs and EKG and stuff so he's ready for the OR. We also have gotten an abdominal X-ray. There's no free air, and I'm not sure, but I think the label reads,* "Grey Poop-on,"*"* as he bursts in a gleeful bout of self-satisfied laughter.

I chuckled along with him and told him I'd be right in. The ER added, *"We're all having baloney sandwiches for lunch later on and if you're successful with the extraction, you could just bring it along."*

*"Aw clam up,"* I joked.

I went to the ER and approached the clerk, *"I understand we have a case of misplaced condiments."*

She gave me a knowing wink and a blushing smile and directed me to the patient's room. I went in and introduced myself and I told the patient I was the surgeon and I was there to help, without getting into the specifics. I am a lady surgeon, and I'm sure I was the last person he wanted to get into the details with.

I had him roll over, reached up there and sure enough there was a stout, glass jar rather firmly tucked where the sun don't shine. I tried to get my hand around it to pull it out, but it basically filled up the pelvic outlet and there was no getting a proper grip on it.

I told him we needed to go to the OR and do this under general anesthesia. He agreed without hesitation. Interestingly he suggested, *"Maybe you could use those tongs they have to get the babies out."*

*"A valid suggestion,"* I replied. *"I shall keep it in mind."* It made me wonder if this was the voice of prior experience.

I went to the front desk at the OR to add on my case. "Millie," the OR secretary, is as straight and serious as employees come. The look of shock on her face was absolutely priceless. While everyone else was bantering about, Millie just shook her head, repeating, *"My Lord, my Lord,"* like a prayerful mantra.

When I got to the OR, the nurses had basically prepared for a delivery. He was up in stirrups, and the baby tongs (called Elliot forceps) and the suction thingy that goes on the baby's head were readily available.

I sat on a rolling stool between the legs, said a brief prayer, and got to work. First I tried the Elliot forceps, but they were hard to get around the jar because, as I said, the jar filled the pelvic outlet and there wasn't much room. I finally got them around the jar, but there was no pulling it out. I tried the suction thingy, but as one might guess, it wasn't exactly designed for **mustard** jars, and I couldn't get a good seal. Thinking maybe I just wasn't strong enough, I asked one of my male partners (who was getting ready for an ordinary, boring old gallbladder operation) to take a walk on the wild side and try his hand at my case. He couldn't do it either. I tried again with the Elliots, but I was really concerned the metal forceps squeezing on the glass jar could shatter it and we ALL would be in a world of hurt. It was a tough decision, but it was clear: We had to do a C-section.

I made a small, vertical, midline incision in the lower abdomen and put my hand down in the pelvis. Luckily, he had left the lid on the jar, so there was no sharp edge to push on, and I could apply steady pressure on the lid to help push it out. I had the nurse push on the lid, while I got down on the butt end with the forceps again. I braced my foot up against the OR table, leaned back with the whole force of my body, and heaved and hoed with the nurse pushing from inside. The circulating nurse braced herself behind me, as she was sure when this thing eventually broke loose I would go flying across the room. The nurse anethestist, whom I will call "Frank" watched from his safe vantage point on the "easy side" of the ether screen. He was absolutely in hysterics at the colorectal circus unfolding before him. Like people watch with excitement during deliveries, *"Is it a girl or a boy? What color eyes? What color hair?"* he was wondering aloud, *"Hey, you think it's* Grey Poop-on*? Hot and spicy?* Gulden's *with horseradish?"* Finally, the jar popped out. It was a healthy, empty, 9 ounce jar of ***French's***.

The nurse asked, *"Do you want me to send it to pathology?"*

I laughed, *"No, that won't be necessary."*

Another victory for modern medicine. The operation was a complete success. ✚

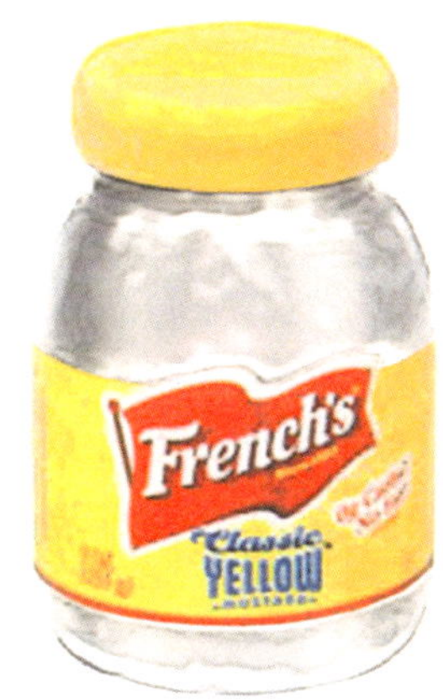

# Welcome to medicine. You are now a doctor.

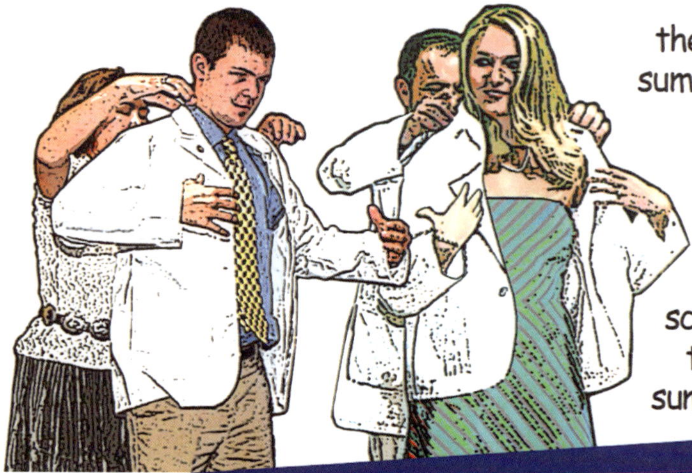

This will be the most amazing summer of your life.

To make it even more enjoyable, here is a scrapbook guide to track your summer activities.

## Make Your Own

# SUMMER SCRAPBOOK

## for Medical Interns

You'll need:

- scissors
- stapler
- markers
- clear tape
- glue

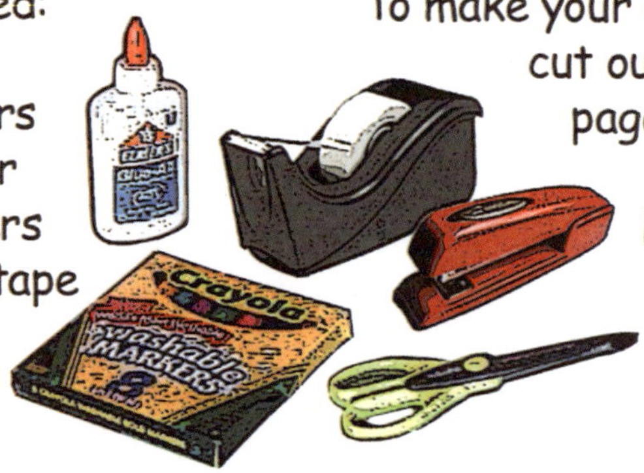


To make your own scrapbook, cut out the next few pages, staple them all together like a book. and you're ready to begin . . .

# MY FIRST SUMMER AS A NEW DOCTOR

## WHAT THE F#CK!!

Draw a silhouette of the first rectal foreign body you removed.

## HA. HA. YOU MISSED ME!

Tape the blade of a scalpel thrown at you by a surgery attending HERE.

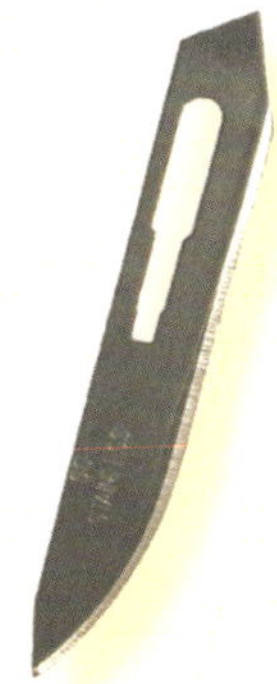

## OUCH!

Glue the first hepatitis-positive needle you were stuck with HERE.

## SCREW 'EM!

Make a list of all the spouses/significant others who left your fellow interns for never being around.

____________________
____________________
____________________
____________________
____________________
____________________
____________________
____________________
____________________
____________________
____________________
____________________
____________________

## LIFE SUCKS!

Glue in a picture of yourself at the exact moment you lost your idealism and became jaded.

## MY FIRST POSITIVE GUAIAC CARD

Glue your first + guaiac card HERE.

## A SAD DAY

Tape the first tissues you cried into as a new doc HERE.

## SOMEDAY I'D LIKE TO KILL . . .

Write in names of your attendings or residents,

## FOR ME? FREE?

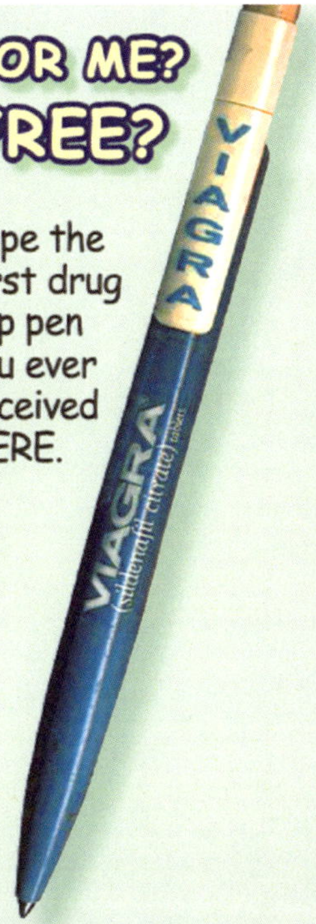


Tape the first drug rep pen you ever received HERE.

## I SAVED A LIFE!

Tape or glue a copy of the EKG strip or actual electrode from the first person's life you saved during a code HERE.

## MUST . . . STAY . . . AWAKE . . .

Tape the first empty NoDoz packet you used to stay up 36 hours straight HERE.

## AVERAGE NUMBER OF HOURS PER WEEK I WORKED THIS SUMMER.

Circle one.

40 60

100 130

150 175

200

## AHH, SOME ZZZZZZZ!

Glue a feather from the pillow that you slept on the one night this summer that you actually got more than two hours of sleep.

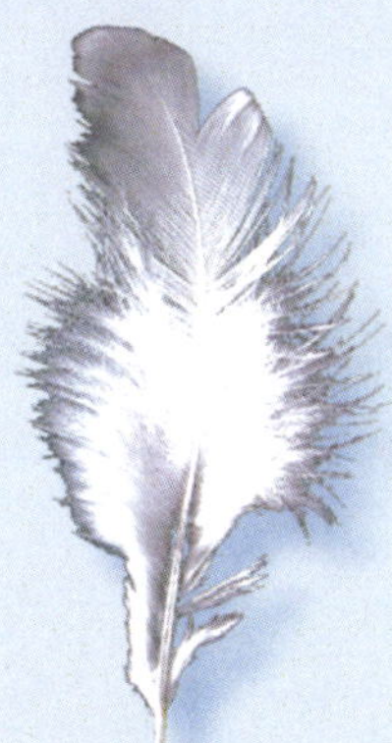

## #%*@$ Attending!!

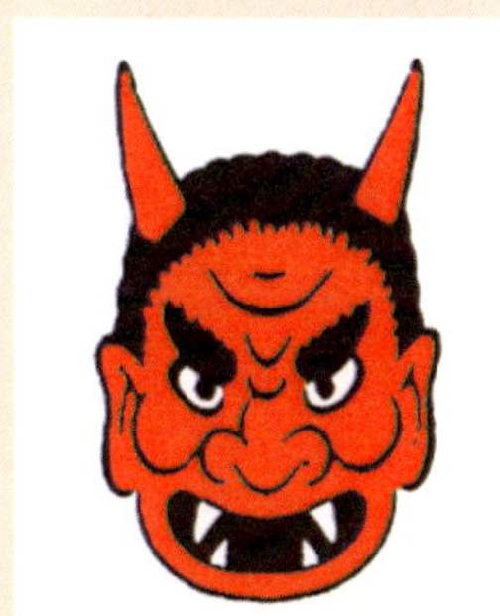

Using markers, draw the face from your imagination of the attending who you never even met, who was your ICU supervisor when you had 80 patients simultaneously coding.

## SAY AAA DAMMIT!

Tape the first tongue suppressor "Ha ppy Face Puppet" you created to calm an irate child.

## IF ONLY . . .

Make a list of all the different careers you would now like to pursue.

## I MADE IT THROUGH MY FIRST SUMMER AS A NEW DOCTOR!

## ANOTHER TRUE STORY OF MEDICINE
# ANESTHESIA ROUNDS

I am often asked to give sedation for upper G-I endoscopys. My usual practice is to spray a topical anesthetic on the patient's throat before we begin the procedure. Recently I told my patient, a young woman, that I need to squirt a little something in her throat before we got started. She smiled and said, *"But doctor, I hardly know you!"* I had to leave the room to try to control my laughter before we could begin.

While "on call" I was paged to labor and delivery to top up an ongoing epidural for a pending forceps delivery. I asked the R.N. if they had Nesacaine (chloroprocaine- a local anesthetic) there, thinking that I would stop by the pharmacy on the way if they didn't. After checking, the R.N. replied, *"There is no Miss Nessie Cain on L and D and there is no Ms. Cain in the entire hospital."* I told her to look for her brother Mark Caine (marcaine-bupivicaine, another local anesthetic) and that I'd be right there.

A young lady scheduled for minor gynecological surgery asked me to give her "that new anesthetic." I was puzzled by what she wanted and asked her to explain. She told me her friend had surgery here and was put to sleep using electricity. The anesthesiologist placed three electrodes on her and as he placed the third one, he said, *"you are going to sleep now"* and so she did. The hypnotic was obviously injected as the Doc placed the last of the EKG electrodes, and she thought the electrocardiogram machine was there to produce anesthesia. ✚

*PJ Adams presents the tastiest blend of all the seasonal beers with its*

# FALL "Out of Your" GOURD Anemic Ale

**Not too bitter and with just the right amount of spices, our Fall "Out of Your" Gourd Anemic Ale is the perfect flavor for the season.**

*"This is great stuff! The gourd flavor did not disappoint. All of us here – actually it's just me – can't wait to get more!"*
Jason, a happy customer

**PJ Adams combines hemp, Mezcal worms, and psilocybin-rich mushrooms with the goodness of fresh New England-grown gourds to produce the beer of a lifetime.***

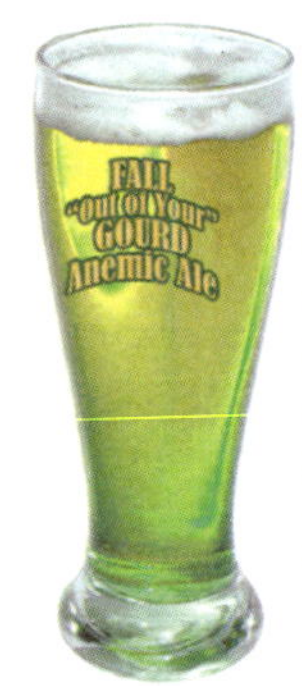


See why PJ Adams' Fall "Out of Your" Gourd Anemic Ale has **grown to be one of the year's most anticipated beer releases.** Each 12-oz. bottle of our Fall "Out of Your" Gourd Anemic Ale pours out with a nice pale greenish-yellow color and a thin foam that loses its head quickly – *just like you!*

**Next time you want a road trip to see the colors of the foliage, just purchase a six-pack of Fall "Out of Your" Gourd Anemic Ale and let its mind-altering properties do their trick. You will never have to LEAVE your home!**

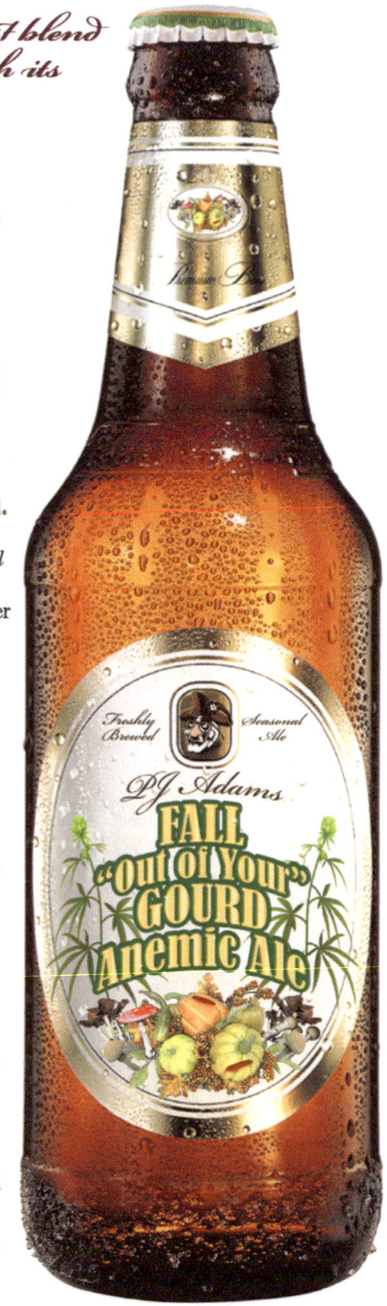


* We highly recommend you drink this product if you are on a MAO inhibitor.

## PJ MEDICAL ALGORITHM OF REALITY

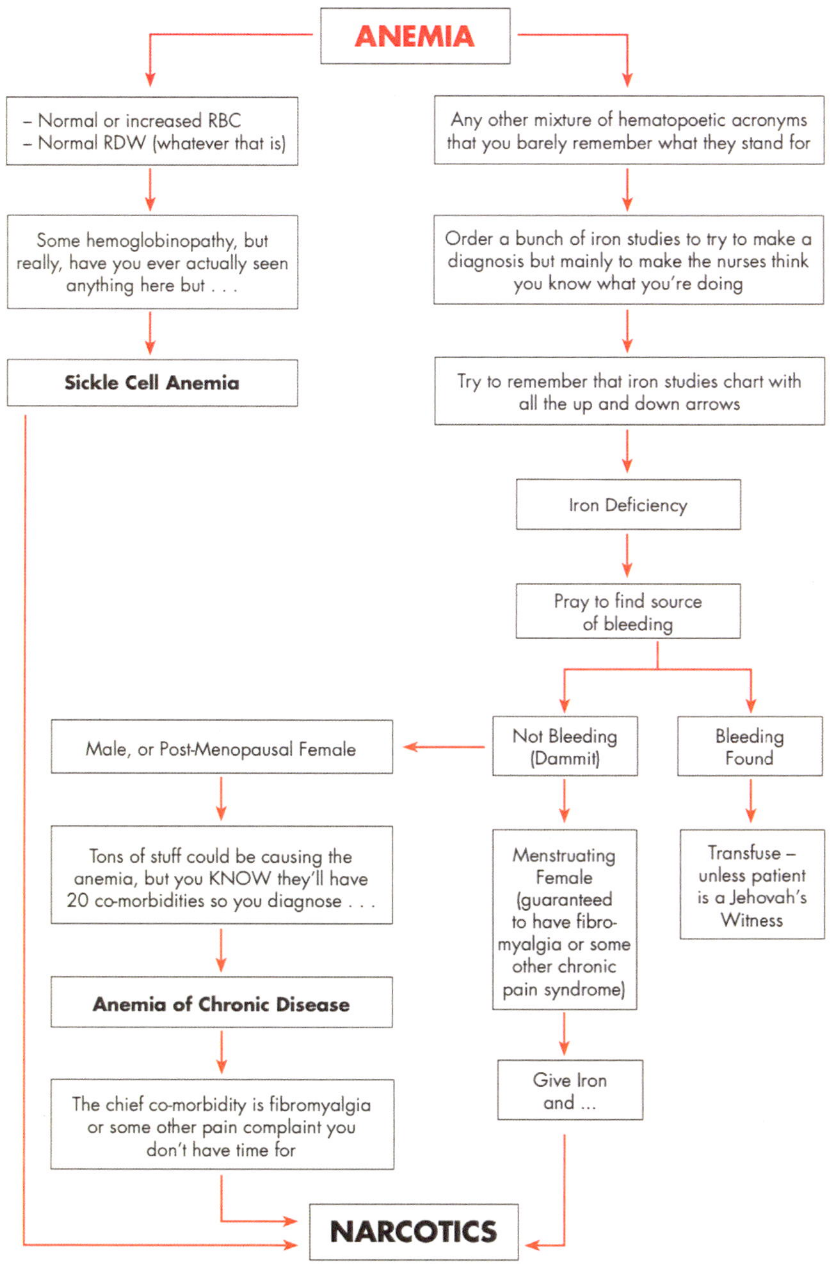


# MEDICAL HALLOWEEN COSTUMES JUST FOR YOU!

***Looking for the perfect costume for your hospital's Halloween party?***
Look no further. At Placebowear Costumes, we know what's funny – or at least in bad taste.

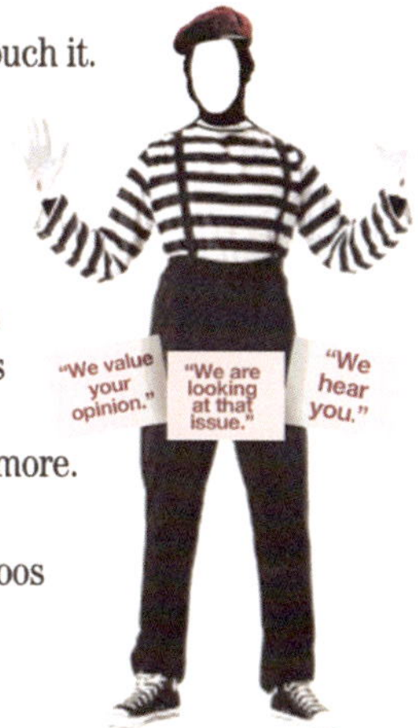


1. **FIBROMYALGIA SUIT** – goes "OwwWW" every time you touch it.
2. **LABOR AND DELIVERY NURSE** – scrubs and a scrub jacket over a fat suit.
3. **MIDDLE MANAGEMENT MIME** – comes with makeup for a white face, mime gloves, and placards that say such things as, *"We are looking at that issue, We have the system's overall health to consider, We value your opinion, We hear you,"* and more.
4. **NARC SEEKER** – skin-tight garb with needle marks and tattoos and a fake ultrasound showing a kidney stone.

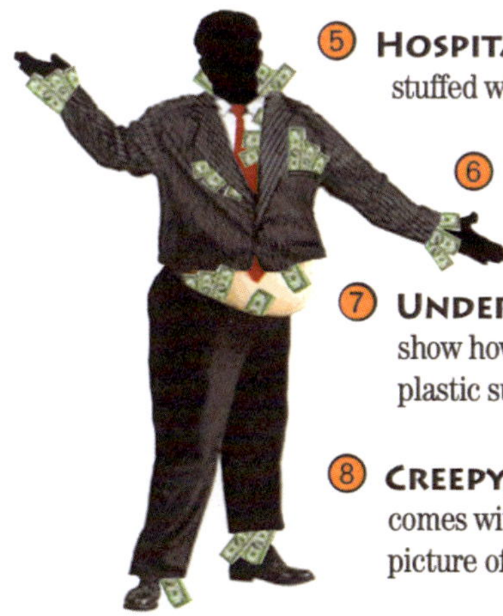

5. **HOSPITAL CEO** – poorly fitted suit stuffed with money.
6. **MALPRACTICE ATTORNEY** – comes with a target on his back and a *Nerf* gun for everyone to shoot.
7. **UNDER-REPRESENTED MINORITY HOUSEKEEPER** – show how plugged in you are when you show up at the local plastic surgeon's Halloween party as the African-American janitor.
8. **CREEPY, HAPPY RETIRED VOLUNTEER** – comes with a pink smock, a shoulder hump, and a picture of a deceased husband.

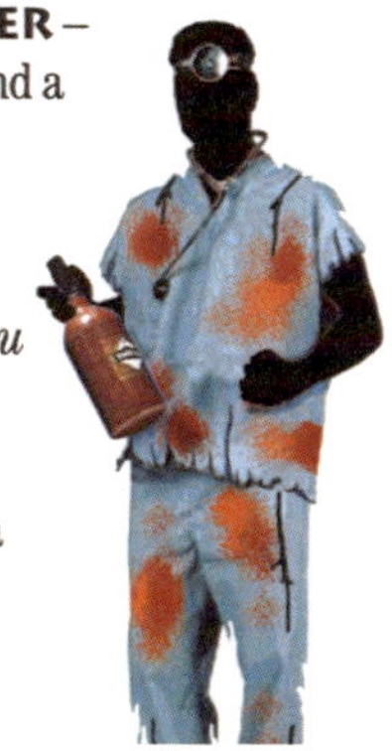

9. **FOREIGN LOCUM DOCTOR** – comes with a beard, a lunch box, and an English translation dictionary. *Stay in character all night as you speak a language no one understands!*
10. **DRUNKEN SURGEON** – ripped up and blood stained scrubs with a big bottle of hooch. *Scream orders and curse out everyone you see!*

**HOPAMAX®**
**(hopeitworksmate) Tablets**

For many patients, their diseases can be a constant cycle of disruption.

Hopamax's off-label use stops their symptoms before they start.

**Are your patients still suffering from something?**

**Do your patients want fewer and fewer worries from their syndromes?**

**Hopamax is your off-labeled answer.**

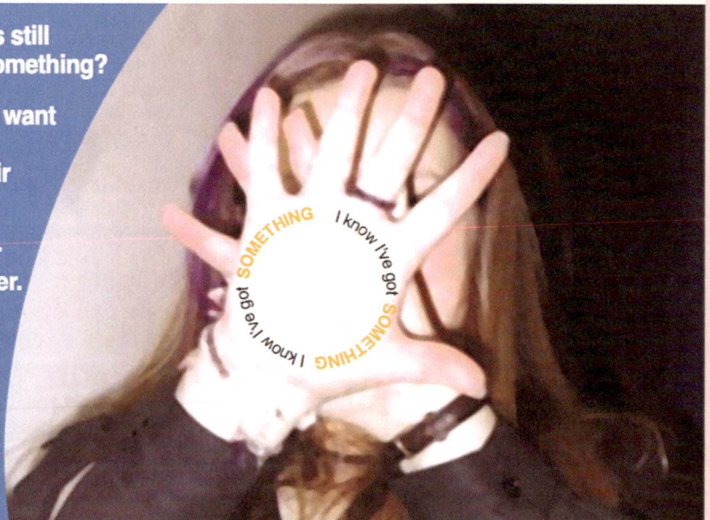
SOMETHING I know I've got SOMETHING I know I've got

**Here is hoping that Hopamax works for you!**

**Hopamax. Indicated for: nothing. Used for: everything.**

Hopamax is the first medication that is used for medical problems it was never intended for. In the hope of making a large profit, PJ Pharmaceuticals has done away with boring "indications" and "clinical usefulness." Now with Hopamax, doctors are able to try it for just about anything and get some results they were looking for or they were not looking to help.

Hopamax has been studied for a lot of things, but due to cost and ethical hurdles its use has been left up to the individual physician's discretion.

Isn't it time for the physician to be back in charge?

**PJ PHARMACEUTICALS**
*The Realistic Drug Company*

Hopamax tablets can cause bloating, syphilis, and alopecia in a lot of people. Do not use contraceptives, tequila, or aspirin with this product because we think bad things could happen. Avoid confusion with similarly named medications such as *Holyshititstings* and *Hobegone*.

### ANOTHER TRUE STORY OF MEDICINE

# NEEDED THE MONEY

I was interviewing a patient for the first time at a mental health clinic. She complained of anxiety and depression. She said he wanted some kind of medication to help her through this tough time. There were many things on her mind which were upsetting to her and she *"didn't know where to start."* To help, I said, *"To start, just tell me the two main things that are bothering you."*

She began by relating a conflict with one of her children and how this grown child would be getting married in a month. She went on about their complex relationship and their frequent ups and downs. She blamed her ex-husband for coming between them. Gradually, she seemed to feel better and we talked about her symptoms of insomnia, anxiety, and her deep wish to repair her relationship with her child. She also complained of being treated unfairly by her child, for whom she had done so much over the years. She said she *"was careful with her health"* and didn't want any habit-forming tranquilizers and we discussed a possible medication for sleep. I also referred her for psychotherapy. I found myself feeling empathy for this well kempt older woman who seemed like a warm and caring mother. She added that she loved going to the theater and that this relaxed her. I found myself warming to this person who seemed like a victim of life's inevitable injustices.

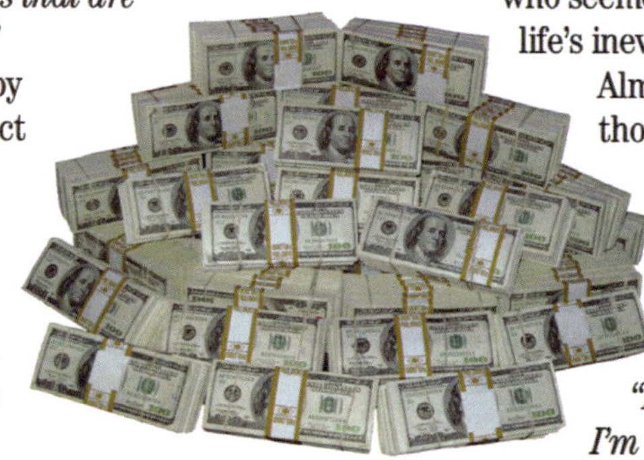

Almost as an afterthought, I reminded her to mention the second thing that was bothering her. She said, *"I don't know if I'm a sociopath or not. I hope not, anyway. I stole a few million dollars from my company. I'm going to have to go to jail. I don't know if I can do the time. I asked my lawyer to try to schedule the hearing after my kid's wedding."*

I asked her why she'd done it. She said calmly and simply, with a shrug, *"I needed the money and I thought I could get away with it. It was dumb. I shouldn't have done it. My kid is really pissed off at me."* ✚

# A WEEK IN PRACTICE WITH A Bitter Family Doc

*Our guest columnist admits to being a bitter family physician in the "Gret Stet of Looooziannna." She sees only a handful of patients a day because her partner is beloved by all, a million years old, a workaholic, and apparently immortal (and not because she is lazy or sees "more complicated patients" like some gal docs claim).*

## MONDAY

Receive a phone call from a young patient who was placed on antibiotics a few hours ago. They *"aren't working yet."* Try to explain pharmacokinetics and bacterial life cycle to patient. **Give up.** Call in unnecessary med.

## TUESDAY

Neurotic hypochondriac adult male patient comes in with *"painful mass in belly."* Anatomy lesson ensues – this is your liver, these are your ribs, this is your poo, none of it hurts when I press it. **You're fine.** Blank stare from patient. *"But there's something wrong. I'm really worried,"* he says. **I give up.** Order unnecessary lab and imaging tests that will all be normal. He is terrified of the needle in the lab. Consider benzodiazepines. One for him, **one for me.**

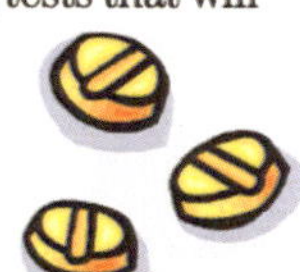

## WEDNESDAY

Drug seeker. **The answer is no.** If you leave now, you might make it to the next town before that doc's office closes . . .

## THURSDAY

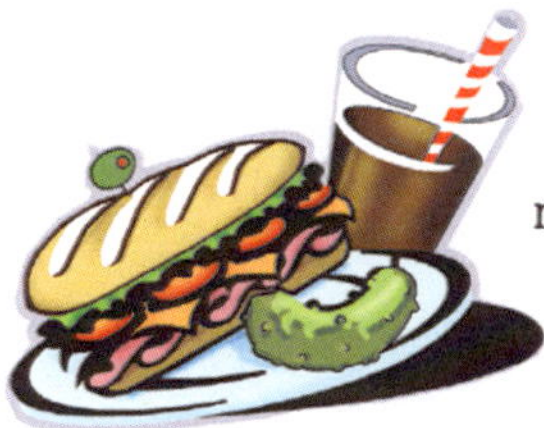

Doctor's Day. Fake show of appreciation at my local hospital. **Good food, though.** I'll be labeled a "disruptive doctor" any day now for complaining about my lack of patients.

Drug rep utters a sentence about how increased protein binding *"may be"* related to patient outcomes. **And monkeys *"may be"* about to fly out of my butt.** Do a randomized, placebo-controlled study on THAT.

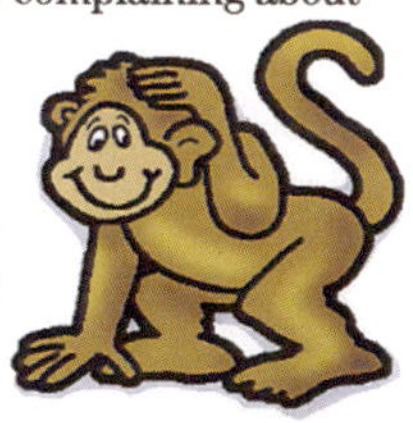

## FRIDAY

Diabetic Medicaid patient with HgbA1C of >13, on multiple oral diabetic meds. Refuses insulin, despite explanation of risks of elevated glucose over time. Wants to try diet for a bit longer. ***Suuuuuuuuuure.***

New patient wants med refills – *Lortab, Soma, Xanax.* ✚

**TGIF**

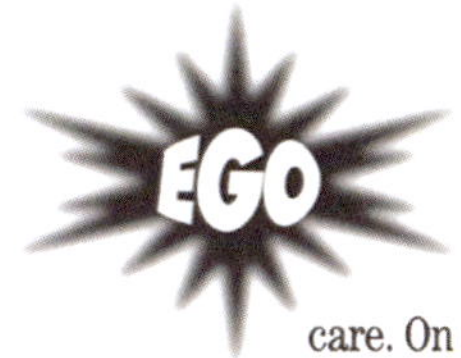


## BURST EGO

Alice was an elderly lady who was seen occasionally for routine care. On one visit, she kept telling me, ***"You really look good!"*** I politely thanked her, but she wouldn't stop. It became rather embarrassing as she continued to praise me, but we eventually concluded the visit.

As I walked out of the examining room, my secretary said, ***"Alice's daughter wanted to talk to you about how confused her mother has been lately!"*** ✚

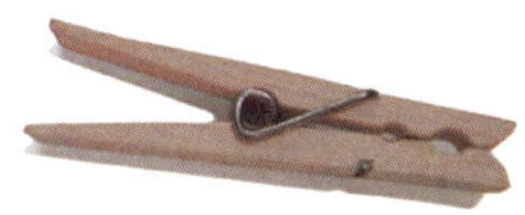

## WHOOPS!

Laura was a very pleasant and likable octogenarian with diabetes. The diabetes was never well controlled. On each office visit when she was told of the latest blood sugar read (*always bad*), she would confess that it was probably because she had eaten (*choose one*) half of a small cookie/a small bite of cake/a small piece of candy at a wedding, birthday, or anniversary four weeks earlier.

One day she arrived for a routine visit and announced that she should have a Pap smear. No, she wasn't having any gynecological problems. She just thought she should have one. When it was time for that part of the exam, she was given the "standard" instructions to "scoot down to the end of the table." This was somewhat difficult for Laura because she had only one hand to assist her in this movement, the other hand being firmly planted on top of her head to hold her wig in place. She accomplished this feat with a series of "bumps" as she would raise her hips, move forward slightly and then repeat. Each "bump" was accompanied by the unmistakable sound of flatus passing, followed by the exclamation of, *"Whoops!"* Her trip to the end of the table thus became ***BUMP – FLATUS – WHOOPS***, but her wig happily stayed in place. We both shared a good laugh when she finally arrived in the correct position. ✚

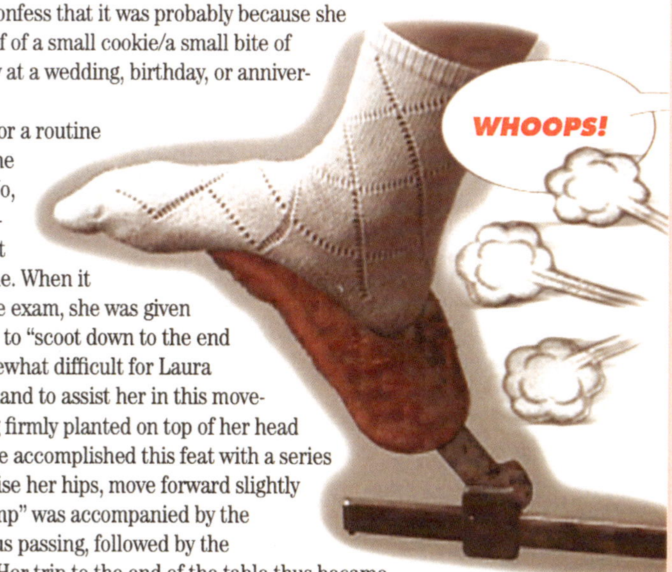

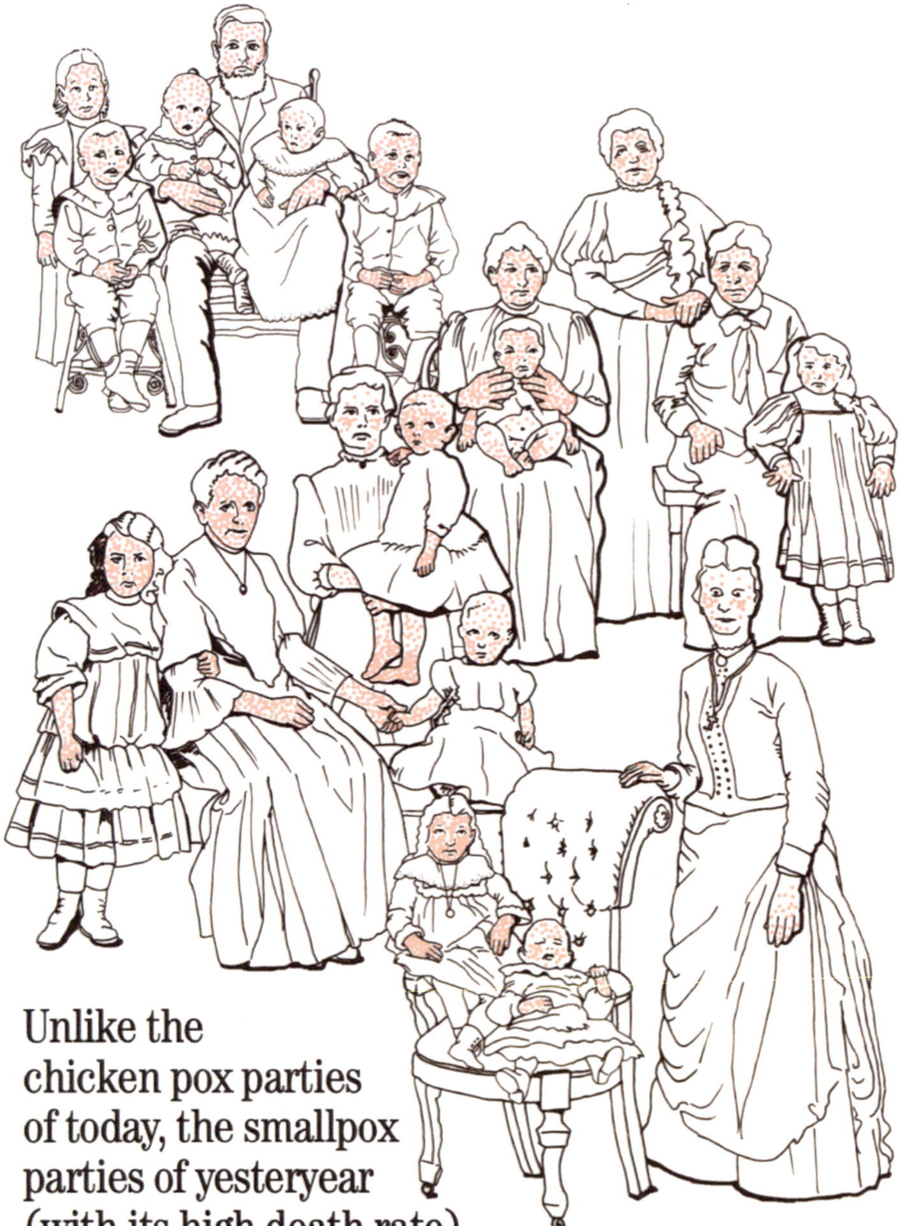

Unlike the chicken pox parties of today, the smallpox parties of yesteryear (with its high death rate) weren't nearly as popular. +

# TOP TEN

## True, But Least Effective Narcotic-Seeking Stories

**THOSE DARN NARC SEEKERS**

**10. Waitress must have taken it in restaurant . . .** *"It was a real dive, Doc."* (like I have never eaten at a truck stop, yeah, they must steal narcotics all the time.)

**9. House burned down** – asked for police report, none forthcoming.

**8. Dog ate it** – no veterinary report forthcoming either.

**7. I forgot the combination to my safe and I have to hide the meds from my girlfriend, who is a drug addict** (but then you didn't really lose it, did you?)

**6. Fell out of motorcycle jacket pocket** (from patient with intractable back pain that prohibits him from working.)

**5. Flushed down the toilet by 2-year-old child --** but the *Naprosyn* was saved. Hooray!

**4. Pharmacist stole it --** (yeah, right! Its a conspiracy!! Oh, please – and at 4:00 p.m. on a Friday . . . I just know Bin Laden is behind it somewhere.)

**3. Husband ran off with girlfriend and *Vicodan* prescription.**

**2. Girlfriend kicked me out of apartment and threw all my clothes on the street that had my *Norco* in it . . .**

**1. I had to sell my *Vicodan* to get gas money just to make it to this appointment.** +

PHOTOCOPY THESE PAGES AND HAND OUT TO YOUR PATIENTS

# American Family Practitioner

## INFORMATION FROM YOUR FAMILY DOCTOR

## Hair Loss and What It Means To You

### Is hair loss normal?

For many men, hair loss is normal. In fact, it is even normal to shed some hair each day. But that's not what you are asking about is it? No, you are wondering if you are going to go bald, aren't you? Well, the answer is, in a nutshell, yes.

### What is causing my hair loss?

A lot of things can cause hair loss. Such diseases as hypothyroidism, lupus, and diabetes can cause it. Hormone problems or anabolic steroid use may be the source. Even medicines for gout and antidepressants can be the problem. Is there a chance that any one of these is the reason you are going bald? Not likely, chrome dome.

### Is there something I am doing with my hair that is causing my problem?

If you are wearing cornrows or using tight hair rollers to bed then we may have something to talk about. If you answered yes that question then this education form really isn't for you. Also, if you are so vain that you use certain hot oil hair treatments or chemicals then maybe you are in luck. The odds are that you are destined to look 10 to 15 years older than you really are. Sorry. Someone had to say it.

### What is male-pattern baldness?

Male-pattern baldness is your father's way of getting back at you for being a prick during adolescence. Remember the times you snuck out at night or stole his car? It's payback time. Your father knew that genetics are nothing to fool with and his baldness was destined to be your curse as well. Your only saving grace is that you have this to dangle over your own son's head as well. Pun intended.

### Can my doctor do something to stop the hair loss?

Yes!

We're kidding. You're screwed. Sure you can go to your doctor and cry that it isn't fair. He may even run some tests or try to quell your fear with some advice. The truth is that you are what they call SOL or "shit out of luck."



**Please note:** The information presented is the best we could make up. Depending on our mood, this could always change. Some of this material is not suited for anyone.

### Is there any treatment for hair loss?

Here is the good news. There is a whole bunch of hair loss treatments that are now available. Now for the bad news: none of them work. You can get the ones by prescription or the ones over the counter but you are just pissing your money away.

### Seriously, there must be some treatment for hair loss?

You're not listening, are you? No, you are just going to use your credit card after be snookered by some infomercial, radio ad, or web cure just to make sure. Here is a little secret for you: unless they create a medication that will shrink your head so that the hair you already have looks normal then you may have a chance. I heard scientists are working on this around the clock. Until then you are doomed.

### What should I do?

Have you considered shaving your head completely? It may make you look tough like a motorcycle gang member? People may believe you weren't going bald but just wanted to look tough. Okay, that was a joke. Sorry to rub it in.

#### Your options are:

- Trying different hairstyles like the comb-over or Bolivian sweep
- Getting a toupee or a wig
- Getting artificial hair replacement and look like a doll's head
- Pretend your black (they look cooler bald)
- Sucking it up and coming to grips with never getting laid again

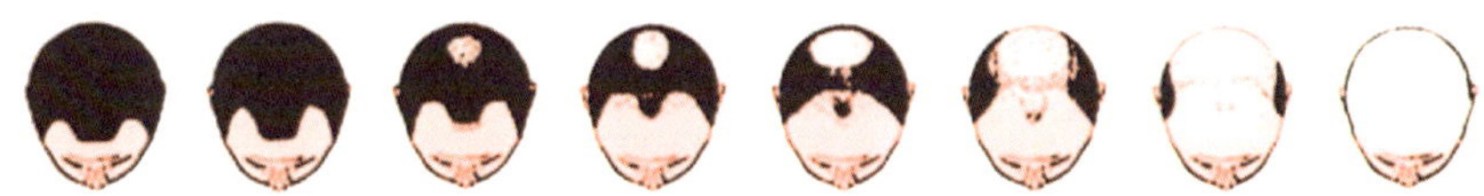

*This handout provides a general idea of this topic. Not everyone will like what they read. For those people, we recommend talking to your own family doctor.*

# PJ Stencils wants you to have some fun this October!

Whether it's simply carving a pumpkin to put in the exam room or to place around the waiting area, this age old tradition is a great way to decorate your office this Halloween.

These templates fit right in with your medical office setting. Use these easy patterns for carving some super, fancy pumpkins. *Your patients will love it!*

Purchase your stencils today at any fine Halloween retail store and receive a FREE set of pumpkin scalpels and pickups!

**Only $22.57**

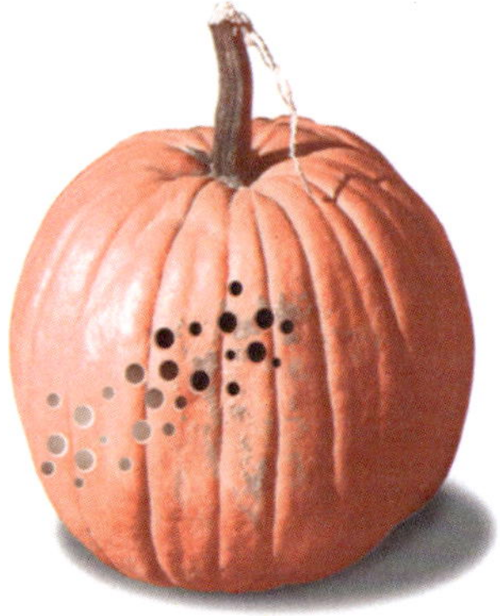

**Shing-O-Lantern**

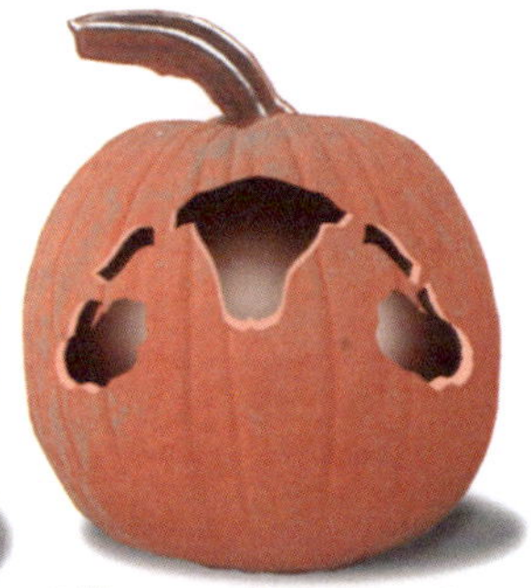

**Bilateral-Tube-O-Lantern**

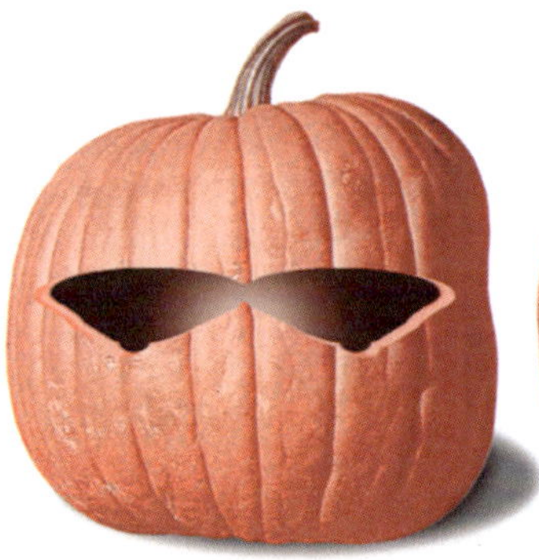

**Mamm-O-Lantern**

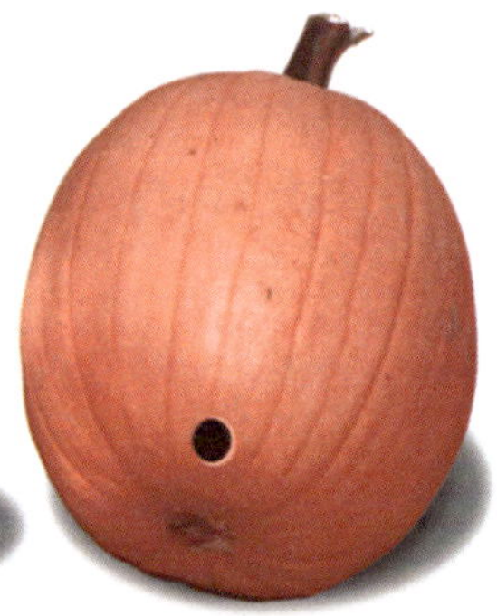

**Rect-O-Lantern**

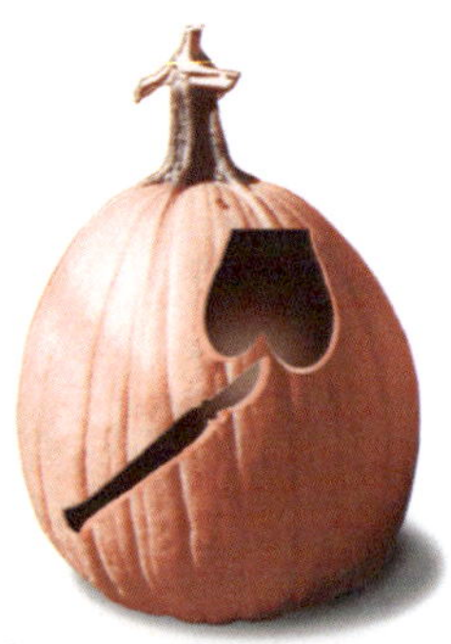

**Vasect-O-Lantern**

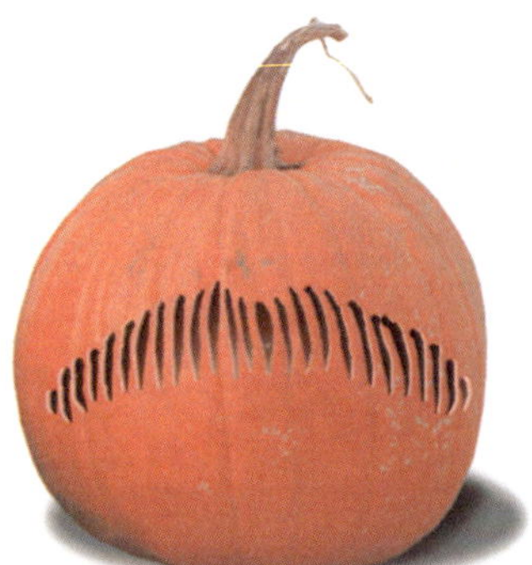

**Hirsut-O-Lantern**

# MENTAL STATUS CHANGE

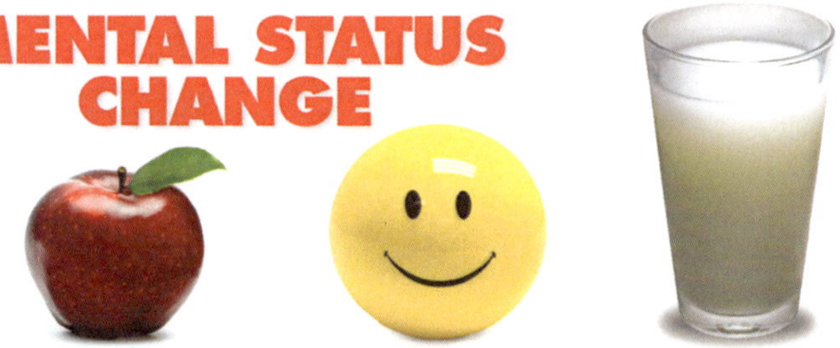

During my neurology residency, I had a two month rotation through psychiatry. One month of this was at a large public hospital, whose third floor became well known as the psych ward. There was a separate psychiatric emergency room, and on nights on-call I got to spend my evenings and much of the night there. The setup was a large waiting area, with perhaps 100 or 200 patients and family members waiting, and a group of small rooms at the front of the area, with a desk, and open door (for security), each with a resident (this was late 70's, staff were home sleeping).

As part of the mental status exam, I would ask the patient to remember three words. So I wouldn't forget the words, I always used the same three words: **apple**, **ball**, and **milk**.

I was seeing a lady who, when I asked her to remember three words, began repeating them over and over again. Then she began shouting them, and interspersing them with whatever else she was saying. So, everybody in the whole area heard her shouting: ***"Apple, ball, and milk, apple, ball, and milk,"*** then she was yelling, ***"apple, ball, and mother f*cking milk"*** over and over again.

Needless to say, I had to pick three different words to use for the rest of my exams that night. ✚

---

**MORE TRUE STORIES OF MEDICINE**

# A LITTLE BIT OF EVERYTHING

This week after a 53-year-old patient, new to our practice, told me he was disabled from a stroke he'd had eight years ago, I asked him what he did before the stroke.

*"Oh, I did a little bit of everything,"* he replied, *". . . cocaine, marijuana, whiskey . . ."*

**Postscript:** He then assured me that he had eliminated those things, except for an occasional joint, and had cut back to just two packs of cigarettes a day and half a case of beer on weekends. ✚

## Finally, a birth control system that is made 4 you!
## Finally, a birth control system that fits your active lifestyle!

Forget patches. Ignore those uncomfortable IUDs.
PJ Pharmaceuticals is proud to introduce the newest and most exciting birth control pill ever –

# Ortho Erupta

## Finally, a convenient, easy-to-use birth control system that causes a menstrual cycle **only once every four years!**

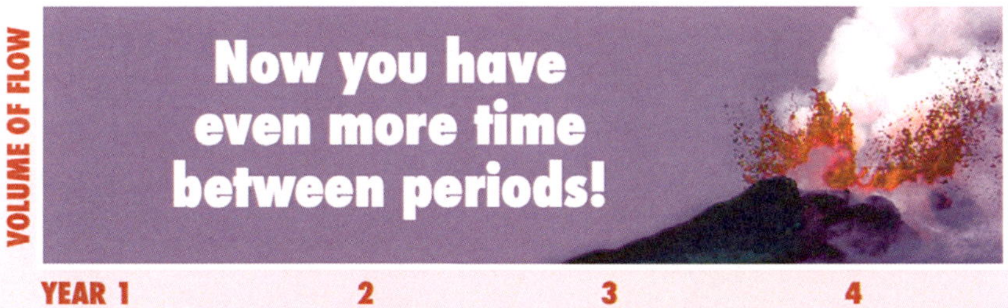


**Ortho Erupta works just like any other birth control that you may have used in the past. It contains similar hormones, is 99% effective against pregnancy, and uses the same once-daily routine. The only difference is that when you do have your period you will bleed like a stuck pig.**

**Ask your doctor if Ortho Erupta is right for you.**

Ortho Erupta is not for everyone. Along with the other serious risks of birth control hormones like blood clots, stroke, and heart attack, Orho Erupta has a slew of its own. These include: • Extremely painful menstrual cycles • Need for transfusion of at least two units of packed red blood cells • Basically, in four years you will have the largest freaking period you have ever seen.

*PJ Pharmaceuticals Women's Health Division*

Pushing chemistry to its limits and manipulating hormones more than a company has a right to.

# Woo Hoo

As a female pediatric intern, I was taking an outpatient internal medicine rotation to keep my skills sharp in case of a military recall. (I had taken a Navy scholarship to pay for medical school and could have been pulled for service at any time.) I knew I was in trouble when the attending handed me a new patient's chart and asked me to give her a "complete overhaul."

The patient (we'll call her Dorothy) was 63 years old, 61 inches tall, and weighed 309 pounds. She had not been to a doctor in 15 years (why now, lady?) and was concerned about a plethora of things, including some vaginal bleeding.

I took a deep breath and decided that I'd better get started if I was planning on eating dinner. (It was 9:00 a.m.)

After recording Dorothy's health history (complete with a positive review of symptoms), I struggled through a basic physical exam. Because the patient was almost spherical, the exam involved a lot of physical exertion on my part. I worked up a sweat as I pushed, mashed, maneuvered, manipulated, prodded and palpated Dorothy's flesh on the exam table. I needed a step-stool to do Dorothy's breast and abdominal exams, and I'm 5 foot 8!

The nurse who subsequently accompanied me into the room for the PAP and pelvic (which was part of the overhaul because of the vaginal bleeding) stifled a laugh as Dorothy slid toward the stirrups. The nurse was safe by the head of the bed, while I was not so safe in the nether regions.

Dorothy's buttocks were so enormous that, when compressed downward by the weight of the rest of her, they made a shelf of bum between me and her vaginal orifice.

The nurse snorted as I surveyed the situation and realized that the speculum wouldn't even reach Dorothy's vaginal lips, let alone her cervix – there was just too much bum in the way.

I sighed and stretched my glove as far up my arm as it would go, and gripping the speculum handle, buried my fist and entire forearm to the elbow between Dorothy's cheeks. Silent tears streamed from the nurse's eyes as I handed her each vaginal specimen while trying to ignore the fact that my arm was slowly going numb in someone's butt crack.

I completed the pelvic only to face the last portion of the "overhaul." It was time (of course) for the rectal exam. I positioned Dorothy on her side, and watched in horror as her gluteal muscles settled into two thick slabs. After gloving up, I tried to lift the top cheek so that I could find her anus. I didn't have the upper body strength, even after putting my shoulder into the effort.

It was then that I inadvertently invented the "positive woo hoo" sign – a method for doing a blind rectal. I lubed my entire right hand, front and back (again pulling my glove as far up my arm as it would possibly go), and placing my extended index finger at the top of Dorothy's crack, I slid my hand (and the majority of my forearm) down between her cheeks in search of the sensitive little dimple we call the anus. ***"Woo hoo,"*** she yelped, as I apparently hit my target. I took a chance and lunged forward, my arm buried past the elbow in Dorothy's folds as the muscle ring I was in search of relaxed before my probing finger. *Jackpot!*

The exam completed, I left the room and collapsed in the attending's office amid applause from the nurse and medical students. ✚

## PLACEBO JOURNAL ALGORITHM OF REALITY

### Initiating and Monitoring Coumadin Therapy

Obtain baseline INR value

↓

Determine Target INR

**Option A**

↓

**INITIAL DOSE**
<65yo – 5 mg
>65yo/frail or <50kg – 2.5mg

↓

**Monitor and Change Medication Per Chart Below*:**
Week 1: Arrange 2-3 times
Week 2: 2 times
Weeks 3 & 4: 1x/week
Week 5: Skip
Week 6: 1 time
Thereafter monthly if stable

**Option B**

↓

Pick a dose out of thin air

↓

Wait a couple days and check INR

↓

Wing it with another dose or ask your kid to hold up his fingers and use that as a milligram dose

↓

Recheck in a week or so and then pull another dosage out of your ass

↓

Check monthly thereafter

| *INR | Action |
|---|---|
| >10.0 | Stop coumadin. Contact patient for examination. |
| 7.0-10.0 | Stop coumadin for 2 days; decrease weekly dosage by 25% or by 1 mg/d for next week (7 mg total); repeat PT in 1 week. |
| 4.5-7.0 | Decrease weekly dosage by 15% or by 1 mg/d for 5 days of next week (5 mg total); repeat PT in 1 week. |
| 3.0-4.5 | Decrease weekly dosage by 10% or by 1 mg/d for 3 days of next week (3 mg total); repeat PT in 1 week. |
| 2.0-3.0 | No change. |
| 1.5-2.0 | Increase weekly dosage by 10% or by 1 mg/d for 3 days of next week (3 mg total); repeat PT in 1 week. |
| <1.50 | Increase weekly dosage by 15% or by 1 mg/d for 5 days of next week (5 mg total); repeat PT in 1 week. |



# MY FAVORITE MUNCHAUSEN

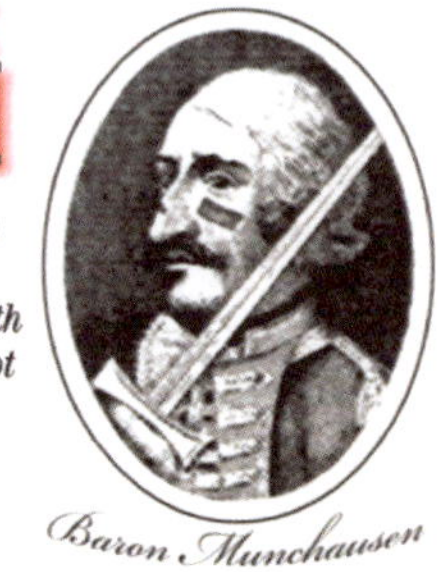


*EDITOR'S NOTE: The editors find the **Munchausen Syndrome** intriguing in an odd way. Publishing these stories may aid some physicians to diagnose these patients with a factitious disorder. We in no way want to make fun of people with psychiatric disorders. Munchausen By Proxy is child abuse and thus we will not publish any of those stories for that reason.*

## Over Easy

Drew was a 37-year-old construction worker who had terrible abdominal pain. His story began when he showed up at a hospital in need of antibiotics. This relieved his symptoms for a while. Unfortunately, he then began having a fever and joint pain. With this he also had some crazy looking tumors that were starting to grow under his skin. Drew was sick. The doctors had no idea what was going on so they did what all good doctors do; they gave him some prednisone. It didn't help. Then they did the next thing all good doctors do; they transferred him to another hospital after being unable to figure him out after three months. Fortunately, the new doctors started to look at Drew a little closer. He did have a history of some minor surgeries and illnesses but nothing that was too impressive. His family history was unknown because they had cut off communication with him years ago. There had to be more to his story. There was.

What really intrigued the new doctors about Drew was his egg-sized tumors on each elbow as well as his swollen ankles and wrists. This was not normal. What was even weirder was that right after the patient was admitted to the new hospital his egg-sized tumors began to disappear. Even weirder. Even after the doctors did all sorts of funky lab work to figure what was going on with Drew, they were still baffled. Almost all of the findings were negative except the ones that came up high for inflammatory reaction. *Hmmm.* This is when they started trying to culture everything. They checked his blood, his sputum, and even his stool but still nothing grew out in the Petri dish. Soon thereafter our little friend began to get sicker. He started having headaches, fatigue, abdominal pain and a whole bunch of other things. *What the heck was going on here?* Our heroes finally decided to do a biopsy at the site of the egg-sized tumors and it revealed a foreign body granuloma. Everyone (including a pathologist, a parasitologist, and other research scientists) was called in to figure what these results meant. At first, they thought it was something rare like Bechet's disease or Weber-Christian disease. *Nope.* It turns out it was something else; a plant root.

Now why would a plant root be in someone's body? Because Drew was a Munchausen with nothing better to do but cost the medical system thousands and thousands of dollars and drive everyone crazy. When the doctors confronted Drew about this possible diagnosis, he went ballistic. *How dare they question him?* Luckily, the nursing staff found an old syringe on Drew with a cloudy material in it. *Whoops.* Though Drew gave some shoddy excuse for possessing it everyone knew the jig was up. It seems that our good friend was injecting himself with two different types of drugs to make himself appear to be sick. Drew was subsequently shipped off to a psychiatric hospital where he will no doubt leave against medical advice only to torture a new set of doctors another day. Good luck to you, Drew, because you are this month's My Favorite Munchausen.

Liberally embellished from Mod Rheumatol (2004) 14:66-69. ✚

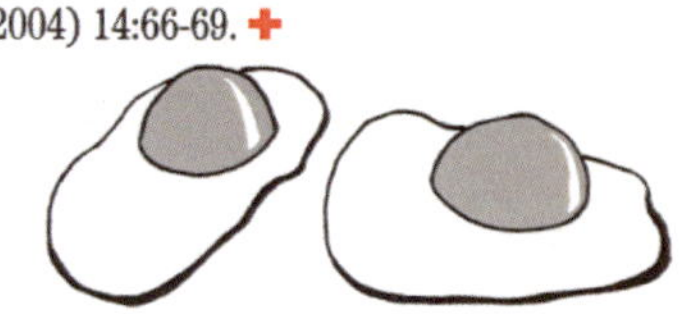

## TRUE STORIES OF MEDICINE

# THE TOILET MONSTER

It was on a typical night that I was scheduled to work with a new nurse and an aide in a small rural hospital. I was returning to the nurses' station with my fresh cup of coffee preparing to settle in for a quiet night, when suddenly the quiet rural air was filled with horrific screams. The new nurse came running out of the ER with eyes wide as saucers and a bewildered look on her face. Her reply to my puzzled look was, *"I don't know what to do for this woman!"*

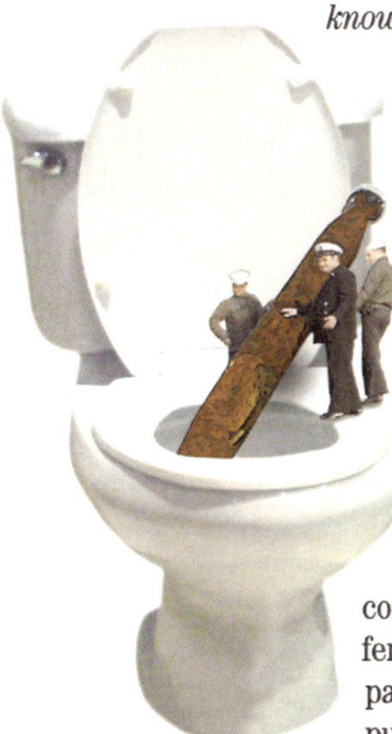

I went into the ER expecting a mortally wounded patient, but what I found was a 30-something constipated female. Her pants were pulled down, and let's just say that this non-pregnant woman was crowning. She was screaming and crying and would/could not hold still for vitals.

I grabbed a handful of *KY Jelly* and led the distraught woman to the bathroom. She sat gingerly on the toilet as I explained the delicate process of fecal disimpaction.

As I stimulated the rectum, she let out a very unique and nearly indescribable sound. My best description of this utterance would be to call it a war whoop. As I instantly discovered, the war cry was a proclamation of successful anal lubrication. A giant torpedo splashed down into the toilet sending water spraying everywhere. She jumped off the toilet and grabbed onto me in a frantic hug, crying, *"Just let me hold you for a while – I LOVE YOU!"*

She was overcome with relief. Soon she was showing off her prize to her family, who did not believe that her extreme discomfort was from constipation.

***"I TOLD YOU DAD – COME IN HERE AND LOOK AT THIS!"***

The younger nurse escorted the patient back to the ER, leaving me to deal with the monster in the toilet. Knowing this thing would never flush, I reluctantly removed it with care, and placed it into a secure biohazard bag. And, yes . . . I weighed it. *Why?* Maybe it was out of sheer morbid curiosity. Maybe it was because I knew I'd be telling this story for years. Maybe it was for accurate documentation, I don't know. I think that anyone else would have done the same. The result: **two pounds.**

A co-worker made a victory ribbon and gave it to the patient, who was excited to take it home and add it to her scrapbook. Once again she hugged me and told me how much she loved me. **Nursing is truly a rewarding career.** ✚



# X-Ray Files

***If we show you ours, will you show us yours?***

## It's Sci-FI Time!

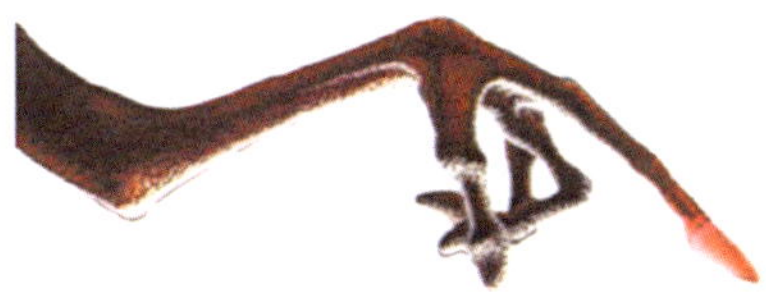

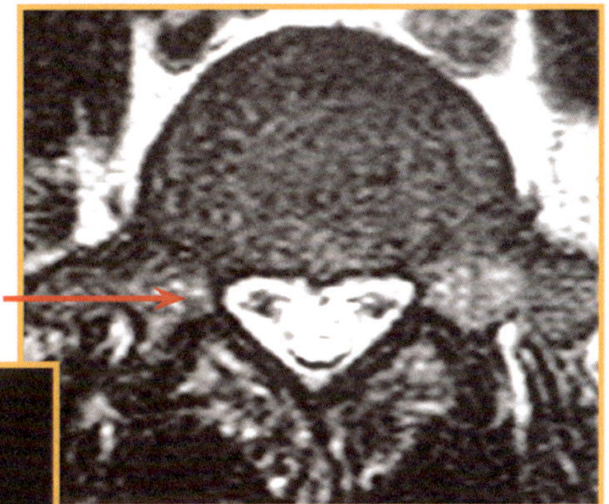

**E.T.** in an MRI of the spine

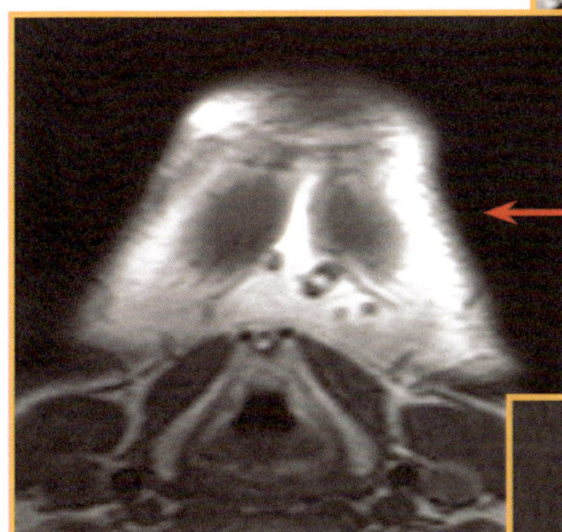

**Darth Vader** on an MRI of the neck.

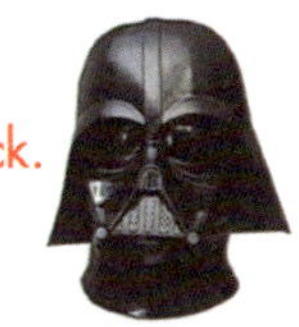

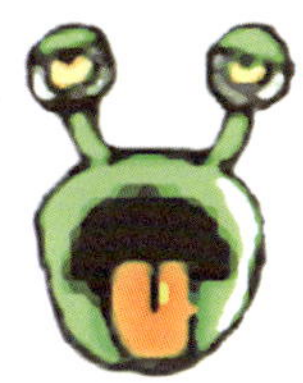

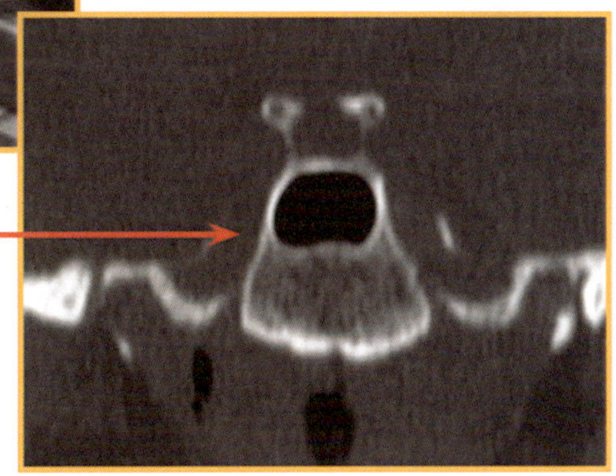

**And another alien!** (It showed up on the skull base of a CT scan of the brain.)

*Introducing the*

# "I Want To Be In Healthcare!"

*Birthday Party Theme*

*Your children love playing doctor or nurse! Now you can make their whole party into a medical theme.*

Our kit will give your kid a taste of what it is like in today's healthcare system. Our full selection of products makes planning your child's party a piece of cake.

*Get your child ready for his future!*

**Your "I Want To Be In Healthcare!" Birthday Party Theme Deluxe Pack for 16 includes:**

## DECORATIONS:

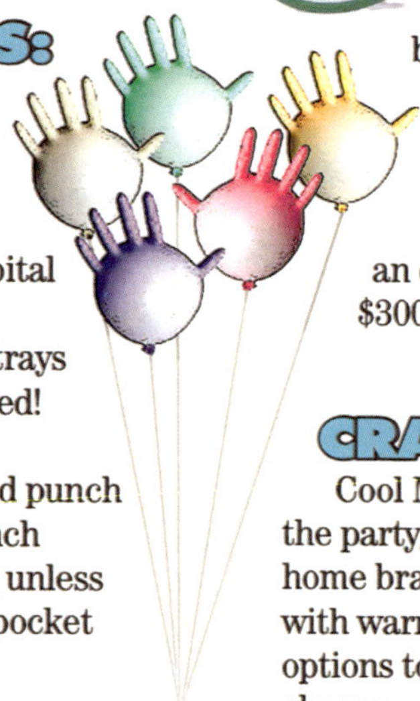

- 16 rubber gloves to inflate for balloons
- 8 surgical caps for party hats
- 8 cheap backless hospital gowns for the others!
- 6 replicas of hospital trays and cups; already pre-stained!
- 16 insurance cards:
  - i. 8 will get cake and punch
  - ii. 6 will just get punch
  - iii. 2 will get nothing unless they pay out of pocket

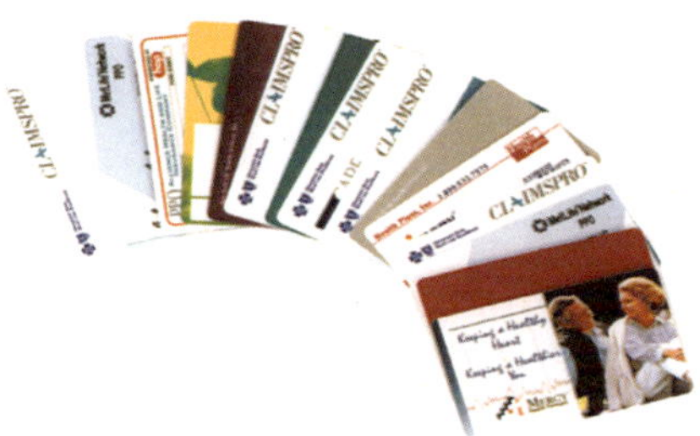

## GAMES: (pick two)

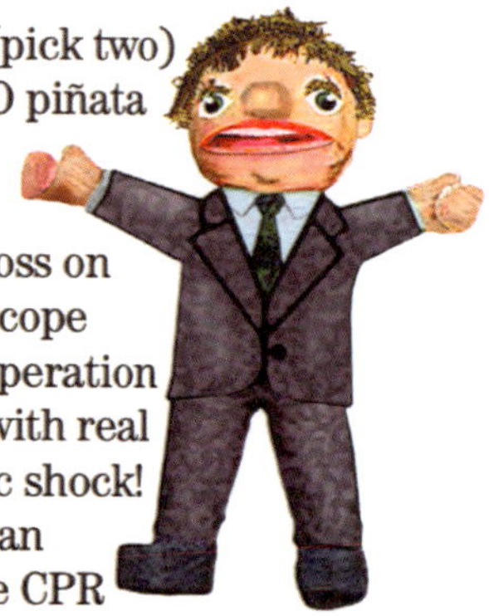

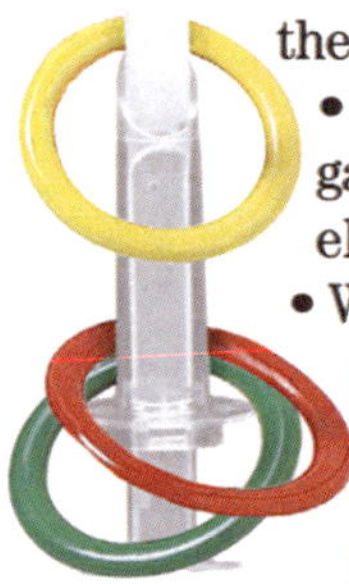

- Hospital CEO piñata
- Pin the Tail on the Lawyer
- Ring toss on the anoscope
- Co-Operation game with real electric shock!
- Who can revive CPR Annie? Includes Ambu bag, intubation kit and defibrillator. This costs an extra $3000.

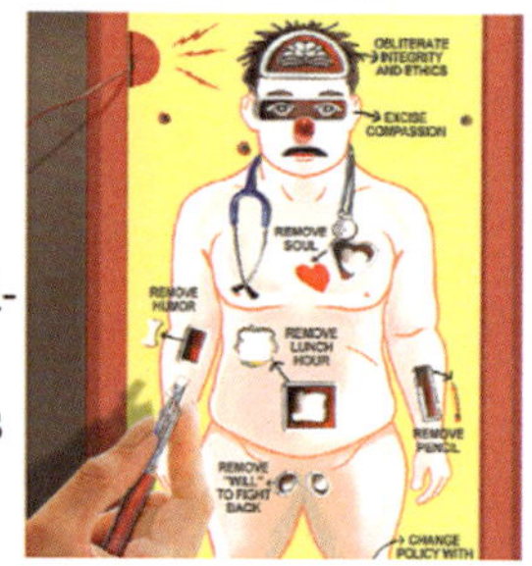


## CRAFTS:

Cool Medical Alert ID Bracelets – the partygoers can build their own take-home bracelets with warning options to choose from such as diabetic, senile, highly infectious, and much more. *WARNING:* removal of these bracelets is next to impossible (just like the real thing).

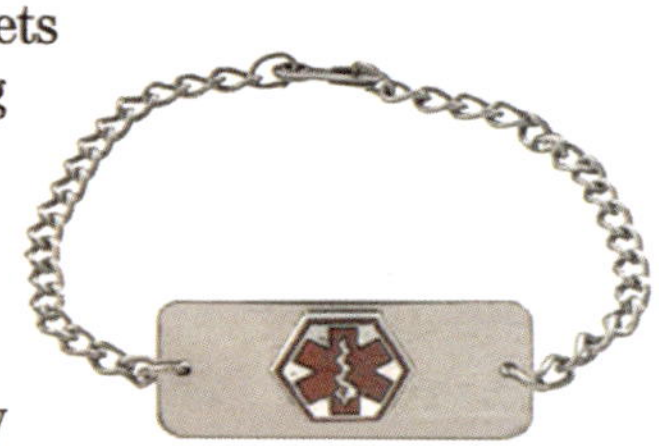

## FOOD: (pick one)

- Diabetic and tasteless cake
- Low salt, low protein ice cream through an IV bag

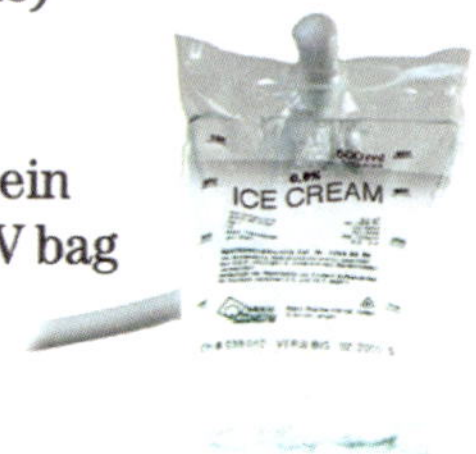


## PARTY FAVORS: (pick one)

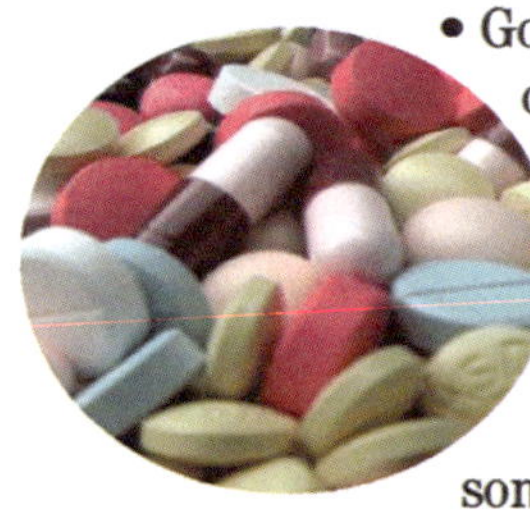

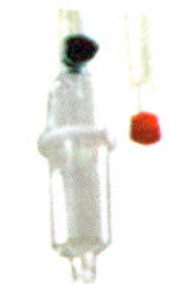

- Goody bags of candy pills that looks just like the ones you'll use or take someday (valium and antidepressants).
- Fortune cookies:

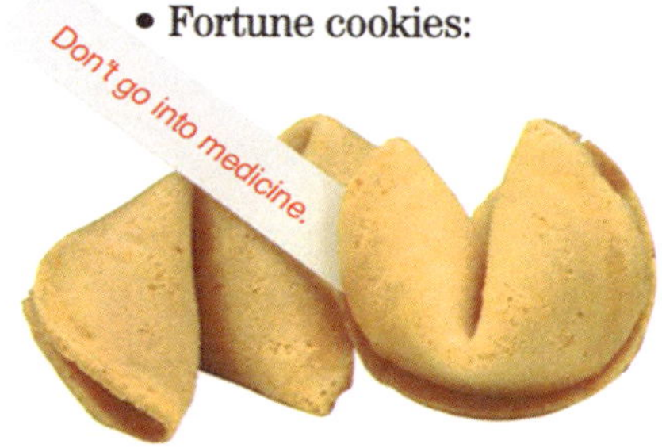


  - i. "Don't go into medicine."
  - ii. "Become a specialist."
  - iii. "Don't sleep with the staff."
  - iv. "Don't forget the pre-nup."
  - v. "You will have an MI before age 45."
  - vi. "You'll someday find happiness in a bottle."
  - vii. And much, much more! ✚

**PJ PARTY GEAR – MEDICAL FUN FOR EVERYONE!**

# "Get your dreams back"

with

# Zerorem

Can't sleep because your EMR is a piece of crap?
Are you up all night because your account receivables are a lost cause?
Does your mind race at night about the good old days of medicine?

If you answered yes, like over 90% of today's physicians do, then *Zerorem* is for you.

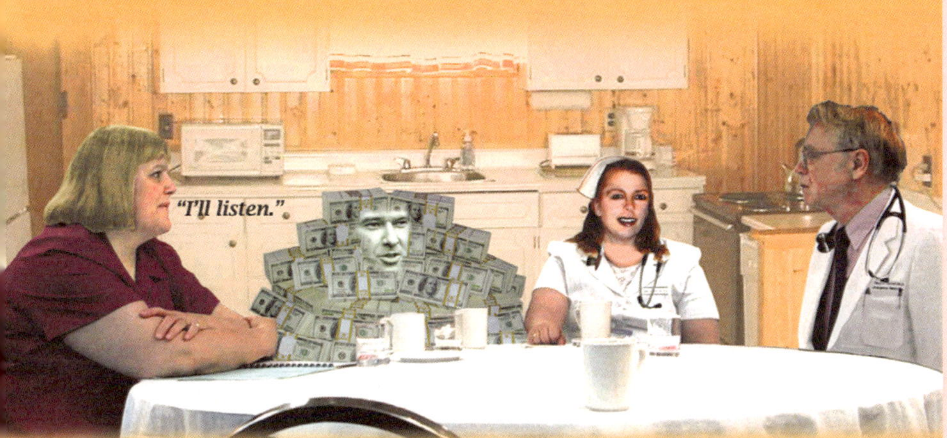


***Zerorem is the first sleeping aid for physicians.***

No one knows how hard it is to be a doctor like you do . . . and *PJ Pharmaceuticals*. That's why we have come up with the only sleeping pill guaranteed to make you enjoy your life again. At least while you're asleep, that is!

**IMPORTANT SAFETY INFORMATION**
Don't drive, drink, drink and drive, or do surgery while you are taking *Zerorem*. Normally, we would ask you to consult your doctor if you are having any side effect, but since doctors don't go to doctors then we recommend winging it on your own.
Side effects may include a sudden urge to quit your profession.

**PJ PHARMACEUTICALS**
*The Realistic Drug Company*



# Complications

A 57-year-old man came to the ER with dizziness. After examining him, I determined that he had vertigo. He had positional dizziness, a spinning sensation, mild nystagmus and nausea. He didn't have a headache, so he didn't seem like a guy with a subarachnoid hemorrhage.

I discharged him home on some Antivert. An hour later, EMS was called to a rural part of the county for a gunshot wound. Back came Mr. Dizziness, with an entrance wound in the left buttock, no obvious exit wound, and severe abdominal pain. It turns out that the round went all the way up through his pelvis and abdomen and entered his transverse colon. Obviously, he went to the OR.

I happened to learn later that he was a known Meth manufacturer and dealer, who had once threatened to kill his wife, forcing her to dig her grave before she escaped. *A real stand-up kind of guy.*

However, I often wondered if his inability to stand up that night, due to vertigo, resulted in a worse or better outcome. Was he unable to run when he heard the slide fall down and chamber that bullet? Or, did his vertigo cause him to stumble and make his assailant change targets, so that he shot his bottom instead of his head?

In the end, I have to wonder, how often is a gunshot wound a complication of vertigo? Not often. But it couldn't have happened to a nicer guy ✚

# Constriction

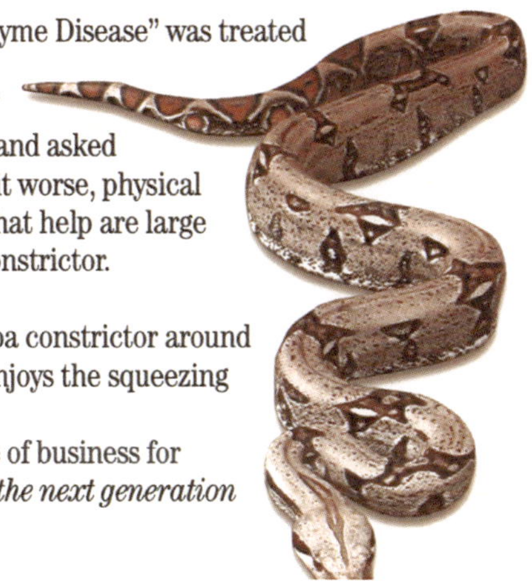

A former patient of mine with "Chronic Lyme Disease" was treated with high doses antibiotics by the local "Lyme Disease" expert. He came to me complaining of chronic neck pain. I did the regular evaluation and asked all the right questions (what relieves it, makes it worse, physical therapy, etc.). He told me that the only things that help are large doses of *Oxycontin* and *Percocet* and his boa constrictor.

*"Boa Constrictor?"* I asked.

He responded by saying that he puts the boa constrictor around his neck three to four times a day because he enjoys the squeezing sensation.

He got me thinking about a whole new line of business for various musculoskeletal complaints. *I could be the next generation of snake charmers!* ✚

## ANOTHER TRUE STORY OF MEDICINE

# NEED TO BLOCK MY CALLS

As an extremely earnest and well-meaning third year resident, I had been working very hard to get one of my chronic pancreatitis patients to understand the error of her ways and quit drinking. After her third admission in five months, we had had many long talks about not drinking alcohol anymore, going to rehab, going to *AA*, taking naltrexone, taking antabuse, going to counseling, taking SSRIs, and her potential for upcoming liver failure. She was only 27, and I was naïve enough to think that the hours that I spent with her during her month-long hospitalization would be the thing that finally got her to give up her three pint a day vodka habit.

She was doing a bit better after about a week in the hospital without food or liquid (just IV fluids). We decided that she could advance her diet to what we call ***Sips and Chips*** which is small amounts of water and ice chips. The order was written and I went on with my day. At about 2 a.m. I received a page; she was vomiting again and in severe pain. I trudged up to the fourth floor to see her. After examining her, I noticed a huge bag of *Cool Ranch Doritos* and a *Mountain Dew* next to her bed. Upon questioning, she confided how excited she had been to get the go-ahead to advance her diet. She had made the trek down to the vending machines in the cafeteria to pick up some ***Sips and Chips*** (which in her mind was *Dew* and *Doritos*). She assured me that she had definitely not gulped the *Mountain Dew* and instead just sipped.

It took many weeks later to finally send her home. After that is when I received a call at home. It was her. She had managed to con the hospital operator into giving her my home number. She had called to ask me what to do as she was having severe abdominal pain again. I asked her what she had had to eat and drink.

*"Just one beer. My friends talked me into celebrating my discharge from the hospital . . ."* +

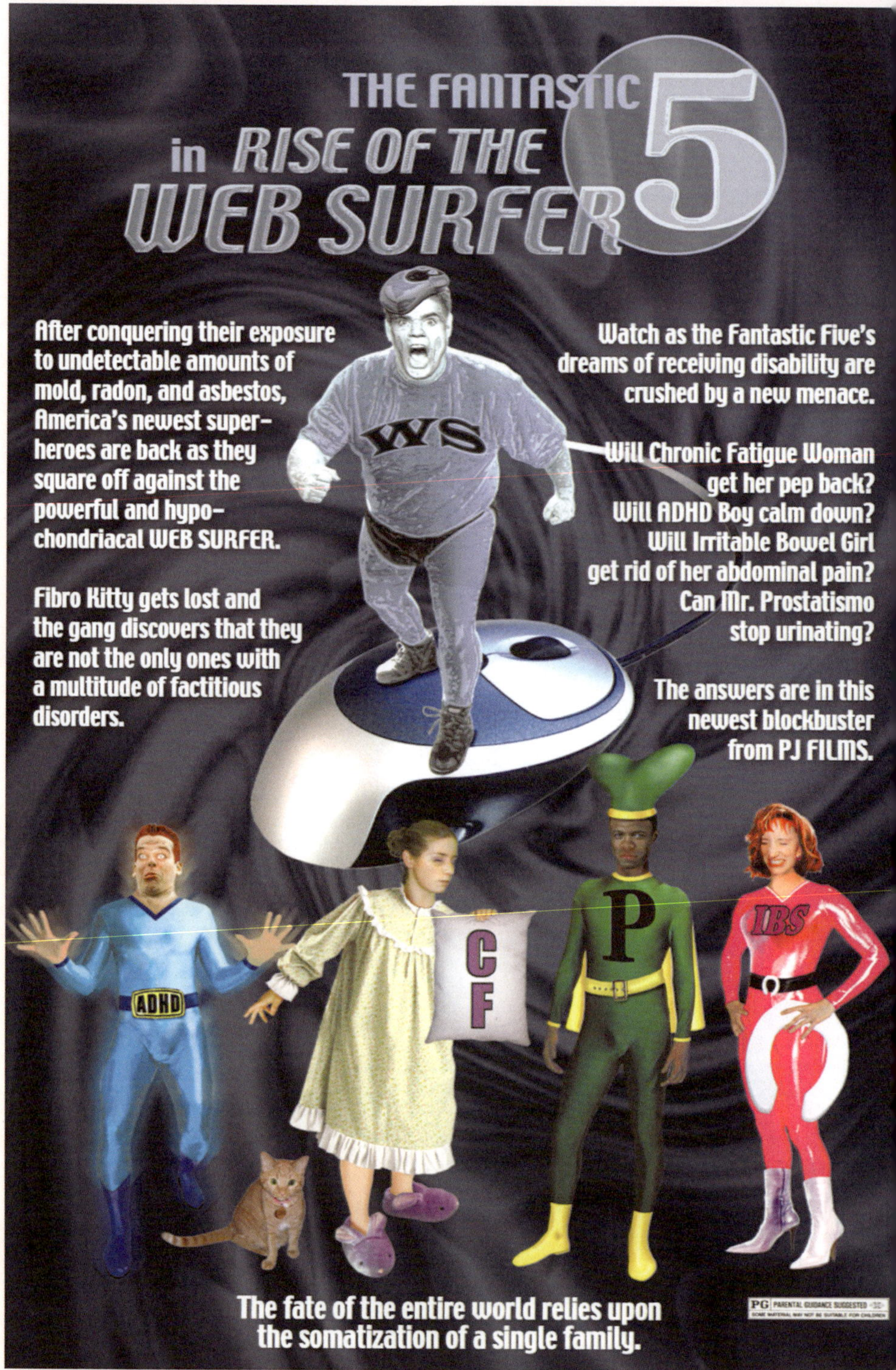
THE FANTASTIC 5
in RISE OF THE WEB SURFER
After conquering their exposure to undetectable amounts of mold, radon, and asbestos, America's newest super-heroes are back as they square off against the powerful and hypo-chondriacal WEB SURFER.
Fibro Kitty gets lost and the gang discovers that they are not the only ones with a multitude of factitious disorders.
Watch as the Fantastic Five's dreams of receiving disability are crushed by a new menace.
Will Chronic Fatigue Woman get her pep back? Will ADHD Boy calm down? Will Irritable Bowel Girl get rid of her abdominal pain? Can Mr. Prostatismo stop urinating?
The answers are in this newest blockbuster from PJ FILMS.
WS
ADHD
CF
P
IBS
The fate of the entire world relies upon the somatization of a single family.
PG

*Now available in bookstores*

# WHAT TO REGRET WHEN YOU'RE EXPECTING

By Cornelius Parody MD and Aristotle Jones PhD

*Here are some examples of some of the questions that come with comforting answers:*

Will I ever have an intelligent adult conversation again – you know, like, umm, about *American Idol* contestants or my favorite kinds of chips?

My boobs are great but they're going to shrink again aren't they?

My husband wants to have sex with me but all I want to do is kick him in his balls. Is that wrong?

These stretch marks aren't going away after I deliver are they?

Who the hell is going to pay for this kid?

Am I still allowed to drink a fifth of vodka a few times a week?

I felt my baby moving again. Does he need to be on ADD drugs?

Can I still go clubbing? What about after my water breaks?

My work may involve a sticky three-inch brass pole. Is that bad for the baby?

Should I get paternity testing now or after I deliver? Is there a way to fake this to get the one who has the most money?

I noticed that they checked me for STDs at my first visit. If I'm re-exposed once or twice a week with different guys, should I get this testing repeated often?

My baby keeps kicking me. Is it mad at me?

The pregnancy is going great and I love the doctors at the medical office. Which member(s) of the health care team is the best to sue after the delivery?

*Also contains:*

- A new section for moms who live off the system
- A new section for hillbilly pregnancies
- A new section on breastfeeding with implants

***Order Now and Receive A Coupon for Free Tanning Booth Lotion!****

*Not to be used during pregnancy – may harm you and your child.

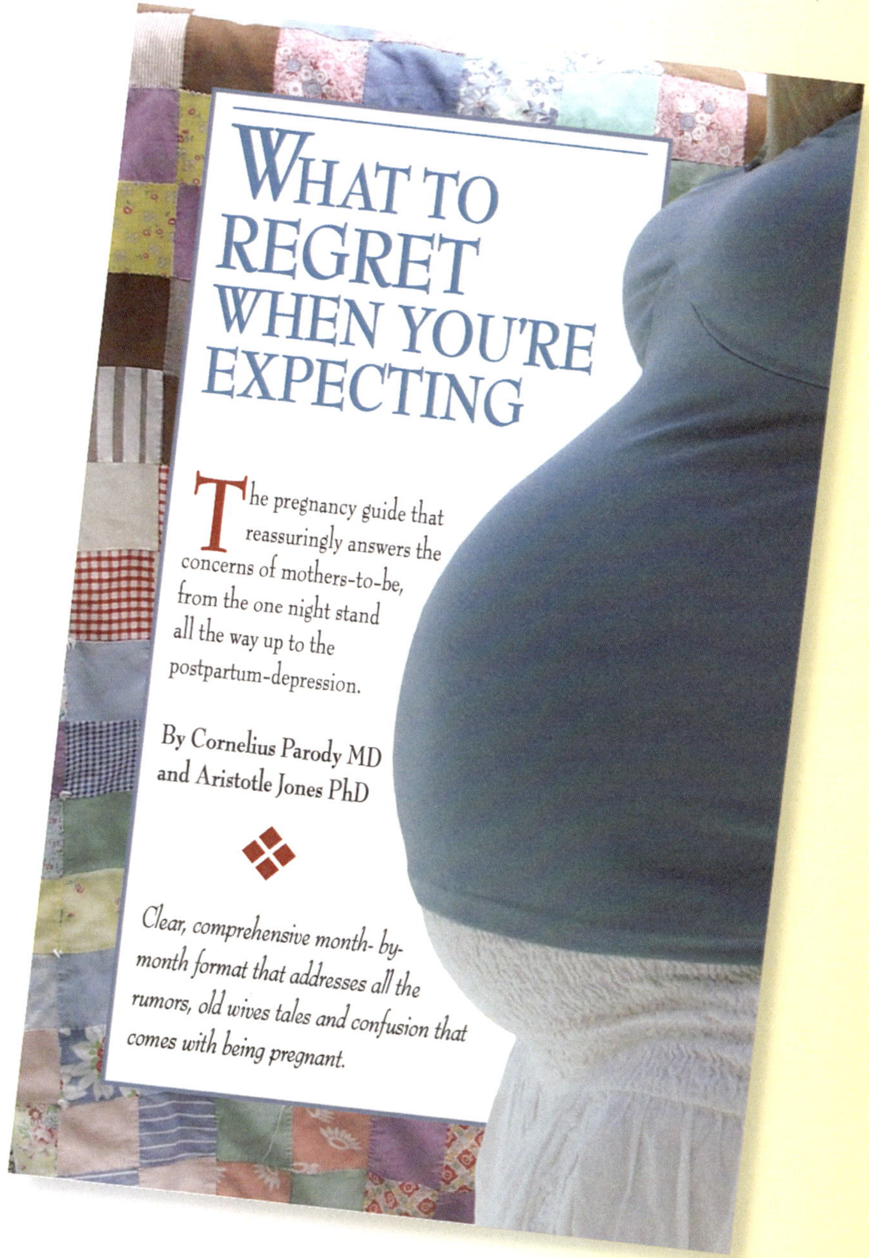


*"After my sixth kid, this book is the only thing that kept me sane. Well, that and my cigarettes."*

Brandi, age 18

# NEW! FROM PJ PUBLICATIONS

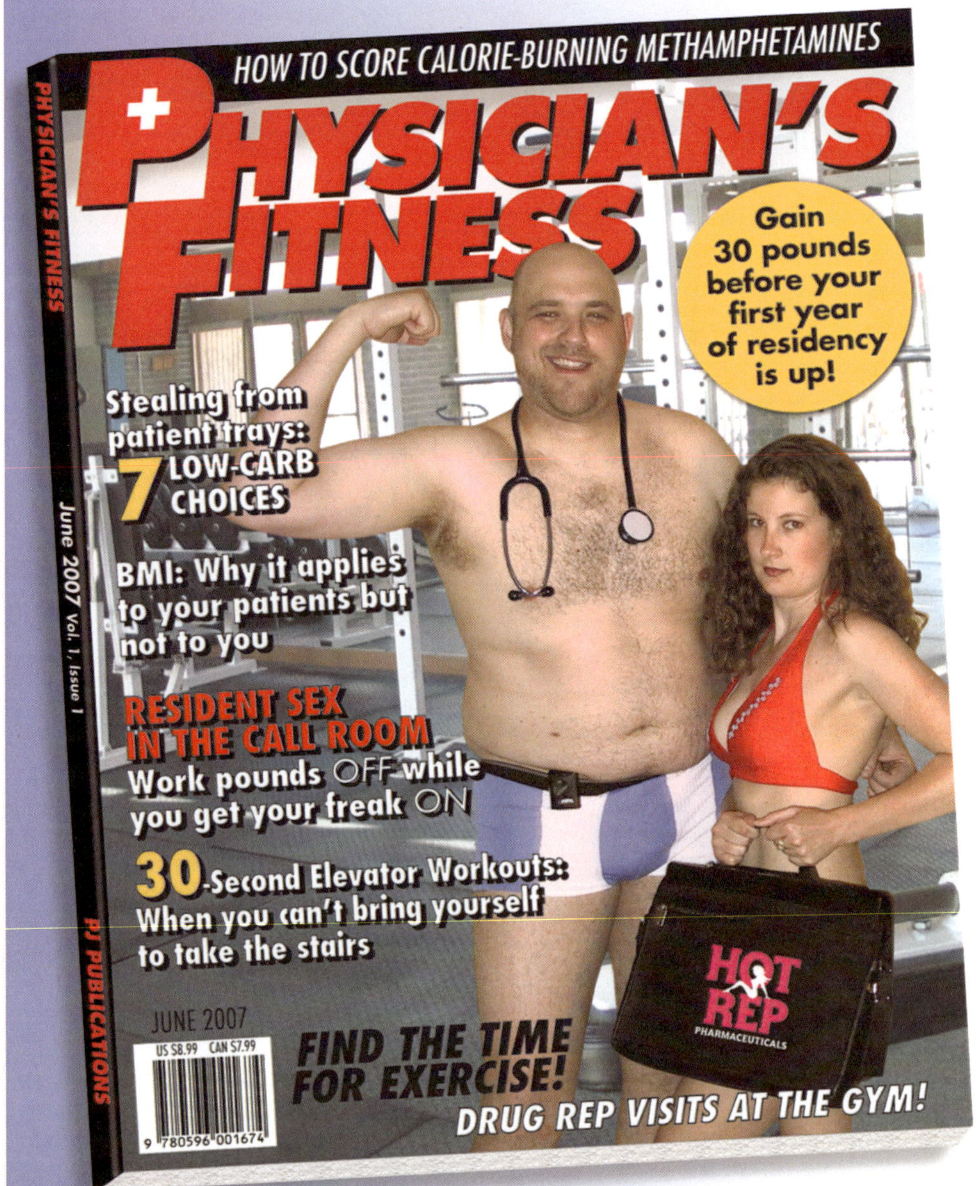


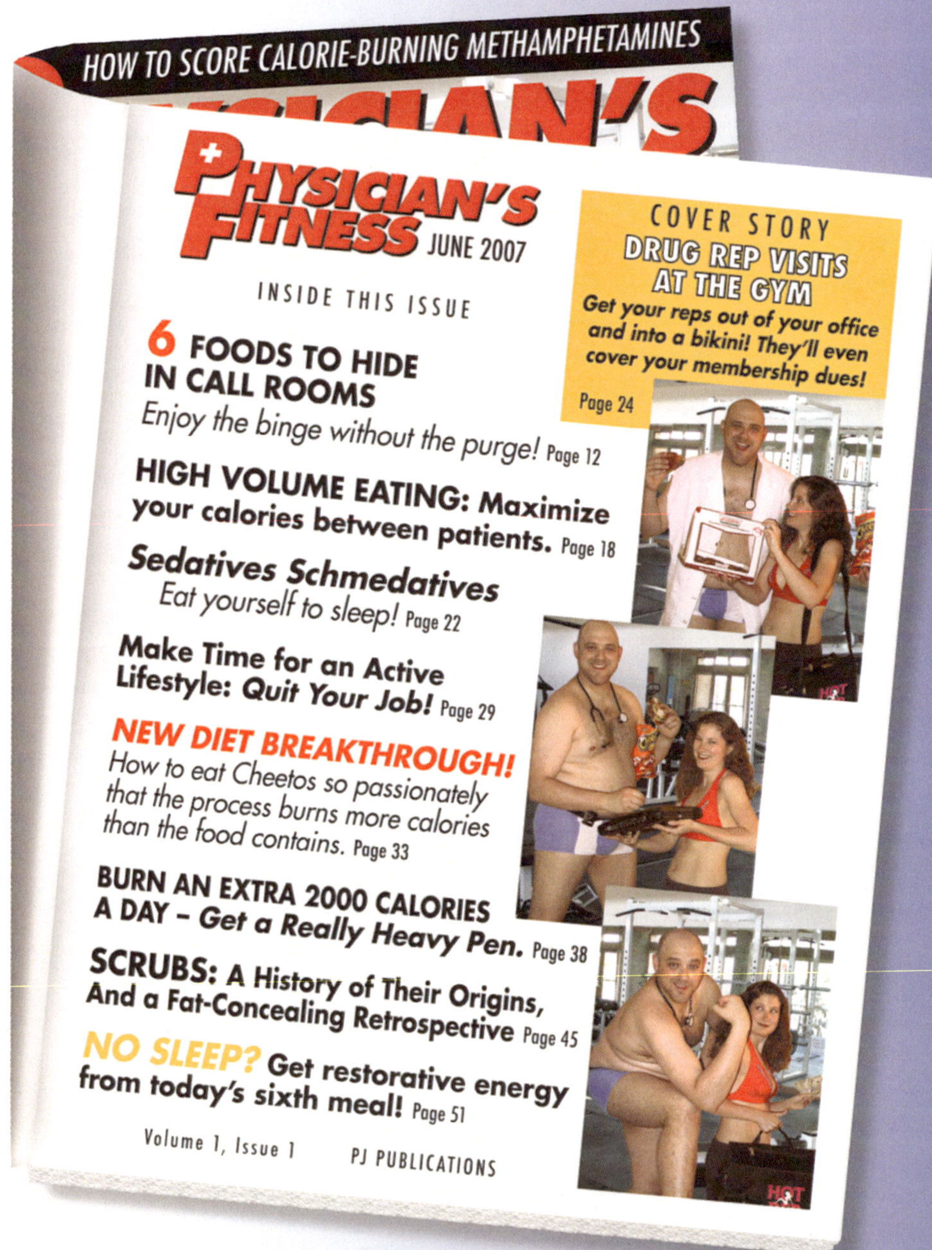


# ON NEWSTANDS NOW!

# Occupational and Environmental Medicine
# + BOOT CAMP +
## *LOCATED IN CHARMING TIKRIT, IRAQ*

*At this unique conference (and environment), workers' compensation and occupational health professionals will be provided with an in-depth learning experience covering the most common issues plaguing the profession.*

*The learning methodology is interactive and exciting, plus there is plenty of sun!*

*You will never think about disability and workers' compensation the same way again.*

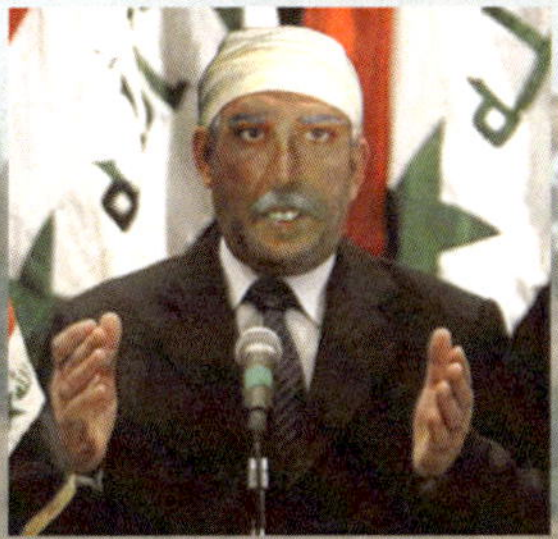

### SPECIAL LOCAL KEYNOTE LECTURE

In your country you get free money for not working? Are you shitting me?

*Dr. Abdi Hussan Mahammad, Occupational Health Minister and Café Owner*

### OTHER TOPICS INCLUDE:

***Why do I still hurt?*** How to maintain composure when your patients look better than you do.
*Dr. Phuk Yuen, MD*

***FMLA:*** A new way for your patients to spell VACATION.
*Dr. K. Illme, MD*

***Acute and chronic attorney exposure:*** Management strategies to minimize physician suicide.
*D. Pression, DO, MPH*

***How to burn out and make a living as a pot-prescribing physician:*** Same patients, better reimbursement, and cool weapons training.
*Dr. Chong, PhD*

***Toilets, dogs, open car windows, and restaurants:*** Teaching patients how to prevent these narcotic-stealing offenders.
*Yur Ryte, MD*

***Cash Cows:*** How you can capitalize when your patient wins the workers' compensation lottery.
*Dr. Alexander Slacker, MD*

***When the Candyman can't:*** What to do with the patients your narc-dealing partner left after he got arrested.
*Ralph Ng MD, PhD*

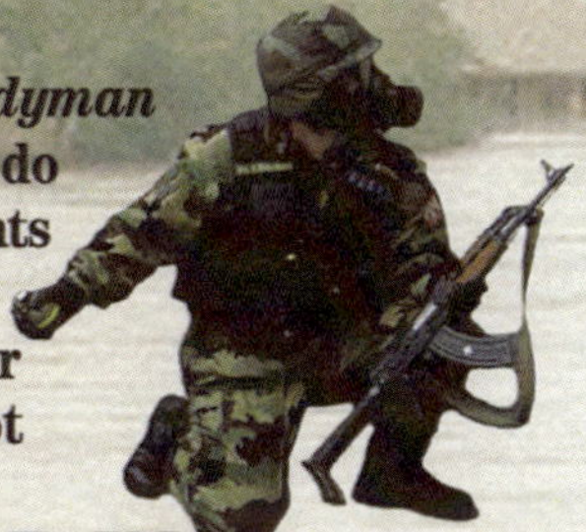

***The EMR solution whose time has come:*** How to get carpal tunnel syndrome and file a workers' comp claim against yourself.
*Myand Hertz, MD*

***"I'm sorry to tell you this Ma'am but your lumbosacral MRI is normal:"*** Strategies for delivering bad news.
*V. Cationzover, MD*

***Overabundance of symptom magnification, malingering, and fraud:*** How to bring closure to your choice of profession.
*Luke Eng-Forachob, MD*

### TUITION

The $13,395 tuition includes a continental breakfast, breaks, lunch with faculty, a detailed manual, and a complete set of body armor.

### CONTINUING EDUCATION INFORMATION

Participants who somehow can survive the whole conference will be credited with 16 hours of CMME.

### ABOUT TIKRIT

Tikrit, Iraq is a small town located 140 km northwest of Baghdad on the Tigris River. The town had an estimated population in 2002 of about 28,900. Today, that number may or may not be less. This "northern angle" of the Sunni Triangle is known for its beautiful scenery, majestic history, and coalition occupation.

### ACCOMMODATIONS

Sunubar Resort and Bomb Shelter offers beautiful waterfalls and 12-inch reinforced walls. Call ahead for reservations. If no one answers, keep calling or check the network news.

### ACTIVITIES

5K Fun Run along the minefield next to the Tigris River on Saturday.

Enjoy family swimming in Lake Saddam.

Watch the local soccer team play (subject to cancellation at a moment's notice).

*All transportation provided by Blackhawk Choppers: "When you really need to get there alive, it's the only way to go!"* +

## MORE TRUE STORIES OF MEDICINE

# Real Doctor

As an ophthalmologist, I frequently deal with patients who mistakenly think I am an optometrist. There is nothing wrong with being an optometrist, but it's not what I trained to do.

One day I was seeing an older woman for a comprehensive exam and, after finishing, I told her I didn't see any signs of cataract, macular degeneration, or glaucoma. She was relieved, and I asked her if she had any questions. She started to say something, and then said, *"Oh, never mind."*

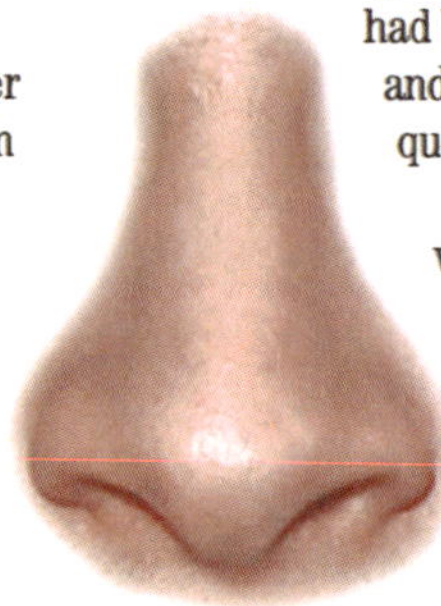

I told her it was okay to ask, and she said her question was for a *"real doctor."* I told her I was a real doctor, and she said, *"No, like someone who has been to medical school, not just eye doctor school."*

My chest puffed out slightly as I explained to her that I was a real doctor, had been to a real medical school, and could probably answer her question.

She relaxed, and I prepared to wow her with the depths of my clinical and diagnostic knowledge.

When she asked, ***"Does it smell to you like I have a yeast infection?"*** I visibly deflated and mumbled something about her needing to see her real doctor. Sometimes we all need to be put in our place. ✚

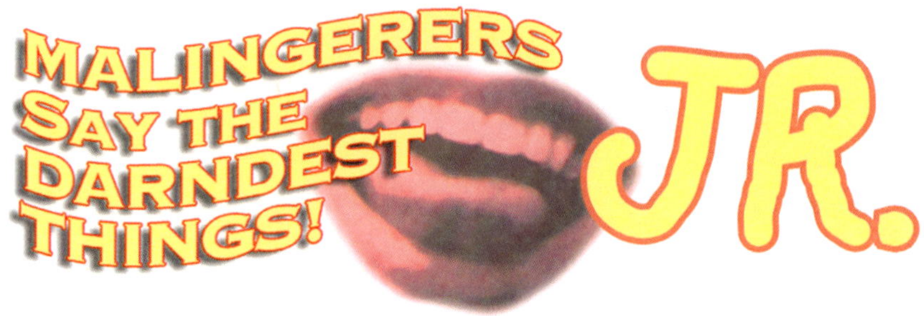


**Ever wonder where malingerers come from? They start early. *Bless their little hearts.* Here's one who gave this note to his 5th grade physical education teacher . . .**

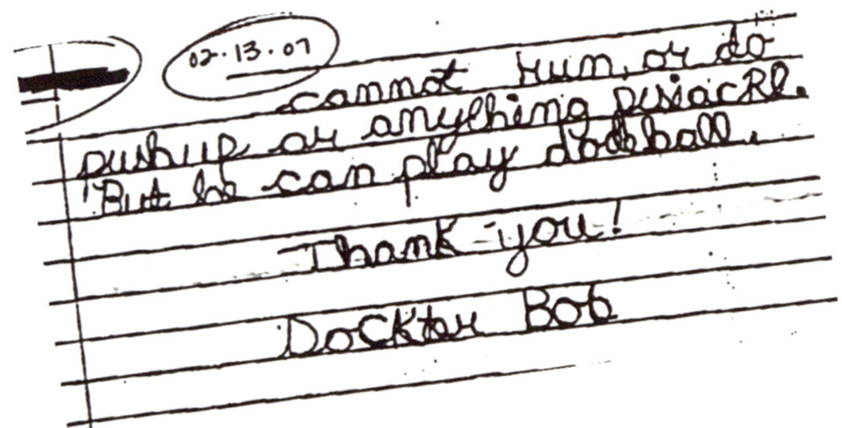

02.13.07
cannot Run, or do
pushup or anything physicRl.
But he can play dodgball.
Thank you!
DocKtor Bob

**It was supposed to say:**

***Cannot run, or do pushup or anything physical. But he can play dodgeball.***

***Thank you!***

***Doctor Bob***

✚

# Compassion Meter

You start the morning psyched up – it's a new day. We are going to help people. And we do . . . we have a lot of very nice patients and the compassion meter is right up there. Then . . .

A 25-year-old man who had fallen at a restaurant comes in. He slipped and fell on water. He said that after he filed a worker's comp claim, he was fired a few days later. He had only worked there a month. This is a real shame – folks getting fired after filing a claim – but it does happen. A resident doc was with me and we went through his medical history and examined him. He seemed a very pleasant, but quiet, young man. **(Compassion meter: 10/10).**

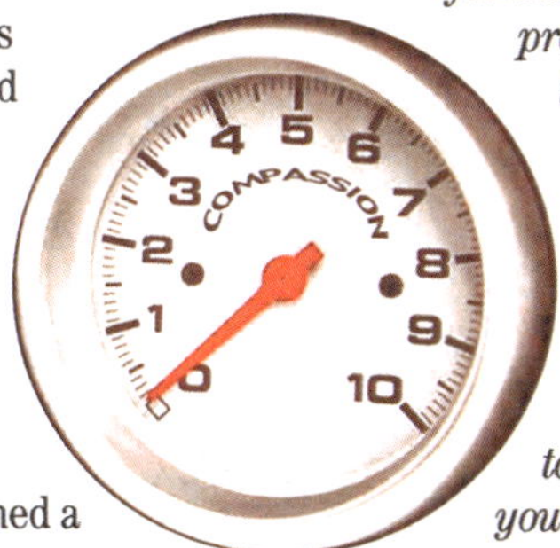


On checking his reflexes, I could see he had a very large scar on his knee from what looked like a pretty extensive, old surgery. Open incision. *"Well, that was when I fell through the floor of a rotted* ***jail cell."*** ***(Oh my*** **– Compassion meter: 7/10).**

*"And I know the docs at XYZ clinic messed up my knee surgery – I'm not even a doctor but I can tell that the screws are all out of whack. They just keep passing me around the clinic. They are supposed to be giving me* Vicodan, *but I just don't have time to keep the appointments and keep going back. Gas is really expensive to keep going back there."* ***(Well, yeah, gas is really expensive*** **– Compassion meter: 5/10).**

*"And I should be receiving disability for that – and for some mental problems . . . although I don't think I have the problem – I think it's everyone else's problem."*

*Do you have a counselor?"* I asked.

*"Yes."*

*"That's good you are taking care of yourself. Are you on any medications?"*

*"Yeah, but I think some of my friends stole them."* **(Compassion meter: 1/10. This is a human being, trying to get by in the world . . . he has an inner child, he just hasn't found his inner adult . . .).**

After a month he missed all his appointments with us and physical therapy. I vented to a doc who works in the prison system who assured me that, even though the incarceration took place in California, the jail cell walls are made out of concrete. No one falls through one of them. **(Compassion meter: 0/10).** ✚

We can only hope that the electrical cord on this

**FISH TANK HEATER**

wasn't plugged in!

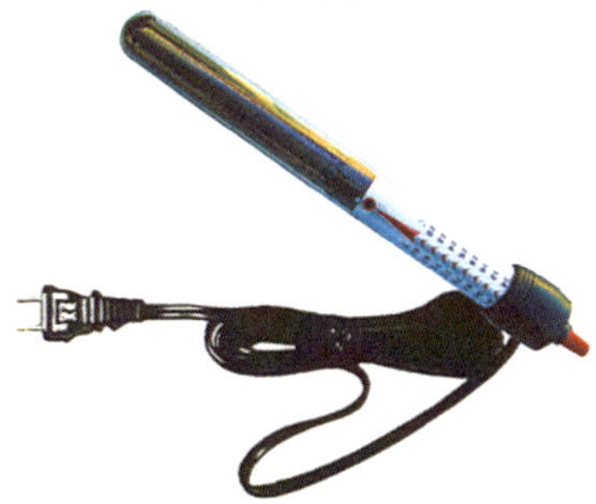

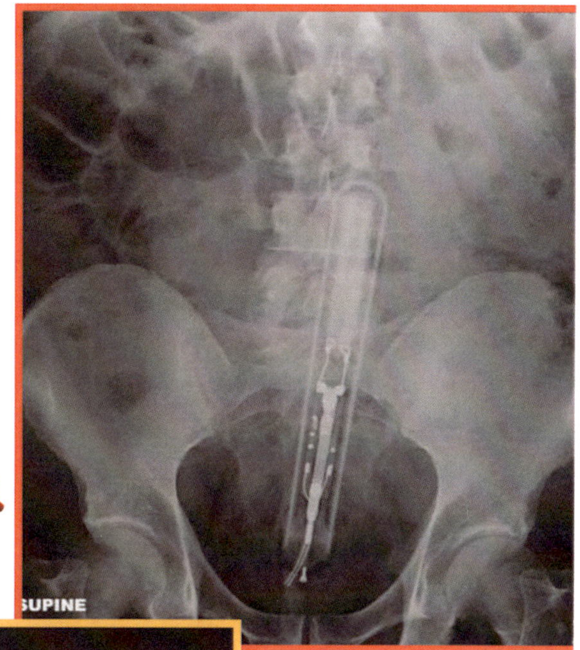


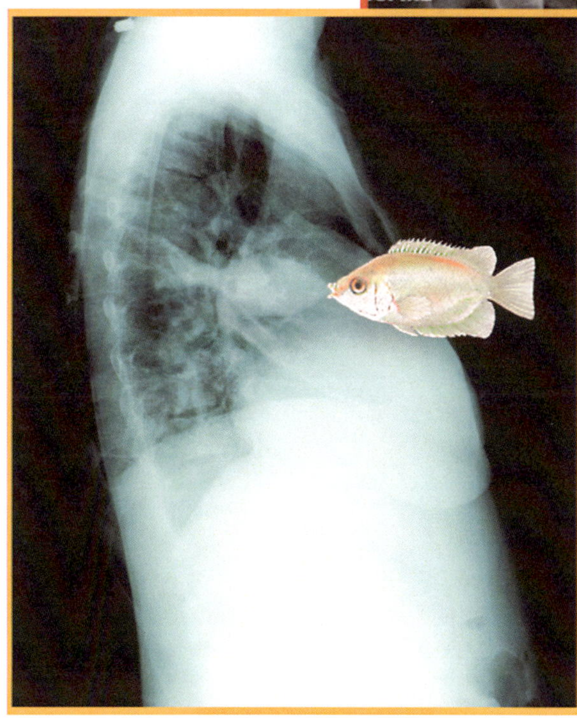

And finally, this patient's x-ray shows a

**FISH-SHAPED TUMOR.**

*Maybe these two patients should get together!*

CONTINUING MEANINGLESS MEDICAL EDUCATION

# CMME

**Fellow Placebians are eligible to receive three hours of CMME prescribed credit that has no meaning at all.** *Please select the most appropriate answer to each of the questions listed below. Check your answers online at* ***www. placebojournal.com.*** *You need to get 80% correct in order to receive your meaningless credit. If you do not get 80% of the answers correct, then we will give you the credit anyway. We really don't care.*

**1. Which one of the following findings is an indication for imaging in patients with acute low back pain?**

A. Crying while in the exam room.
B. Weakness of the legs.
C. Sciatica.
D. Insurance.

**2. You hear a murmur on a 64-year-old male who is in your office for a complete physical. Which of the following would predict whether it is pathologic in nature?**

A. The patient gets dizzy while he takes a deep breath.
B. You hear a midsystolic click.
C. The murmur has a musical quality.
D. You pull out the echocardiogram and find out that the patient has severe aortic stenosis.

**3. Which one of the following reverses the effects of warfarin (*Coumadin*)? More than one answer may apply.**

A. Aspirin.
B. Spinach.
C. Vitamin K.
D. Death.

**4. Which of the following is true about the "Just Wants to Meet You" visit?**

A. It is a nice way to show your personality.
B. The visit is confusing after the initial handshake.
C. You would rather drink a pint of hydrogen peroxide rather than go into the room.
D. You ain't getting paid jack shit for your time.
E. All of the above.

**5. Which of the following will create a welcoming atmosphere in the waiting room?**

A. Putting in slot machines.
B. Providing free "massages."
C. Having a narcotic dispensing vending machine.
D. Allowing the patients to watch OTB (Off Track Betting) races.
E. Allowing the patients to watch OTB races after they place a bet with your front staff.

*Check your CMME answers online at*

**WWW. PLACEBO JOURNAL .COM**

ANOTHER TRUE STORY OF MEDICINE

## With This Stool, I Thee Wed

My cute and sharp as a tack, 93- year-old female patient pulled a ring box out of her purse and set it on my desk saying, *"I have a present for you."*

Her little chuckle told me not to expect an antique diamond ring. The photo shows what her gift was.

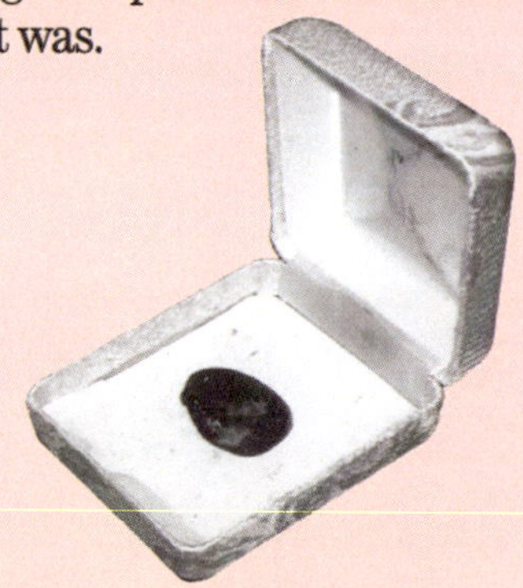

She explained she had been eating "a whole crop" of red beets and her stool looked like this. A negative guaiac test made her so happy she gave me the ring box which was promptly strutted around to all staff to surprise them with my present. ✚

## LONG WAY DOWN

A stripper came in to the ER claiming that she fell 14 feet off a stripper pole. I was last in a strip club 25 years ago and I don't remember the poles being that high. *Them's some strong thighs shimmeying 14 feet up a stripper pole!*

She said she got knocked out and when she came to she couldn't move her arms or legs at first and her ribs and back hurt. Instead of calling 911 she went home and took *Tylenol*, which didn't help her pain but her stepfathers' *Vicodin* worked great.

She asked the registration clerk if she would qualify for workers comp.

When I examined her I found no bruising anywhere on her body from the 14 foot fall. I also noted she was awfully chatty and had methface and pinpoint pupils.

*Let's solve this medical mystery with a tox screen, super sleuthers.*

Vital signs: normal
Head CT: negative
Hematocrit: normal
Chest X-ray: normal
Drug screen: positive cocaine, opiates and benzodiazepines

**The moral of the story:** If you want to screw the strip club owner with a bogus worker's comp claim AND cop narcotics from the naïve ER doc, don't smoke crack and snort oxycontin right before you spin on the stripper pole. ✚

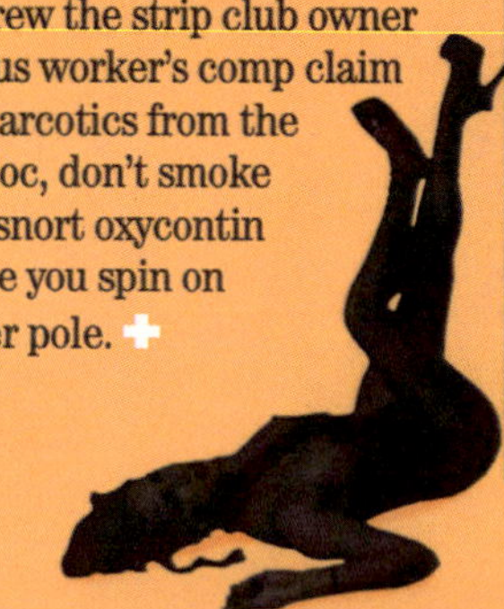

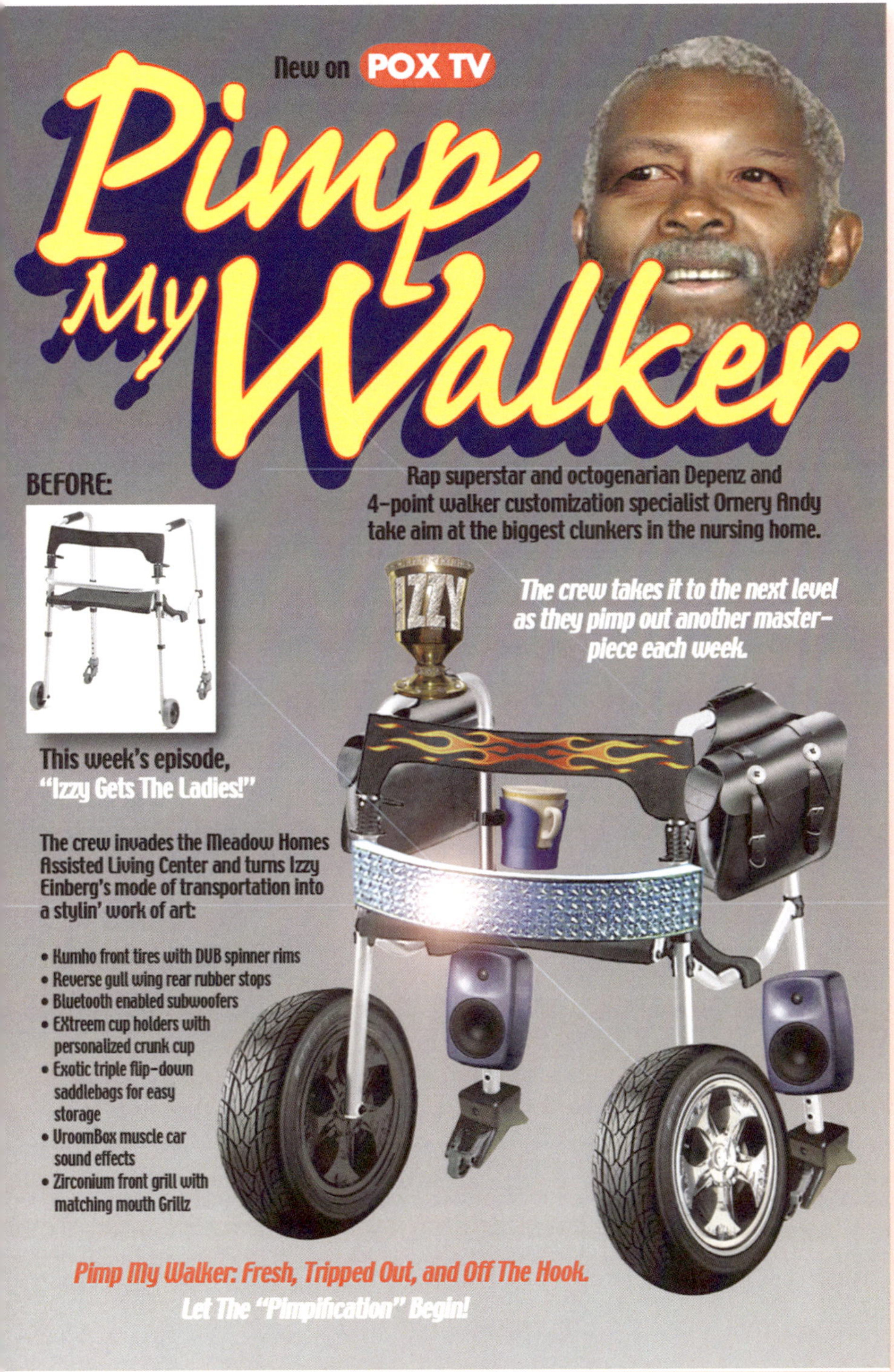
New on POX TV
Pimp My Walker
BEFORE:
Rap superstar and octogenarian Depenz and 4-point walker customization specialist Ornery Andy take aim at the biggest clunkers in the nursing home.
The crew takes it to the next level as they pimp out another master-piece each week.
IZZY
This week's episode, "Izzy Gets The Ladies!"
The crew invades the Meadow Homes Assisted Living Center and turns Izzy Einberg's mode of transportation into a stylin' work of art:
• Kumho front tires with DUB spinner rims
• Reverse gull wing rear rubber stops
• Bluetooth enabled subwoofers
• EXtreem cup holders with personalized crunk cup
• Exotic triple flip-down saddlebags for easy storage
• VroomBox muscle car sound effects
• Zirconium front grill with matching mouth Grillz
Pimp My Walker: Fresh, Tripped Out, and Off The Hook.
Let The "Pimpification" Begin!

# Ditto

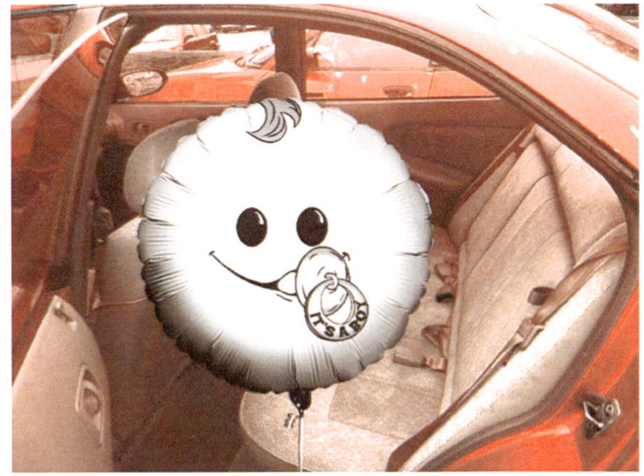

As a young GYN resident I was riding up the hospital elevator on the way to the delivery area. In the elevator was an older colleague and a woman in labor, very advanced labor, who proceeded to deliver right there in the elevator. We swung into action and very soon the baby was born. She was placed on a gurney and both of us surprised docs walked her and the newborn to the delivery room. She kept apologizing for causing so much trouble.

The other doc, an older southern gentleman, assured her it was okay, nothing to apologize for. He smiled down and patted her shoulder and told this story . . .

*"You were at least here in the hospital. A couple years ago I was crossing the parking lot and heard a loud call for help and a commotion. I delivered a baby in the back seat of a car . . ."*

She looked up surprised and said, ***"Oh, about two years ago? Well, that was me too!"***

We all got a laugh out of that. ✚

# All Clear

A daughter brought in her 83-year-old mother whom she thought was having some memory loss. She had been an accountant all her life but was having problems balancing her check book (*like don't we all?*). I gave her the Mini-Mental State Exam (MMSE) and she did quite well, answering the who, what, when, and where questions without difficulty. She did have a problem spatially spelling "WORLD" backwards or subtracting 7's from 100, but overall was doing fine. I gave her the pad and pen and asked her to compose a sentence. She handed back the pad and written on it was . . .

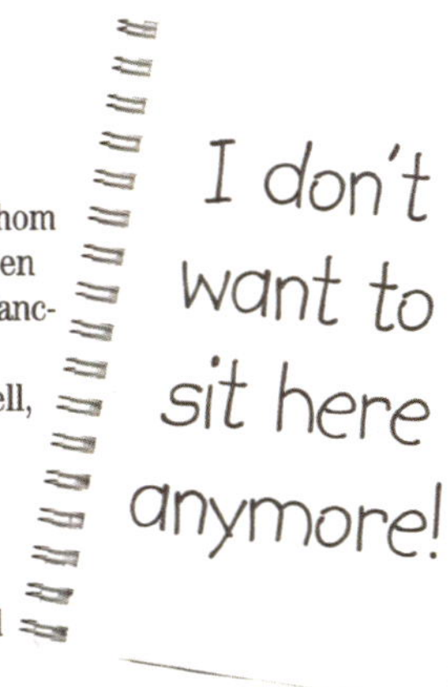


I roared with laughter and declared her mentally competent. ✚

NEW FROM PJ GAMES

# DOCOPOLY

**Going broke as your career progresses.**
**For 2 to 8 players**

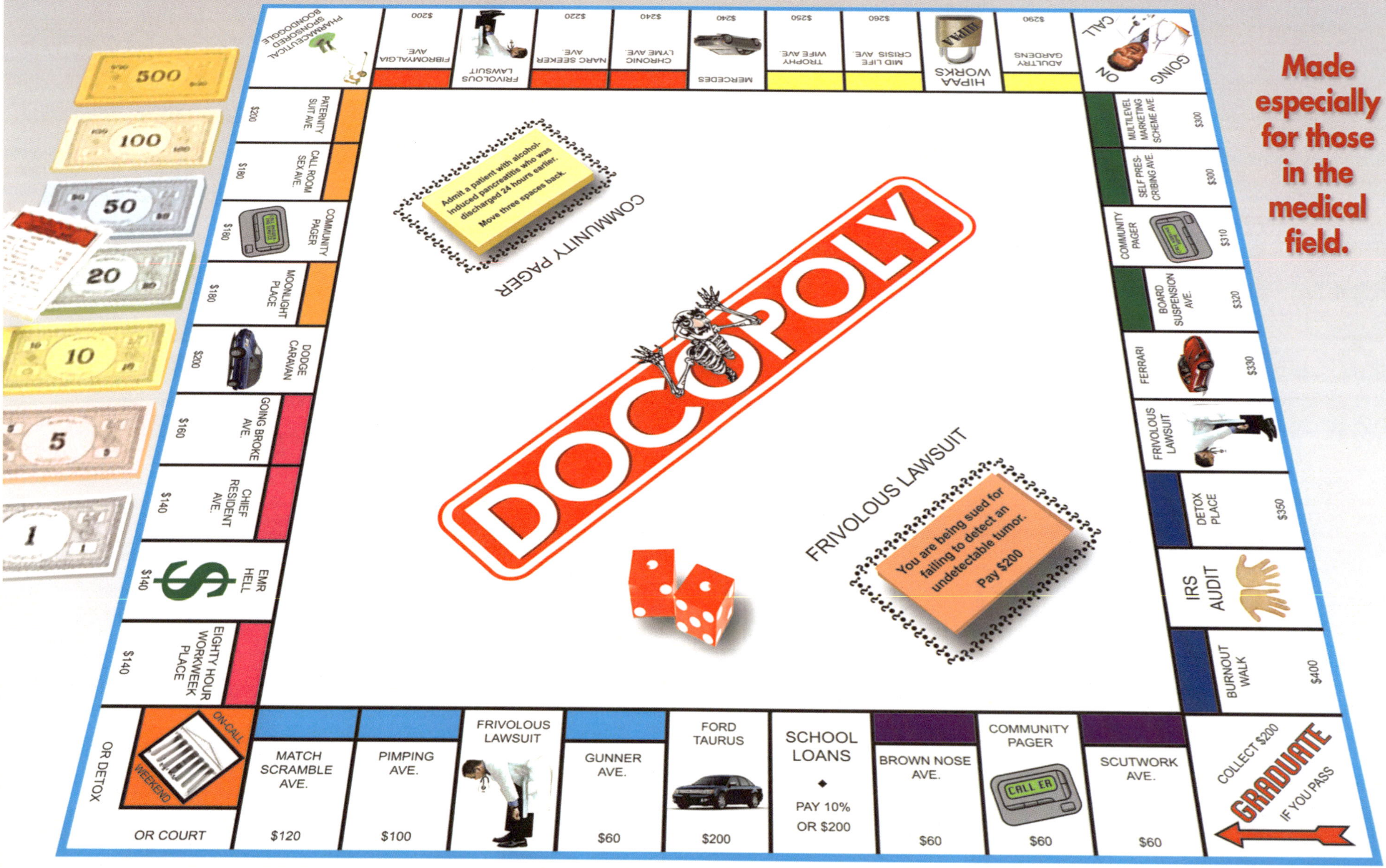


**Made especially for those in the medical field.**

## A TRUE STORY OF MEDICINE

# Letting Loose

As a long time EMT working in the emergency department of a hospital, there are certain types of patients who we dread seeing, and specific patients who cause a great anguished wailing and gnashing of teeth just by showing up on our doorstep.

Let me begin this tale of woe by describing the patient. "Sally" is an obese alcoholic, a chronic smoker, and she is none to careful about her personal hygiene. Her voice can be best described as an irritating whine. It seems that whenever Sally drinks (which is often), her daughter (a miniature version of Sally) feels that it is her duty to call 911 and have Mom hauled to the ED by ambulance. I can understand this in a way because the idea of 350 pounds of drunken behemoth stumbling around the house would scare just about anyone.

This particular day, Sally arrived with a BAC around .20, and was placed in a room where it was hoped (in vain, it turns out) that she would sober up without undue disruption to the staff.

Naturally, if Sally had just spent her visit in a quiet alcoholic stupor, I would not be telling this tale.

It turns out that Sally had a little surprise for us. It seems that in addition to her current drunken state, Sally was also afflicted with a pretty bad case of diarrhea. Sure enough, after just a short time in her room, she hit the call light and announced that she had just soiled the bed. Guess who was sent to clean up the mess? *Yep.* That would be me!

Apparently, every time Sally would cough (which, being a smoker was often) she would lose control of her bowels, and deposit a little "gift" of loose, runny stool on the bed. From the smell in the room, Sally had been living on a diet of *White Castle* hamburgers and cheap beer.

So, here I am, trying to clean up the mess, wiping Sally's great big bum with washrags when suddenly (*you see what's coming here, don't you??*) Sally gives a great big cough, and at the same time lets out a great burst of gas that sounded like a walrus blowing on a huge tuba. I was instantly hit with a foul smelling mist of diarrhea that pelted me over my entire right side. *"Oops. Sorry"*, said Sally.

Well, being the dedicated ER Tech that I am, I quickly finished up with Sally, and then hit the locker room for a shower and a change of scrubs, but I can't help but to think that this was the kind of thing that never seems to cross people's minds when they think about how glamorous it is to work in a hospital emergency department. +

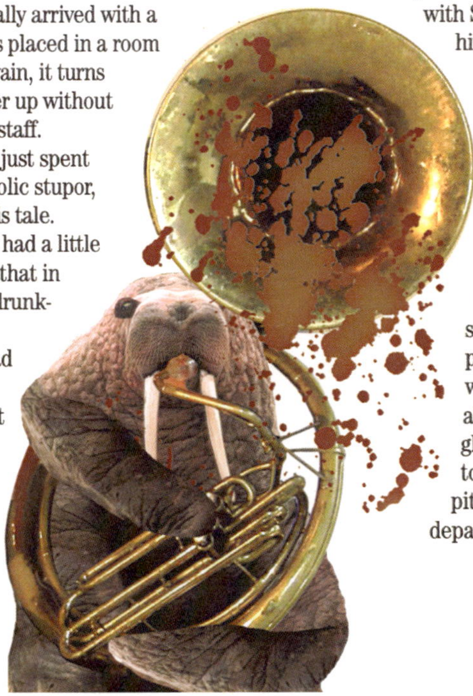

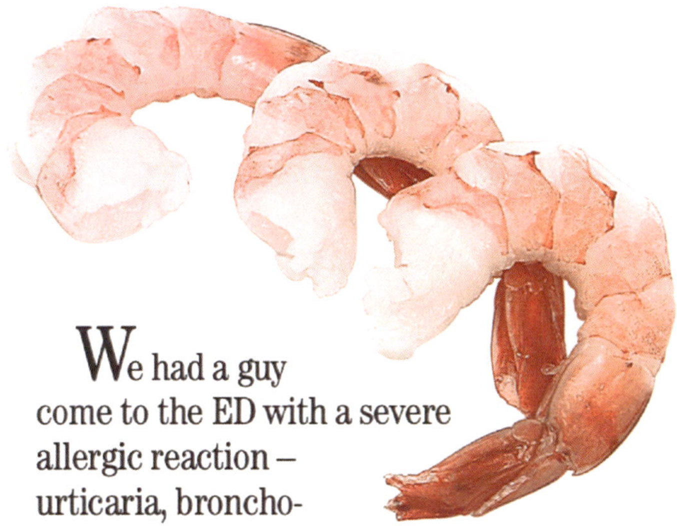

We had a guy come to the ED with a severe allergic reaction – urticaria, bronchospasm, vomiting, etc. When I asked him what might have precipitated this, he replied, *"Shrimp."*

*"Have you had a reaction to shrimp before?"* I asked.

*"Many times,"* he replied.

So I asked him, *"Why did you eat shrimp again tonight?"*

He said, *"But these were popcorn shrimp; I thought that would be different!"*

I told him . . .

**"Shrimps is Shrimps."**

+

# SMILE TAKERS

***Realistic medical stickers for your patients!***

RECORD NUMBER OF COMPLAINTS TODAY
(WRITE NUMBER IN CIRCLE)

I HIT ON MY
(Circle One) RECEPTIONIST
NURSE
PHYSICIAN
FELLOW PATIENT
TODAY!

I JUST STOLE A WHOLE TUBE OF KY JELLY
BUSY LATER ???

I'm An A.D.U.L.T.
(Alcohol and Drug-Using, Lying Teenager)

I KNOW WHAT DRUG I NEED...
I have the same thing my mother's friend's son's girlfriend's nephew has.

SAMPLE WHORE

*My Mom, sister and I got our ears and throats checked for FREE!*
*(My little brother actually had the appointment.)*

The doctor is late getting to YOU because of ME!

Member of V.B.D.T. (Vertical Blinds Destruction Team)

I'LL BREED 'EM SO YOU CAN FEED 'EM
*. . . with YOUR Tax Dollars!*

I'm not saying the doctor is wrong, I just have to confirm it in my chat room.

I always need a same-day appointment... I just don't like paying a same-day co-pay!

I CAN'T AFFORD MY MEDS
because tobacco, alcohol, and bowling are
SOOO EXPENSIVE!

Why pay a prescription co-pay when you can mooch free samples ?

My doctor says that if I no-show for one more appointment I'll get a SPECIAL LETTER!

MUDDIEST BOOTS AWARD

I PUKED
(Check appropriate box)
- ☐ in the lobby
- ☐ in the exam room
- ☐ on the nurse
- ☐ on the physician
- ☐ all of the above

I limited my office visit to what it was scheduled for ONLY.
GOLD STAR PATIENT

I spent my deductible on shoes . . . can't you just write off my visit?

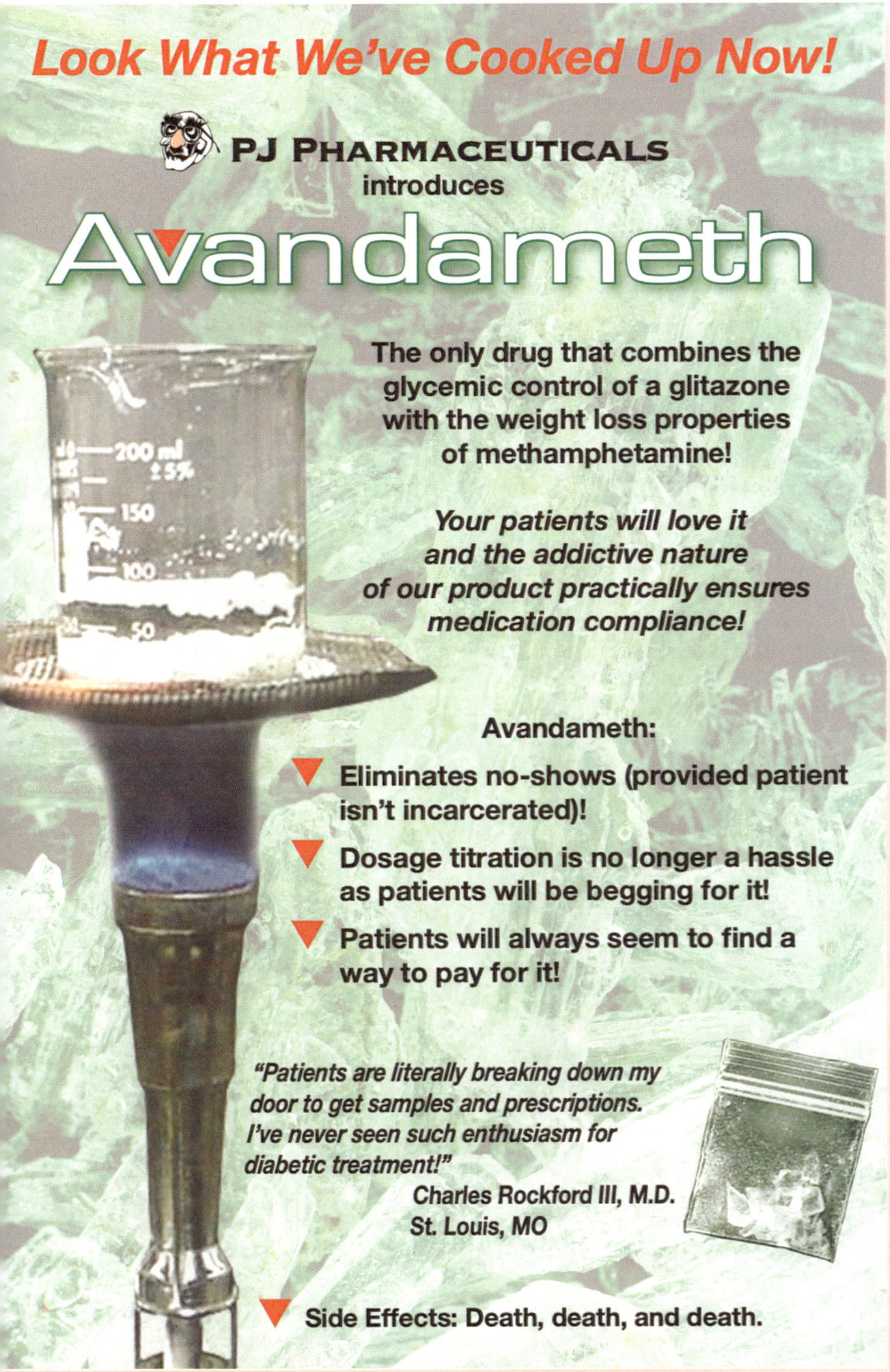
Look What We've Cooked Up Now!
PJ PHARMACEUTICALS
introduces
Avandameth
The only drug that combines the glycemic control of a glitazone with the weight loss properties of methamphetamine!
Your patients will love it and the addictive nature of our product practically ensures medication compliance!
Avandameth:
Eliminates no-shows (provided patient isn't incarcerated)!
Dosage titration is no longer a hassle as patients will be begging for it!
Patients will always seem to find a way to pay for it!
"Patients are literally breaking down my door to get samples and prescriptions. I've never seen such enthusiasm for diabetic treatment!"
Charles Rockford III, M.D.
St. Louis, MO
Side Effects: Death, death, and death.

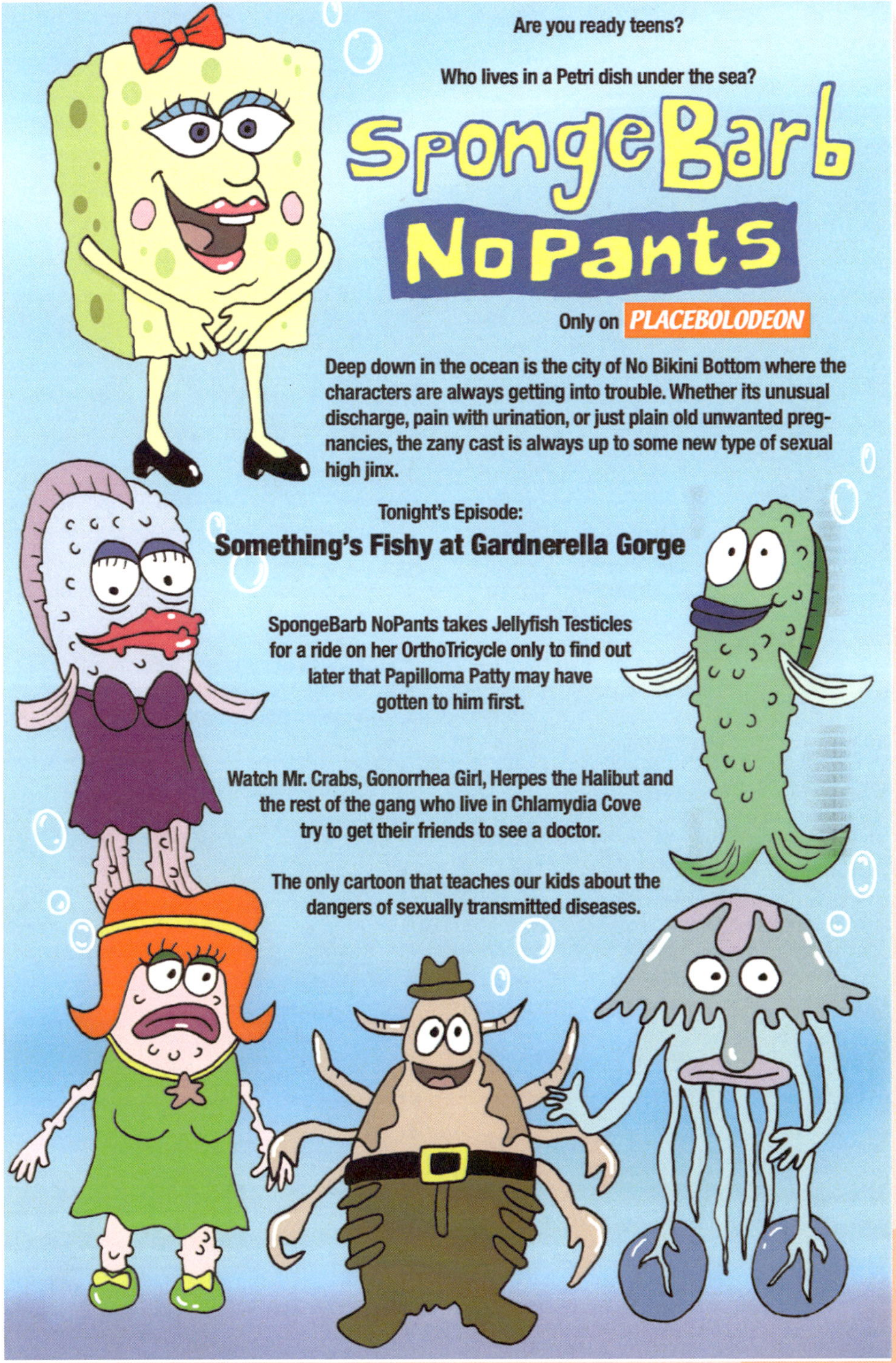
Are you ready teens?
Who lives in a Petri dish under the sea?
SpongeBarb NoPants
Only on PLACEBOLODEON
Deep down in the ocean is the city of No Bikini Bottom where the characters are always getting into trouble. Whether its unusual discharge, pain with urination, or just plain old unwanted pregnancies, the zany cast is always up to some new type of sexual high jinx.
Tonight's Episode:
Something's Fishy at Gardnerella Gorge
SpongeBarb NoPants takes Jellyfish Testicles for a ride on her OrthoTricycle only to find out later that Papilloma Patty may have gotten to him first.
Watch Mr. Crabs, Gonorrhea Girl, Herpes the Halibut and the rest of the gang who live in Chlamydia Cove try to get their friends to see a doctor.
The only cartoon that teaches our kids about the dangers of sexually transmitted diseases.

# CONTINUING MEANINGLESS MEDICAL EDUCATION

**CMME** **Fellow Placebians are eligible to receive three hours of CMME prescribed credit that has no meaning at all.** *Please select the most appropriate answer to each of the questions listed below. Check your answers online at* ***www. placebojournal.com.*** *You need to get 80% correct in order to receive your meaningless credit. If you do not get 80% of the answers correct, then we will give you the credit anyway. We really don't care.*

**1. Which one of the following anti-emetic drugs is the best tolerated?**
A. Metoclopramide
B. Ondansetron
C. Prochlorperazine
D. Ganja

**2. Which one of the following statements about breast examination is correct?**
A. It has been shown to reduce breast cancer-specific mortality.
B. It has been shown to reduce all-cause mortality.
C. It has been shown to increase the number of biopsies.
D. It can get you thrown out of most gentlemen's clubs.

**3. Which of the following comes to mind when a doing a cerumen removal?**
A. You will have better luck with an ear pick.
B. Irrigation with your nurse's help will work best.
C. Trying an ear candle may not be a bad idea.
D. I became a f#cking doctor to do this?

**4. Which of the following is the primary goal of the field of complementary and alternative medicine (CAM)?**
A. To facilitate a broader understanding of healing and wellness.
B. To encourage physicians to adopt Eastern medical practices.
C. To offer less expensive treatment options for patients.
D. To unburden yourself of "impossible to treat" patients and make them someone else's problem.

**5. When going to your next major medical conference, your goal should be to:**
A. Steal as much free stuff as possible.
B. Learn. *Sorry, that was a joke.* To golf, sit by the pool, or forget medicine altogether.
C. Pick up chicks or dudes or whatever suits your fancy.
D. Two words – Escort Service.

*Check your CMME answers online at*
**WWW. PLACEBO JOURNAL .COM**

*Do you want to dine out daily in a four-star restaurant, fly first class, and wear the bling you so desperately desire?*

*Do you believe in the ancient tradition that the world owes you more than you deserve?*

*Are you looking for the secret to change your life forever?*

***Then you need this . . .***

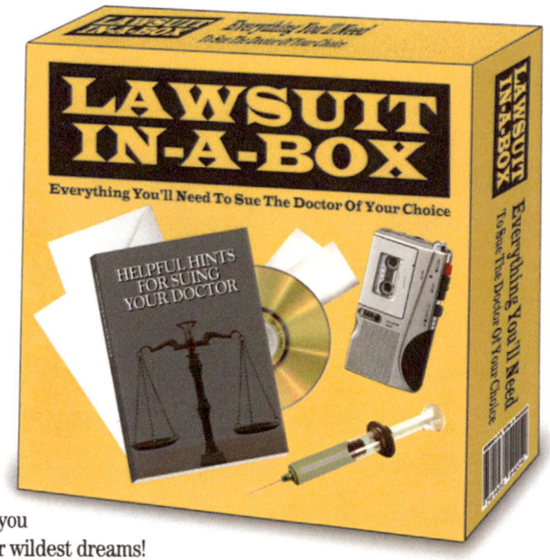


It is so powerful that it will transform you from a failure to a success beyond your wildest dreams!

**The LAWSUIT-IN-A-BOX is the first all-inclusive home business that will allow you to practice* malpractice law right at home! Each kit includes a:**

- discount card to shop for appropriate "testifying" gear at a local **L-I-A-B** approved store
- 32-page information packed booklet with hints on what to sue for and the easiest specialty of physician to win against
- tape recorder to catch your unsuspecting doctor in a trap that you get to set
- local **L-I-A-B** approved attorney's business card
- syringe already pre-filled with toxic material to inject under your skin
- list of medical specialists who will testify on your behalf now matter what the evidence says
- list of **L-I-A-B** approved semi-retired physicians who will give you the diagnosis you need

**We are creating more millionaires than any other so-called "ethical venture."**

***EXCLUSIVE BONUS GIFT:***
Mention this ad and receive a fake finger to help you sue a local fast food restaurant *– all in your spare time!*

**Practicing law is our profession.**
**Settling for millions can now be yours.**

To get your own **LAWSUIT-IN-A-BOX** for a special introductory rate of only **$99.99 call 1-555-GET-L-I-A-B now!**

**Learn the Basics on How To:**
- Make false accusations
- Pit staff members against the physician
- Effectively fake symptoms
- Teach your kids the secrets of how to sue when they grow up.

**Order Now and Get a Free DVD on How To:**
- Get the highest settlements
- Get quick cash for your "supposed" pain
- Negotiate out of court by getting your doctor to say he is sorry and then nail him for hundreds of thousands
- Get creative and start multiple lawsuits at once

*You really can't practice being a lawyer. You still have to call us for the finishing touches.

# A TRUE STORY OF MEDICINE

### Rainbow Room

A few years ago I was hanging around in the hallway of my clinic waiting for my nurse to put in my next patient when I saw a small white woman wearing a yellow sundress. That in itself is not interesting; however, this young woman was wearing her hair in rainbow colored dreadlocks. My nurse rolled her eyes as she went to put the patient back in the room. I chuckled and went back into my office to do some paperwork. A few minutes later I looked up to see my nurse standing there perplexed.

*"Um, Doctor, do you have a copy of the lunar cycle?"*

*"Why in the world would I have that?"* I said.

*"Well, this patient says her period 'was when the moon was last full!'"* Oh brother I thought. When asked what the patient's chief complaint was my nurse stated it was another vaginal discharge. *Great.*

*"So is she undressed?"* I asked.

*"Not exactly,"* my nurse replied. This just keeps getting better I thought.

I entered the exam room to find my patient standing up in front of the door. Once I verified the chief complaint I asked her to undress and told her that I would return in a moment.

*"Don't bother,"* she exclaimed while in one fell swoop she hiked up her skirt, jumped backwards onto the table and spread her legs waiting for the exam. *Okay.*

So I placed the patient into the stirrups and verified that there was definitely a disaster spreading from her southern regions.

*"So when did you start having symptoms?"* I asked.

*"Well, for the last couple of weeks all my girlfriends said I tasted funny when they went down on me."* **Gulp.** I sideways looked at my nurse who was trying not to laugh.

*"All your 'girlfriends'?"* I asked.

*"Oh yes,"* she replied *"it's what me and all my girlfriends do for fun."*

Unable to resist I said, *"Hmm, when I was in college my girlfriends and I just did each other's nails."*

After taking the necessary cultures and wet prep I had the patient scoot back up the table.

ME: *"Well as long as you are here today do you need any birth control?"*

HER: *"Oh no, I'm a lesbian; I won't be needing any birth control."* Hmm, just to make sure . . .

ME: *"So you don't have sex with any men then?"*

HER: *"Just my friend, Billy"*

ME: *"Is Billy a guy?"*

HER: *"Yes."*

ME: *"Does Billy put his penis in your vagina?"*

HER: *"Well, yeah!"*

ME: *"Then you STILL need birth control!!"*

HER: *"Oh!"*

ME: *"Just get dressed, er, straighten yourself up and have a seat in the chair in my office just across the hall. I'm just going to go look at this slide."* Leaving the room I went across to my lab and placed the malodorous slide on the scope. As she walked by, I realized the error of my ways! *"Uh, don't sit down in the . . . never mind."*

**Too late.** The yellow sundress was yellow for more reasons than one. *Damn.* After giving her scripts for *Floxin, Doxy, Flagyl* and OCPs my nurse walked her out of the building. Maintenance walked my chair out to the dumpster.

I never saw "Rainbow" as a patient in my clinic again. I have no knowledge that she and "Billy" ever reproduced. I did however see her years later on our local version of *"Cops."* There she was with her dreads and skirt flying biting an officer. I doubt if she used protection with him either! ✚

# TOP 7 Excuses for Early Refill of Pain Medication

**7. Victim of pill-sucking black hole in the toilet or drain** (see this captured on film at *placebojournal.com*).

**6.** ***"I have a very dexterous and durable dog who can remove the caps from pill bottles and eat all the narcotics without dying."***

**5.** ***"My baby was crying so much in the car that I gave her the prescription to play with to keep her quiet and it flew out the window."***

**4.** ***"I spilled my pills on the floor and my dog has worms so I'm afraid to use the pills now."***

**3.** ***"I had the pills on the front seat of the car and made a sudden stop. The pills rolled off the seat and fell through a hole that rusted through the floor."***

**2.** ***"I got tired of taking pills so I flushed them down the toilet, and then I realized I really do need them."***

**1.** ***"My grandmother died*** *(for the fifth time this year)* ***and I have to go out of town for the funeral, which happens to be when I am due for a refill."*** ✚

# Sameness

Yesterday, we had two patients (a woman and a man) check into the same room in the ED. Here's the nurse's notes:

**Female Patient:** "The patient says she has a different odor from her vagina for two days. She has no vaginal discharge and no urinary symptoms, but when she touches herself and smells her fingers the odor is different and she knows something is wrong."

**Male Patient:** "His girlfriend says she has a different odor in her vagina and he wants to be checked for the same."

This is the job we do. ✚

# MY "REALISTIC" WEEK IN PRACTICE – IN THE STATE HOSPITAL

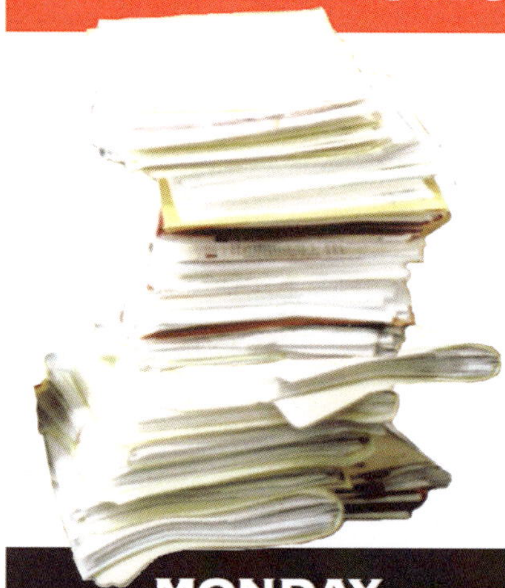

## MONDAY

The day starts with the weekend report of who said what to whom, who was inappropriate with whom, and most importantly, the funniest thing anyone said. One of my patients was the winner – a pleasant man with chronic schizophrenia – who talked about being the next Pope, the world's only 10-star general, and how he went to Iraq on Saturday and came back on Sunday; but is peeing out shrapnel. When asked how he knew it was shrapnel (this time), he talked about seeing blood in his urine. Despite the fact that he's said this not less than seven million times in the past, he said the magic word – blood – and so he goes for a urology consult. They recommend a cystoscopy (surprise!), despite the lack of any blood in the urine. The rest of the day is spent avoiding patients and other staff while I try to get less behind on my paperwork – I'm two weeks behind on my paperwork. By the end of the day I'm less behind by a day or two.

## TUESDAY

A patient who is here because of Not Guilty by Reason of Insanity tells me that we have violated his rights (again). He is going to have his lawyer sue the hospital (again) because of the staff's flagrant and malicious attempt to hold him incommunicado. Translated into reality, he was upset that the staff shooed him away from the telephone so one of the other 45 patients could use it after he monopolized it for over an hour. Since this patient's lawyer has sued this hospital – and lost – more times than I can count, I can only conclude either that A) the lawyer is as paranoid as the patient, or B) he is taking the patient's rich family for the longest ride he can. I suppose that it could be A and B; but who knows? Anyway, the patient frequently uses this threat of a suit more with the aim of cowing staff, but with decreasing effect on staff, sort of like the boy who cried wolf (*or perhaps, for him, cried shark?*). Nevertheless, the commotion that ensues, like clockwork when he says the magic words, *"I'm going to sue!"* takes so much time that even after doing paperwork all afternoon yesterday, not having been able to get to yesterday's and today's

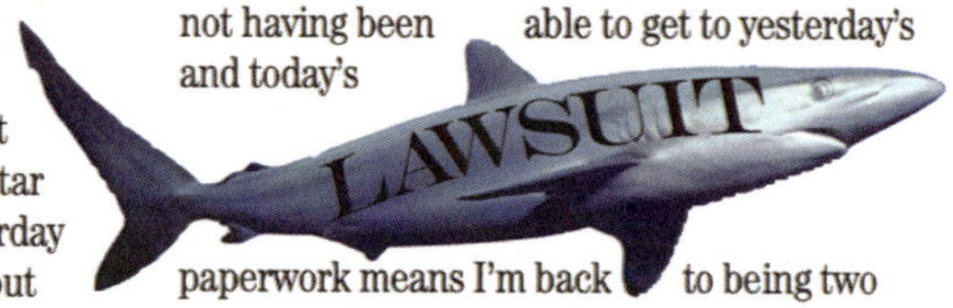


paperwork means I'm back to being two weeks behind on my notes. By the way, we have a pool on who he's suing for the most money. I'm ahead, at $50 million dollars.

## WEDNESDAY

We have a conference about a patient who has been here for many years. He is fairly stable, but being that he has zero or less insight into his illness, we're stymied in going forward with him. He has the pseudological idea that, since someone stole his brain, he can't be mentally ill, because how could you be mentally ill

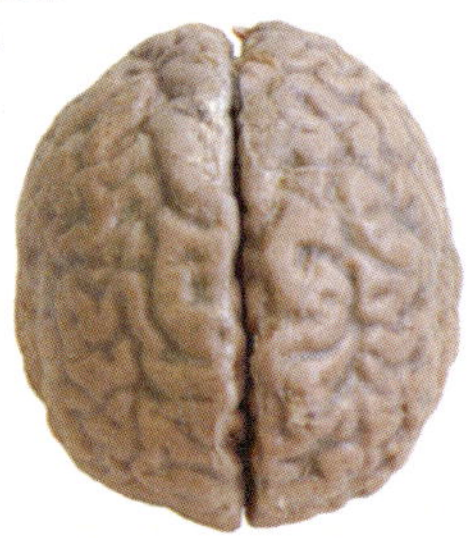

without a brain? He has also changed his story. He used to be a spy for George Washington in the Revolutionary War, but now he is an agent for the local country & western radio station, though what they hope to find out by having him in the hospital is something he can't explain. Needless to say, his *Clozaril* dose was increased.

"Cystoscopy Man" comes back and tells us he peed out all the shrapnel before they did the procedure, but they put in a chip to monitor his whereabouts. This is because he is vital to the war effort. He tells us that Vice-President Cheney came to the procedure room to get advice from him. This caused some merriment amongst the more liberal staffers who wondered if perhaps straightforward psychosis isn't preferable to what passes for rational thought in Washington. I have more time to do paperwork today and I broke the two week barrier. *Hurrah!*

## THURSDAY

One of our sex offenders touched someone inappropriately for the umpteenth time. When confronted on it, he first says he didn't do it (*it was witnessed by staff*) anf he then says the staff really didn't see it, so

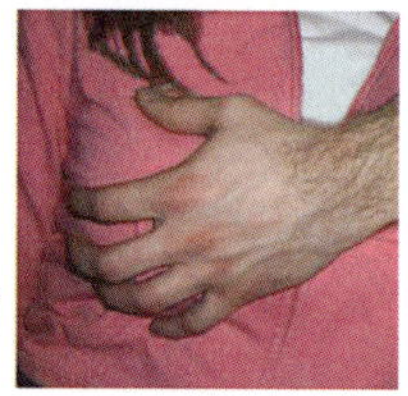

they must have it in for him (*they did see it, and while they do have it in for him - given his PITA behavior - there were too many witnesses to suspect some mean staff people made it up simply to get him in trouble*). He then says that the recipient of his attention asked for it by her behavior, and therefore deserved it (*he can't explain why behavior that has gone on for four years without change suddenly has a different meaning for him*). And finally he admits he did it. He went on to say that he wouldn't ever do it again. This would be a nice outcome, except that this progression – denial of the deed, claim it was trumped up, a reason for it, then admission and a promise of improvement – has been his MO since before I started working at the hospital. I couldn't get any paperwork done today, so now I'm nearly back to being two weeks behind on my paperwork.

## FRIDAY

We have our weekly discipline meeting, where we are told how we're screwing up by administration. We haven't been faithfully filling out some useless form that JERKO - I mean, JCAHO - has decided needs be done. Someone who has not yet given up asks why the focus is on paperwork instead of the clinical work – *those new attendings are so cute!* After the rest of us older (*read: resigned to it*) physicians have finished snickering, the department head kindly explains that what counts in paper work is not what you write but that you write something. Of course this isn't true, with our Health Information Management regularly sending us notices that our last note is no different from the note before - as if there are enough words in the thesaurus to document no change for the past ten years. One of the docs says his aim in life is to write a note that says,

***As above, see below.***

Mr. Lawsuit tells me that because he brought food onto the unit (a no-no) his belongings were searched without a warrant, which is a clear violation of his constitutional rights. Since I ordered the search, I'm responsible. I'm way ahead in the pool now, up to $100 million! Anyway, because of the additional meetings, I could only get some of the paperwork done I had planned, so I'm back to being two weeks behind in my paperwork. I promise myself that, come Monday, I will try to balance - somehow - seeing patients and doing paperwork. In my heart I know it won't happen, but for now, TGIF!!!

# TOP 7 Stupidest Things I Have Heard An Administrator or Admistrative Physician Say

**7.** ***"We aren't about just healthcare anymore, we are managing the healthcare experience."***

**6.** ***"We must see more and more patients, more and more quickly – that's what quality is about."***

**5.** ***"Just telling someone you are working on something makes them feel better, even if you can't do anything."***

**4.** ***"I wish I had the luxury of seeing a patient every 15 minutes when I was in practice."***

**3.** ***"Our outside consultant, Mr. Darkside, said we needed two more staff, however, at this time we cannot budget the two more staff but are looking into it."*** (After they paid the outside consultant the equivalent of the salary of two more staff).

**2.** (The following year) ***"Our outside consultant had some valuable ideas, why don't we ask him to come back again?"***

**1.** ***"I'm so sorry to be leaving but I will be working for the esteemed Mr. Darkside as a consultant."*** +

## LEARNING CURVE

### TRUE STORIES OF MEDICINE

As a second-year medical student in the surgical clinic, I was asked to examine a lady who returned for follow-up after a hemorrhoidectomy. She was extremely corpulent and was positioned on her side with her buttocks exposed. As I proceeded to do my first ever rectal exam, her comment was,

*"Doctor, that is not my rectum."* +

## POINTS FOR HONESTY

We had a fellow the in ED who'd been stabbed in the chest during a drug deal gone bad. After we made sure he was stable, I asked him if he had any medical problems. The following conversation ensued:

Patient: *"Well, I'm HIV positive."*

Doctor: *"I'm sorry to hear that. How long have you been HIV positive?"*

Patient: *"I found out about six months ago."*

Doctor: *"Are you on any medications for HIV?"*

Patient: *"I was on HIV medications, but I stopped taking them about two months ago."*

Doctor: *"Why did you stop taking them?"*

Patient: *"Well, I couldn't afford them and the crack cocaine too."* +

## YOU DON'T GET IT

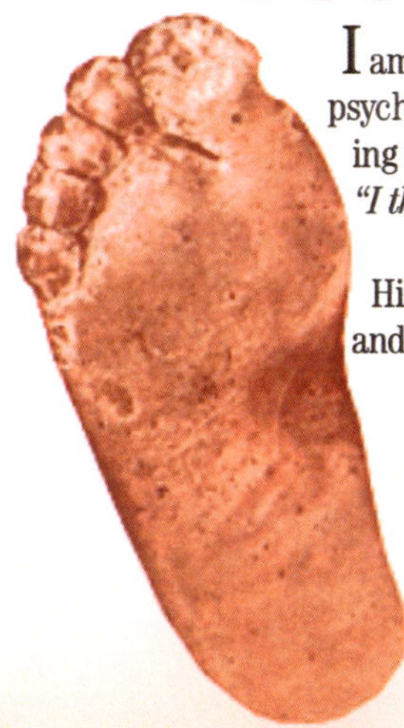

I am a psychiatrist talking to a new psych patient in the ER. He was showing me a rash on his feet and I said, *"I think that's 'athlete's foot'."*

His face clouded up in despair and he said,

*"That's impossible! I'm not athletic!!!"* +

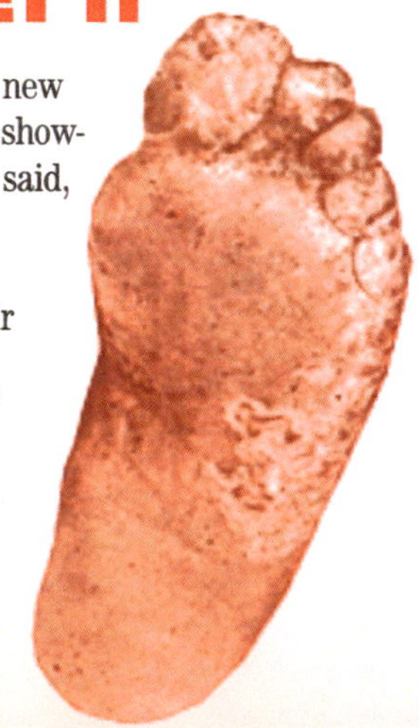

## MORE TRUE STORIES OF MEDICINE

# EMBEDDED

As a PA in practice for ten years, I thought I had a handle on things. Boy, was I wrong. Never sued (that came later), and never fired (still hoping) and never a needle stick. The last was about to change.

I practiced with two internists who hated dermatology, so I got to do all the lesion removals in three practices, which was actually pretty neat.

I was happily draping the patient that fateful morning getting ready to remove another FLB (Funny Looking Bump) thinking about how cool life was. The patient was lying on the exam table while I sat on my nifty rolling stool ready to inject the lidocaine into the side of his chest wall.

As I finished injecting, I fumbled the syringe and needle, dropping it. I immediately realized something was horribly wrong. I looked down to my lap and saw the syringe and needle there, *POINT DOWN,* in my pants. My acute senses told me the rest of the story. *IT WAS EMBEDDED IN MY LEFT TESTICLE!!!*

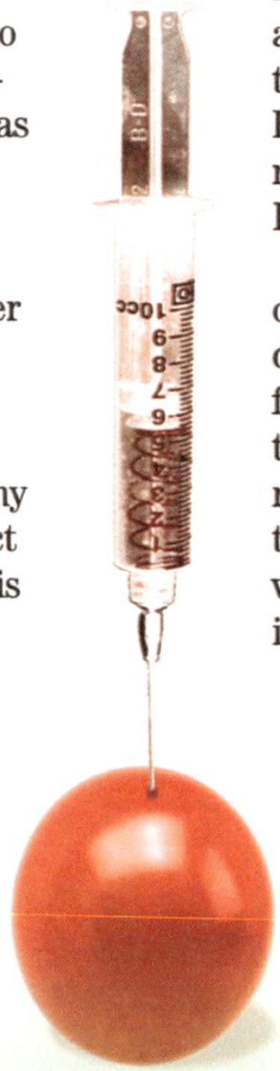

Without saying any of the things I was thinking, I calmly plucked it out, laid it on the tray, got up and closed the door. I then said to the patient, *"We have to talk."* He assured me of his very low risk for HIV or hepatitis and I then proceeded to finish up.

The worst part of the whole ordeal was filling out the incident report and needle stick form for my employer. It seems that we were much better at respecting PATIENT confidentiality than the providers'. I was forever in living down that incident.

And to this day that is why I always want to drape MYSELF with one of those lead x-ray aprons before I do minor surgery.

# THE BIG SHAKEDOWN

## . . . of blood pressure.

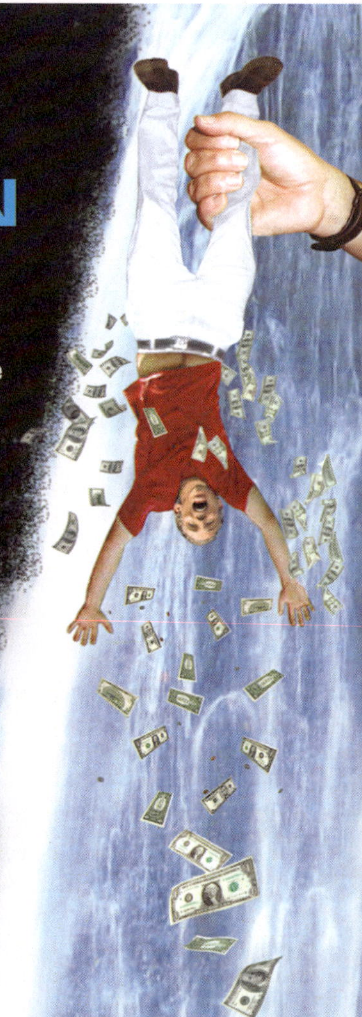

**By manipulating the patent process, PJ Pharmaceuticals is proud to announce a medication that should have come out years ago!**

**Extort.**

**Hypertension is bad.**

**So are some the side effects from the medications used to treat it.**

**Not any longer.**

**Common questions about Extort:**

**Why did it take so long?**
Because we held the patent on the older combination therapy and wanted to squeeze out as much profit as we could.

**Now that the older combination therapy is generic, is it still good?**
No.

**EXTORT®**

**Why is Extort so expensive?**
Due to our proprietary recipe of greed and indifference, we are unable to reveal our secret. Let's just say, our marketing research shows that you will pay an exorbitant price for a cool name like Extort.

*NEW from*
**PJ PHARMACEUTICALS**
*The Realistic Drug Company*

**It's effective, it's expensive, and you can't do shit about it.**

# WELCOME TO THE RINDHOUSE

**DIRECTIONS:** Take the Extrinsic Pathway onto vonWillebrand Highway. Watch for traffic and factor in five or more minutes before you hit Route 81. Take the next exit on Highway 325 and we are on the left at the corner of Warfarin Drive and Salicylate Ave.

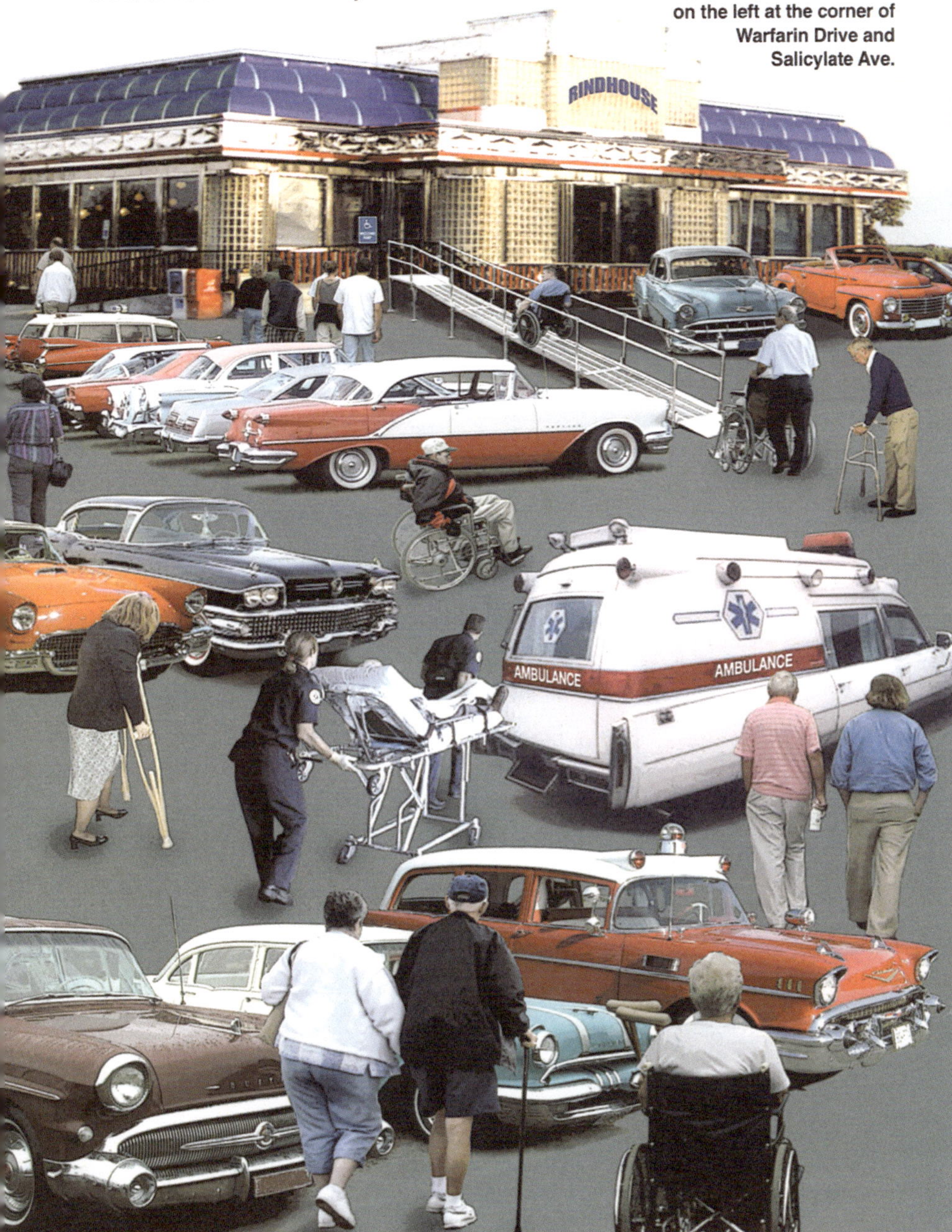


## Different Strokes for Different Folks.

### Some of our special menu items include:

1. **The Ischemic Burger** layered with our special occlusive dressing
2. **Chicken Fried Thrombosis** with extra gravy
3. **Watershed Salad** with crumbled emboli cheese
4. **Locked-In Sandwich** with chipotle sauce
5. **tPAtty Melt** with horseradish sauce
6. **CT salad** with contrast vinaigrette
7. **Arteritis French Frytis**
8. **Wernicke Club Sandwich** stacked high with bacon, lettuce and vasculitis

### Drinks include:

1. **Our world famous Long Island Iced TIA**
2. **Ice Cream Tremor Shakes**
3. **Visit our Old Fashioned Soda Fountain** with home grown flavors like sasparalysis and anoxic ale

### And for Dessert...

1. **Wernicke's Brownie and Caramel Confusion Fusion**
2. **The "Remember When" Banana Split Sundae**
3. **The "Remember Any-thing?" Hot Fudge Sundae**

**Don't forget to check out our Children's Menu (Mini-strokes for Mini-folks)**

**Open 24 Hours a Day Seven Days a Week**

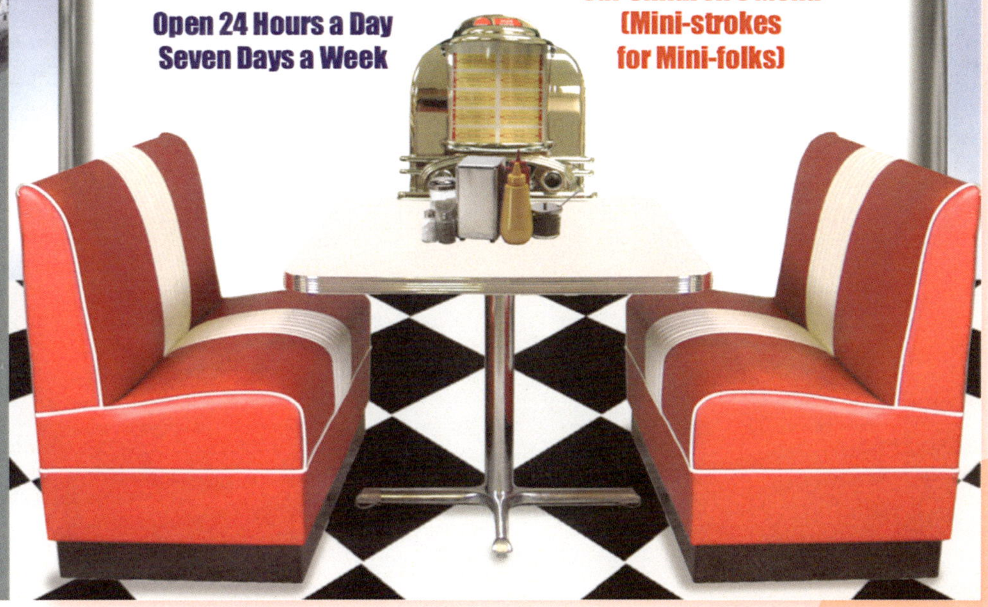

**Now Available at Electronic Stores Everywhere!**

## +DOCTOR REMOTE

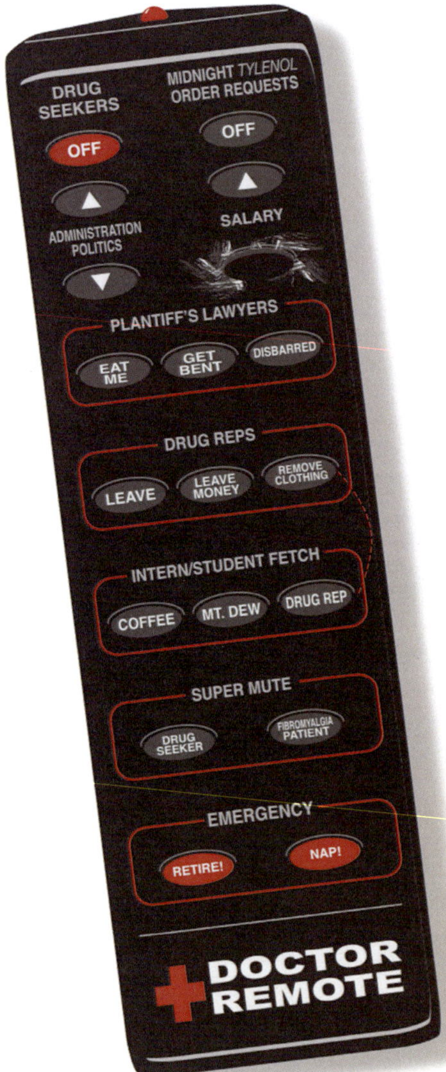


# TOP 7

## Stupidest Things Actually Said To Me By A Drug Rep.

**7.** ***Vioxx*** **rep:** ***"If you don't write for Vioxx, and your patient gets a GI bleed, you'd better have your malpractice insurance in order."***

**6.** ***Mobic*** **rep: (Five years later)** ***"If you write for*** **Vioxx***, and the patient has a heart attack, you'd better call your malpractice carrier."***

**5.** ***"If you take our vouchers, they're just as good as samples."***

**4.** ***"I'm personally taking*** **Cefafreak-inkillsital** ***for my sinusitis right now and I feel so much better." (every time she was taking it – or a close relative)***

**3.** ***"Doctor, I know your time is valu-able . . ."*** **(so why are you barging in here when I have five patients backed up?)**

**2.** ***"I would just hate to have to deal with sick people all day."***

**1.** ***"If you don't prescribe*** **Propulsid***, its not that your committing malpractice, but you're just not giving your patient the best. Don't all patients deserve the best?"*** **(Drug recalled one year later)** +

# OFF THE CUFF

*This was it!* It was the first day of my rotating internship and I was armed with only two years of patient contact, albeit without true responsibility. I was on call for the emergency room and prayed that I would see only a few lacerations and asthmatic attacks. But it was not to be. Within 30 minutes of starting my shift, the telephone rang (no pagers or cell phones in those days.)

***"Possible coronary in E.R. #1."*** My own heart skipped a beat as I reviewed my mandated actions in such a case, while also reviewing how many ways I could screw things up.

The man was large, florid and sweating. He was wearing a tuxedo and I presumed he'd been enjoying himself when tragedy struck. His pants had already been loosened and the tux jacket removed. I rapidly checked his pulse – about 120 per minute. I wrapped the blood pressure cuff around his substantial arm and noticed the chief E.R. nurse observing me. She had the reputation of eating young doctors for lunch and could literally disembowel an intern with a few sarcastic words. I decided I would proceed in a faultless manner.

*What the fu#k?* I noticed the pressure cuff was absent its gauge and tubing. I knew these parts were often interchanged in a busy E.R. Thus, I announced, in my best Doogie Howser voice, *"Nurse, this cuff is faulty, get me another, STAT, before we lose him!"*

Nurse Crachett did not respond as I expected but simply said, *"Doctor, I believe you have his cummerbund wrapped around his arm."* +

## TRUE STORY OF MEDICINE

# TOUCHÉ (or NOSE JOB)

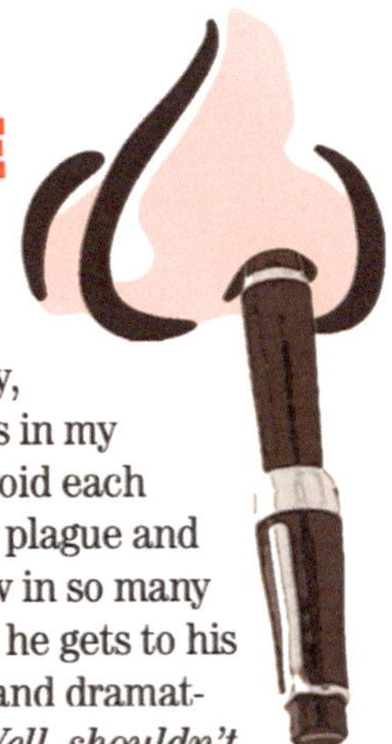

A patient had allegedly committed suicide by shoving a pen up his nose. Of course, in the interest of justice and shotgun lawsuit approach, every doctor who had breathed the same air as him in the last 90 days was being deposed with an eye to a lawsuit. *(Never mind that he had been transferred from the hospital to the inpatient psych unit to discharge to follow up outpatient care with his psychiatrist.)*

The lawyer strode into the room with his $1,000 suit, slammed down his $500+ leather case and prepared to intimidate me. Little did he know that in my previous life I had worked for an orthopaedic surgeon who made his own millions in personal injury and workman's comp cases and I had done dozens of depositions. Plus, after I had left that job, I had tried to expiate my guilt by testifying for employers in ludicrous workman's comp cases and had been raked over the coals by the best scumbags in the legal field.

Anyway, the questions drag on as the lawyer tries to intimate that I am somehow best friends with the psychiatrist and thus am trying to cover his butt as well as mine. Actually, all the doctors in my small town avoid each other like the plague and I let him know in so many words. At last he gets to his dagger stage and dramatically asks, *"Well, shouldn't you, a doctor, have known this patient was going to commit suicide?"*

I shrug and say,

*"I don't know that he committed suicide. There was no note. All we have is a dead body and a potential weapon."*

The lawyer's face goes ashen as he sees his case crumble, all the jury now thinking of *CSI* and related shows. ✚

**SUBMIT YOUR TRUE STORIES OF MEDICINE ONLINE**

**WWW.PLACEBOJOURNAL.COM**

*COMING SOON TO A NURSING HOME NEAR YOU!*

# Wee™

by Intendo

The only video game system made exclusively for the elderly.

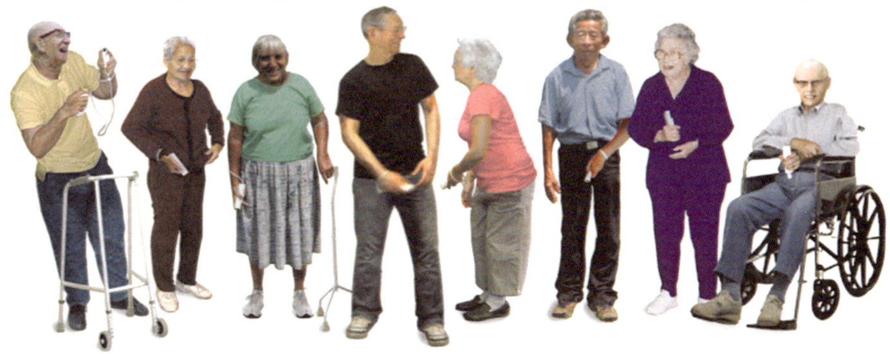

The *Wee* allows the geriatric population to feel what it is like to urinate normally again. *How?* The Wee's revolutionary motion sensor controller lets those with incontinence, BPH, or indwelling catheters pretend their genitourinary system is intact.*

*Wearing diapers?* Get the *Wee.*

*Your sheets a mess?* Get the *Wee.*

*Getting up eight times a night?* Get the *Wee.*

Try using the *Wee* and even pretend to write your name in the snow again! Play online with others and even cross streams!

*"My stream is as strong as a teenager's! I feel like I can cut glass with this sucker."*
Hyram Lepanski, age 91

*"I feel like one of those nerds you see in the movies. You know, like* War Games *with Matthew Broderick. They should call this Leaks for Geeks!"*
Bill O'Callahan, age 83

*The *Wee* is not a medical treatment. It is designed to make us money.
If you are demented, please do not urinate on the *Wee*.

# MY "REALISTIC" WEEK IN RURAL MEDICINE

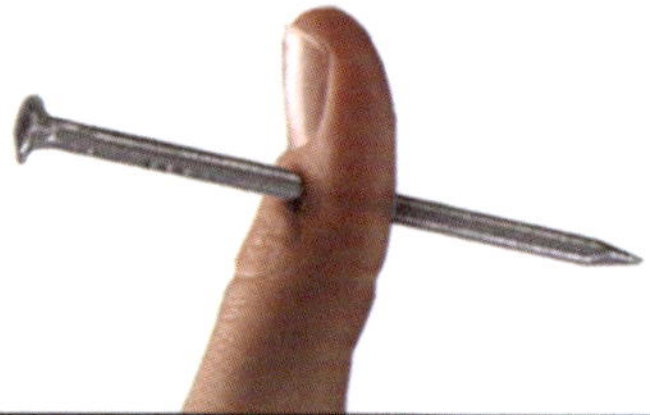

## MONDAY

I've just started as an internist at an underserved clinic in a small southern town. It's my first official day in the clinic after a week long (bloated) orientation. Apparently the last two hires complained about the paucity of their orientation so I was the lucky guinea pig for the new expanded orientation. I'm more of a "learn as you go" type but I suppose getting paid while watching others work isn't too bad.

The midlevel stops by first thing that morning to give me the lowdown on the area specialists. Fortunately there is only one doc on her do not refer list. Unfortunately it just happens to be my new landlord. Something about an ongoing national investigation for insurance fraud. And having already lost his hospital privileges. And having temporarily lost his medical license for sexual misconduct with a female patient. *Exactly what good is a realtor if they don't warn you about your landlord?*

First patient of the day is a man who had put a nail through his thumb two weeks earlier. He had gotten his ER script for *Motrin* filled but just didn't have the cash to get his *Keflex* filled. Apparently that Medicaid co-pay was just too extravagant. The finger has now become more painful, swollen and red. I briefly consider giving him an antibiotic prescription and telling him that only when he returned with the antibiotic pills in hand would I give him a script for pain meds.

At the end of the day, I head home to my lovely brand new townhouse and search all the light fixtures and electrical outlets for hidden cameras and wait for the feds to come and seize it.

## TUESDAY

I see a new female Medicaid patient who reportedly gained 60+ pounds from IV steroids used to treat her post-op respiratory failure. She wants Medicaid to pay for *Meridia* to help her lose the weight. Never mind that she just completed a month of *Meridia* which she paid for out of her own pocket and didn't lose a single pound. I didn't realize that state-funded *Meridia* is more effective than self-funded *Meridia*.

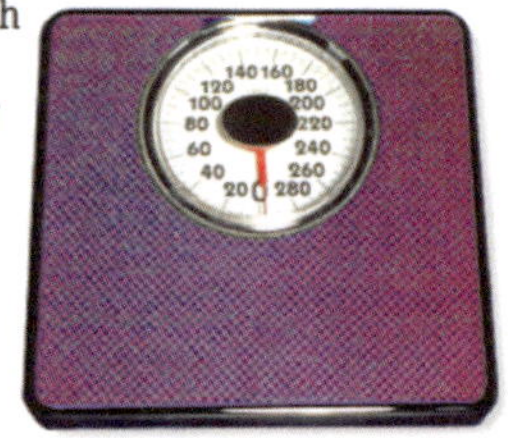

Lunch is provided by a drug rep. An internist from a nearby town is in tow to teach (aka indoctrinate) us on the benefits of their new ARB combo. *How do docs who hire themselves out to the pharmaceutical industry have any self respect?* I hope she at least gets paid handsomely for selling her soul.

## WEDNESDAY

Patient comes in saying, *"Oh, I just have a cold."* One of these days I'll have enough courage to reply, *"And what the fu#k do you expect me to do about it?"*

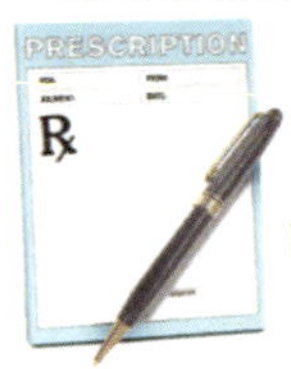


My day is redeemed when a patient tells me kindly that I am too young to be a doctor. Nothing like a little flattery to bring out the old prescription pad.

I discover that evening that the doc living in the townhouse next door to me has apparently realized that I have been borrowing (a kinder word than stealing) his wireless internet signal and has implemented security. Unfortunately, I am not computer savvy enough to hack through his password protection. I would have done the same thing but free high speed internet was sweet.

## THURSDAY

There has been a steady stream of drug reps all week. They all want to say good-bye to the doc I am replacing, a lovely looking, and flirty Hispanic male. The nurse comes by today to tell him a drug rep wants to see him. He doesn't look interested. The nurse says, *"She smells like cotton candy."* His eyes light up. The ensuing flirting makes me nauseous. *Why in the world would a forty odd-year-old woman want to wear the same perfume that her 13-year-old son bought his school sweetheart?* Oh, that's right – she's a drug rep!

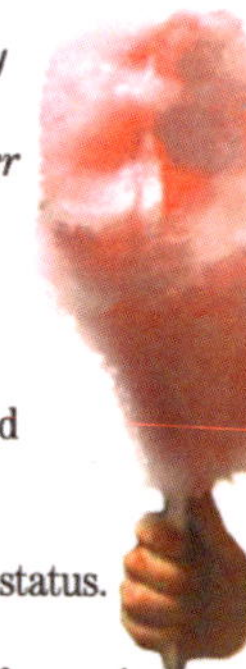

The nurse comes to me about a patient who just stopped by to get more samples of her PPI and *Lexapro*.By now I've learned to ask about insurance status. She has both Medicaid AND Medicare! *Please! No samples for you!*

## FRIDAY

Friday afternoon. Almost done. Patient was told by her psychiatrist to see her family doc after blood work he drew came back abnormal. Patient has no idea what was abnormal, the results were not faxed over, and his office is closed. *Lovely.* Patient to come back.

The nurse comes in to warn me about my second patient, a 26-year-old girl with back pain. Seems that her boyfriend likes narcotics a bit too much and as he has run through all docs, clinics, ERs, and pharmacies in the area he is using her as his supplier. I was standing outside the room reviewing the chart when a second nurse comes up to warn me about the patient. *This is not going to go well.* The pimp, er I mean boyfriend, is in the room but doesn,'t say a word during the entire visit. Seems the poor girl had a fall at work and now reportedly has a herniated disc. Poor little thing was denied disability on her first (sure to be first of many) attempts at getting disability. Poor thing ran out of her *Lortab* and *Soma* on Wednesday. I do not want to get into the narcotic cycle with this girl. So I start with all my usual tactics.

She has already had PT. **Girl 1, Me 0.**

Already seen a neurosurgeon. **Girl 2, Me 0.**

Also already seen pain clinic. **Girl 3, Me 0.**

MRI not in chart, I won,'t prescribe narcotics until I review the results. She doesn't object. **Girl 4, Me 0.**

She must sign a narcotic contract and the first random UDS is right now. She doesn't flinch. *Damn she's good.* **Girl 5, Me 0.** Please, please, please let her have at least some marijuana in her system. *Is that too much to ask?* ✚

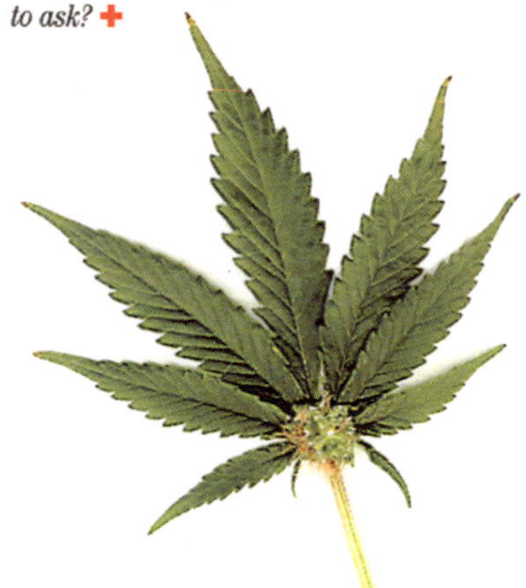

**SEND US YOUR "REALISTIC WEEK" IN MEDICINE TO WWW.PLACEBOJOURNAL.COM**

**IF WE PRINT IT YOU'LL GET A FREE ONE-YEAR SUBSCRIPTION!**

# Administray-Doh

MODELING COMPOUND

The Hospital Executive Game that allows you to spit out the same type of employee drone found all across America.

***Where administrators are taking shape!***

This playset provides dozens of fun ways for your hospital team to never change while at the same time remain mediocre!

When conformity is all you need to keep your own place in the food chain, then the *Administray-Doh* playset is for you.

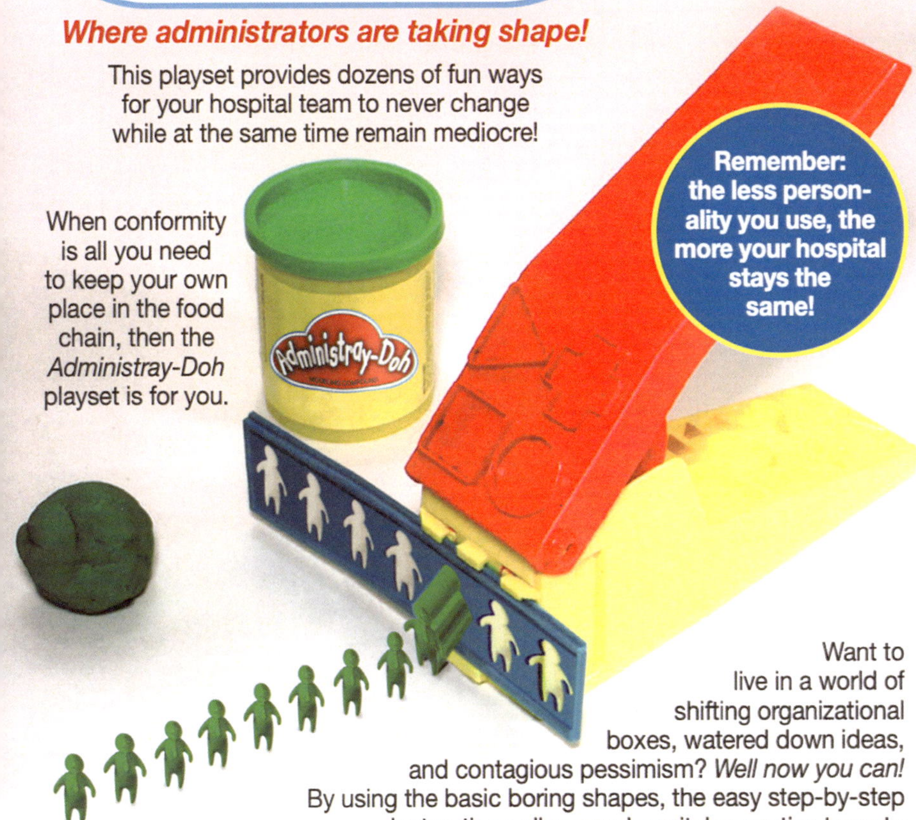


Want to live in a world of shifting organizational boxes, watered down ideas, and contagious pessimism? *Well now you can!* By using the basic boring shapes, the easy step-by-step instructions allow any hospital executive team to create the same employee over and over and over again.

Each one of your creations will learn how to: • generate bureaucratic drag • suppress spontaneity • create unnecessary hurdles and • obliterate enthusiasm.

Each set contains cans of totally limited possibility! No need for imagination with *Administray-Doh.* Our modeling compound leaves little room for creativity which is the foundation of a typical hospital administrator.

***Warning: Extremely toxic to physicians.***



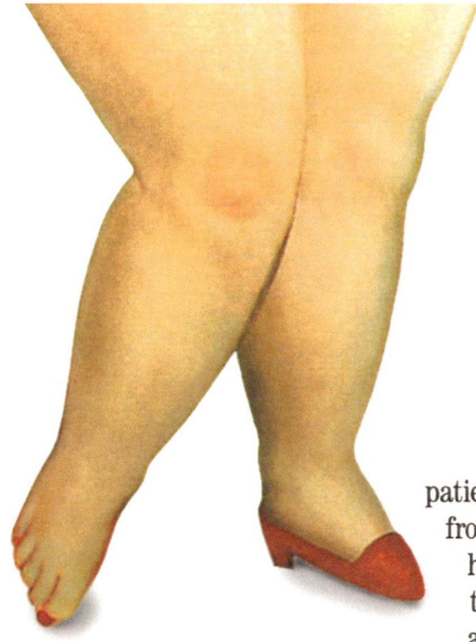

# THOSE DARN NARC SEEKERS

## You Come Highly Recommended

My partner saw an awesome new patient recently. When she checked in, the front desk staff noticed that she only had one shoe on. When she zig-zagged to the desk to speak to them and they asked why she was here, she said, *"I need my medicine."*

They diligently gave her a clipboard to fill out. It took her about 20 minutes to fill out 12 or so lines of personal info, and at one point, she wobbled back to the desk and asked, *"How do you spell hydros?"*

She eventually made her way back. She almost fell off the scale while our nurse weighed her (she was over three bucks). While waiting to be seen, she opened the exam room door two or three times demanding to know when the doctor was going to be in the room. *Remember, this was a new patient!*

Fortunately, the state of Tennessee now has an internet-accessible scheduled drug record, so he was able to research the patient before walking in. *Wouldn't you know it.* Last month alone, she had been given over 300 "hydro's" by three or four different docs.

My partner walked in and politely asked what he could do for her. She first told him that she just moved here from "town x." A second or two later, she mentioned that since she moved here from "town y," she hasn't been able to find a good doctor. My partner started to tell her that he would be glad to help her but he couldn't write her "hydros" or her *Xanax* until he got her medical records. He was about to whip out the printed copy of her narcotic prescriptions, when the patient said,

***"I came to see you because you were highly recommended."***

Being quite quick-witted, he responded, *"Really. Hummmm. What's my name then?"*

He let her stare blankly into space for a minute before he escorted her out the door. ✚

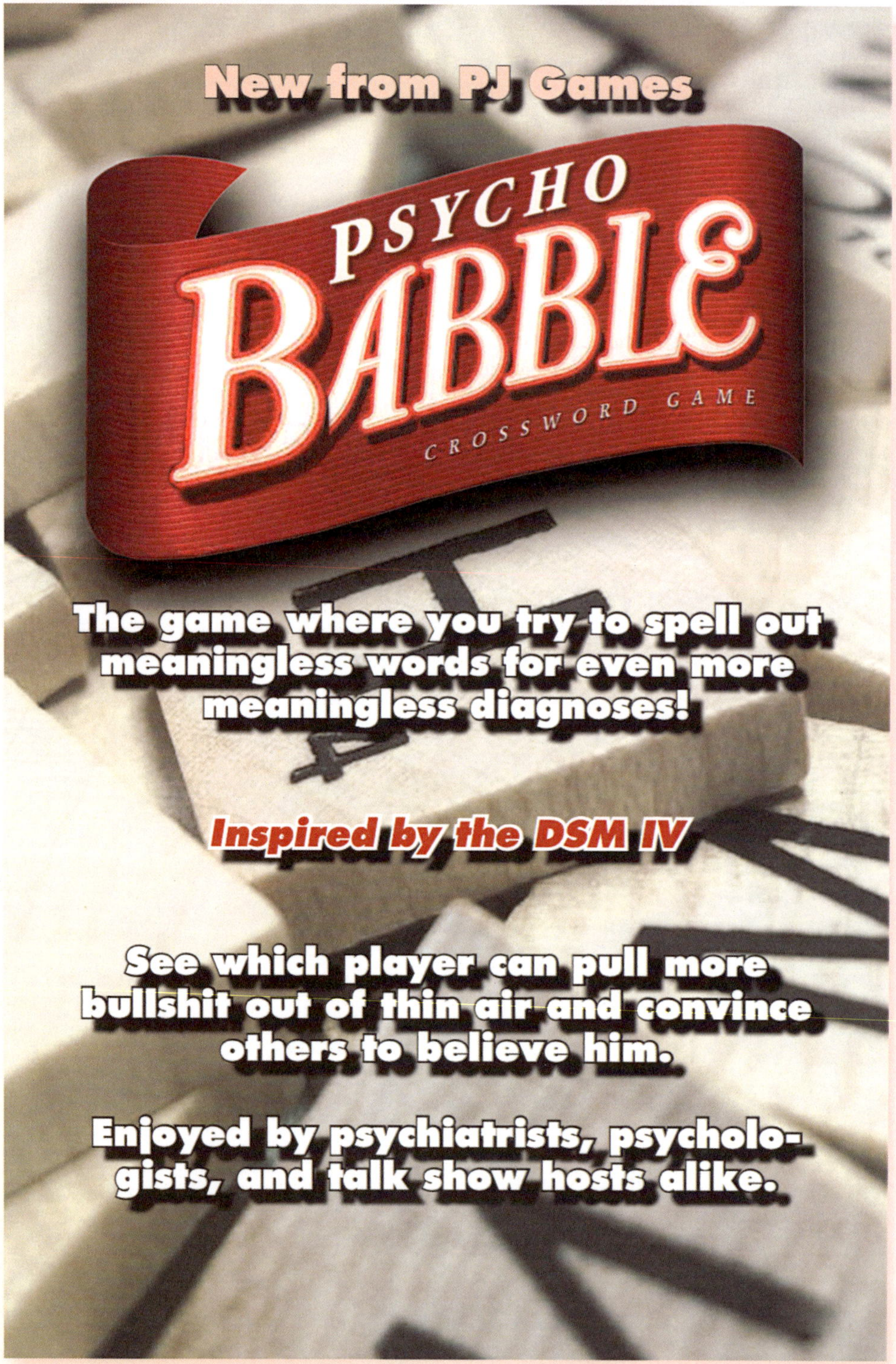
New from PJ Games
PSYCHO BABBLE
CROSSWORD GAME
The game where you try to spell out meaningless words for even more meaningless diagnoses!
Inspired by the DSM IV
See which player can pull more bullshit out of thin air and convince others to believe him.
Enjoyed by psychiatrists, psychologists, and talk show hosts alike.

## MORE TRUE STORIES OF MEDICINE

# SHOULD HAVE ASKED

*I learned a good lesson, the hard way.*

Back when I still did OB, I had a young, rather uneducated patient in her thirtieth week of pregnancy. She had asthma and had gotten real sick, with suspicion of pneumonia. At that time, it was standard practice to admit such patients to the hospital. She grew Neisseria species out of her sputum, and according to the lab, it was only sensitive to penicillin.

**She was allergic to penicillin.**

The OB consultant and I decided that we had to consult with Infectious Disease. The problem was that the only one we had practiced in Grand Rapids, about 45 miles away. He came over, God bless him, and proceeded to do his consult. And me, being the eager young thing that I was, sat in. I figured I would learn something. **And boy did I ever.**

He sat on her bed, and by this time, of course, she was scared to death. After all, she had this "Bad Bug," and we had no way to treat it.

*"Well,"* he said, *"young lady, you have a bad pneumonia and need an antibiotic, I'd say. But you're allergic to penicillin.* ***WHAT HAPPENS WHEN YOU TAKE IT?"***

(Why hadn't I thought to ask that?)

*"I get a yeast infection."*

While I hoped for the floor to open and to fall through to the basement, he calmly suggested IV penicillin and went back to Grand Rapids. To this day I have **NEVER** forgotten this embarrassing moment and I never forget to ask a patient again, *"What happens when you take it?"* ✚

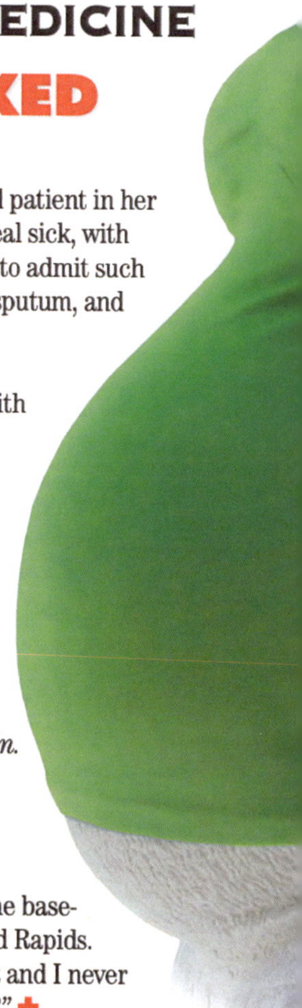

# FUTURE BOYFRIEND

This is another story form my past days of working in the ER. We had a young lady who was two months pregnant come to the ER wanting to be checked for STD's. When the nurse asked her if she had sex with a person of concern recently, she stated, *"No."*

She then asked her why she wanted to be checked for STD's. The patient related that she was at a party the previous evening and that she had put her mouth on a man's penis and that, *"it had the skin peeling off and had a terrible stench."*

When asked if this was her boyfriend, she replied,

*"Well, he was gonna be."*

Well, we swabbed her throat for GC and sent her on her merry way. ✚

# PATIENT DIALOGUE BUTTONS

Your patient population needs to be educated and informed about their healthcare. These "quality" buttons can be worn right in the office and are an excellent way to bring up important topics to your patient.

Here are some examples you can purchase now:

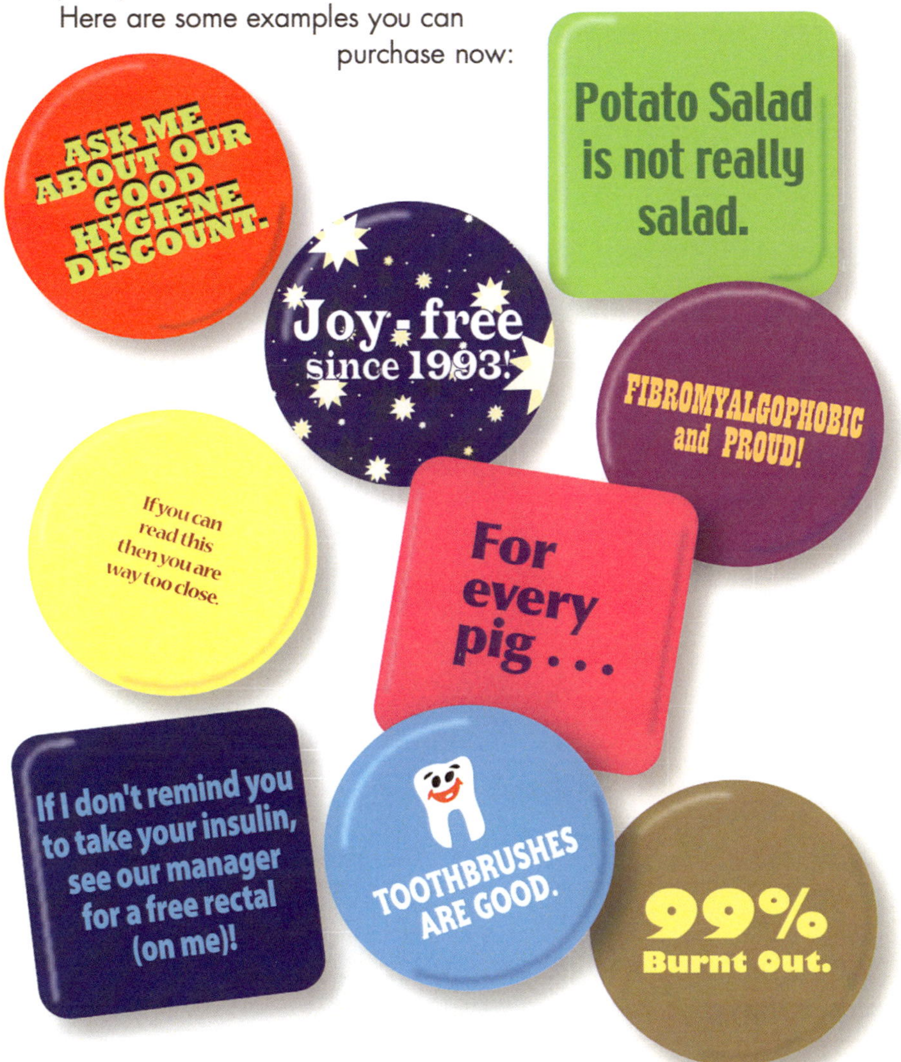
Potato Salad is not really salad.
ASK ME ABOUT OUR GOOD HYGIENE DISCOUNT.
Joy-free since 1993!
FIBROMYALGOPHOBIC and PROUD!
If you can read this then you are way too close.
For every pig . . .
If I don't remind you to take your insulin, see our manager for a free rectal (on me)!
TOOTHBRUSHES ARE GOOD.
99% Burnt Out.

## The future of healthcare lies in the future of buttons!

Wearing these buttons with "flair" will highlight the message that you care, as well as boost your patient education scores.

Each metal pin-back button measures 2.25 inches and feature a mylar/UV protective cover. ***Only $3.24 each!***

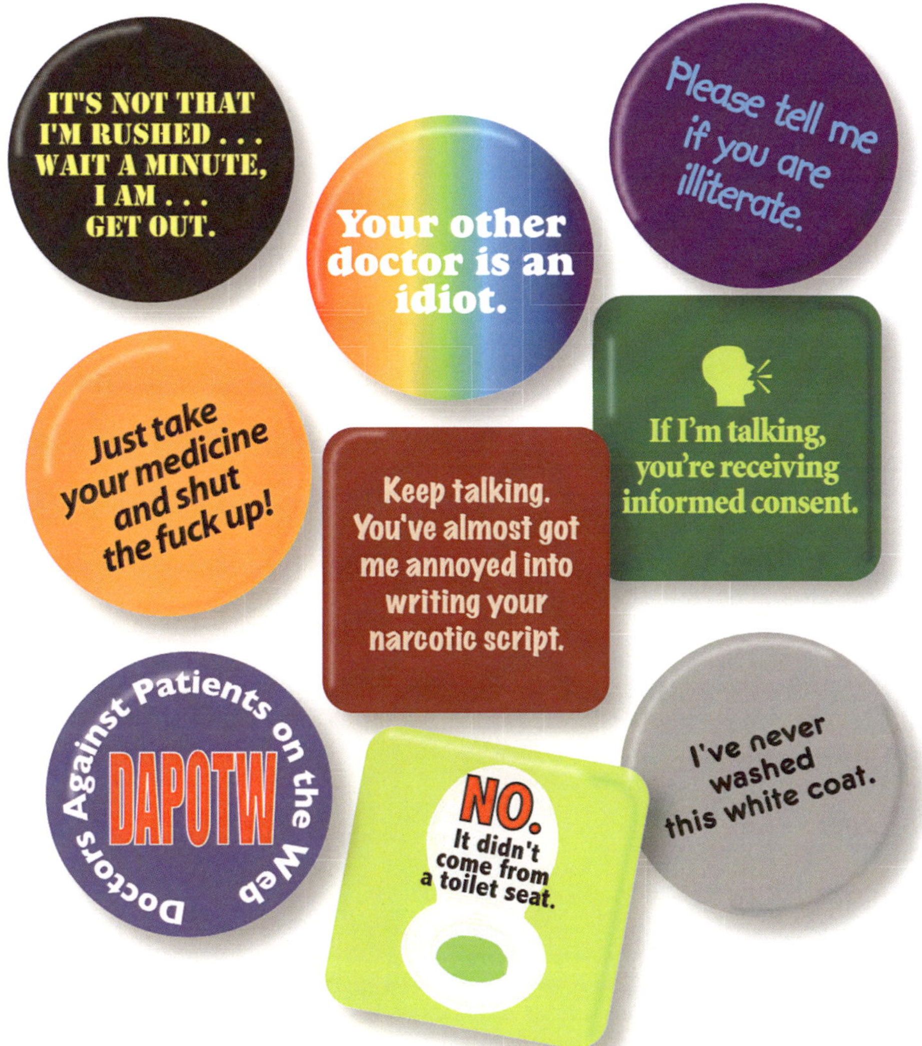
IT'S NOT THAT I'M RUSHED . . . WAIT A MINUTE, I AM . . . GET OUT.
Your other doctor is an idiot.
Please tell me if you are illiterate.
Just take your medicine and shut the fuck up!
Keep talking. You've almost got me annoyed into writing your narcotic script.
If I'm talking, you're receiving informed consent.
Doctors Against Patients on the Web
DAPOTW
NO. It didn't come from a toilet seat.
I've never washed this white coat.

Why spend a lot of money for an electronic prescription service when it may not even work?

*Make life simple with the . . .*

# ez-can PRESCRIPTION service™

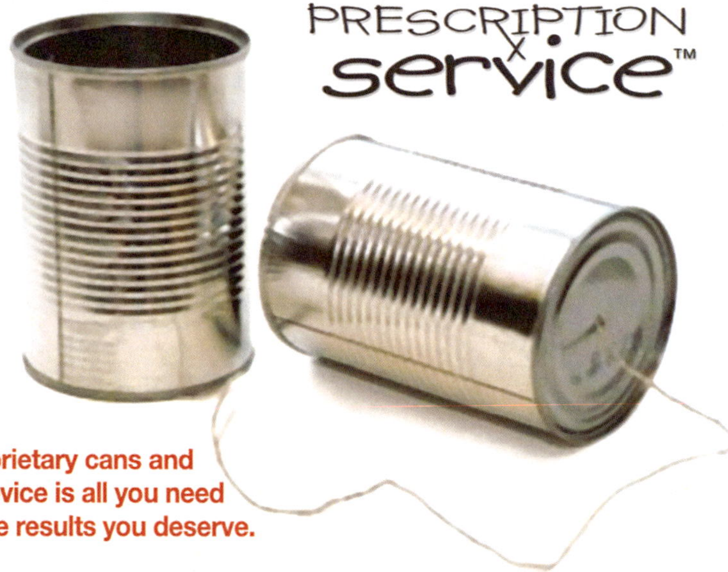

**Our proprietary cans and string device is all you need to get the results you deserve.**

Don't be intimidated by those other high tech companies with their fancy computers and techno-speak.

**Just pick up the can and talk loud. *It's that simple!***

Put the power of the can in your office.

- Save time & money with fewer pharmacy calls & faxes
- Attempt to cut down on medication errors
- Cheapest & most convenient prescription service on the market!
- Have a straight line right to the pharmacy
- Refill multiple prescriptions at a time

*Guaranteed end-to-end connectivity and HIPAA approved.*

Customize your very own EZ-Cans by choosing from the latest fashion colors, request any label you want, or design your own! You can even select the length of the string!

**Save time and money. Enhance practice efficiency.**

EZ-Can Pharmacy Prescription Service provides clinical decision support with a 24-hour phone support team.

***Isn't it time you started c-Prescribing?***

**Sponsored by American Aluminum Inc.**

# X-Ray Files

***If we show you ours, will you show us yours?***

Remember to **SMILE!** Here are some unhappy dental bridges done on a dental patient. ☺

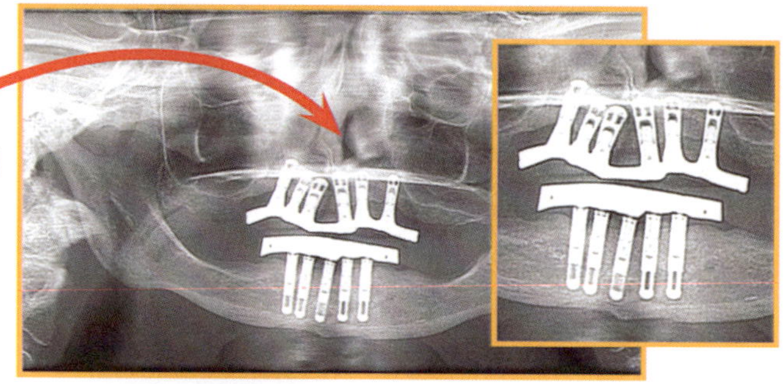

Now this is what is called **A STABBING HEADACHE!**

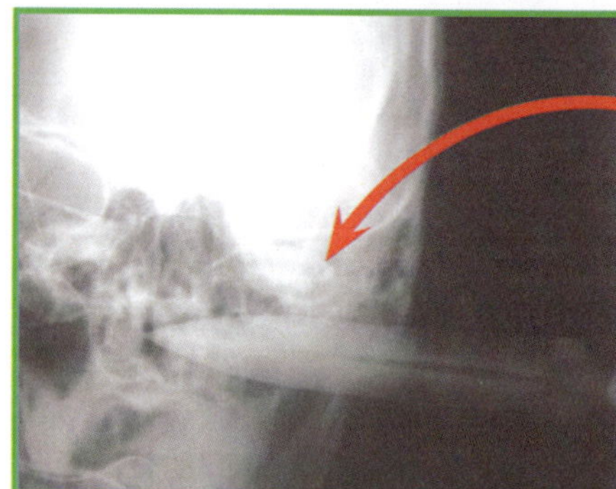

*Clearly a male – with a vibrator stuck in his rectum. It almost* **WRECKED 'EM!**

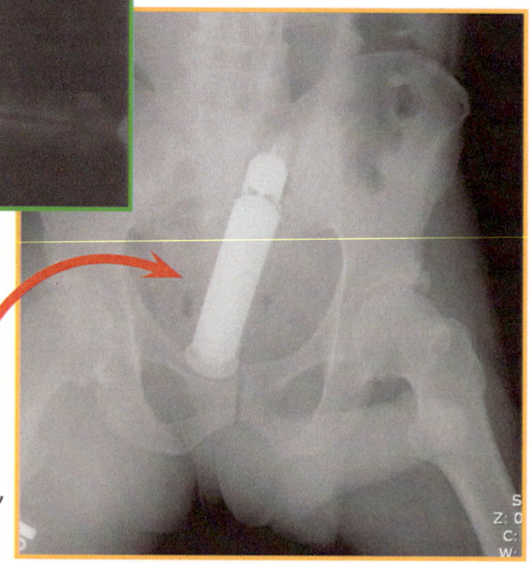

If you're a radiologist, show us your files. If we use them, you will get a **FREE ONE-YEAR SUBSCRIPTION!**

# POKER FACE

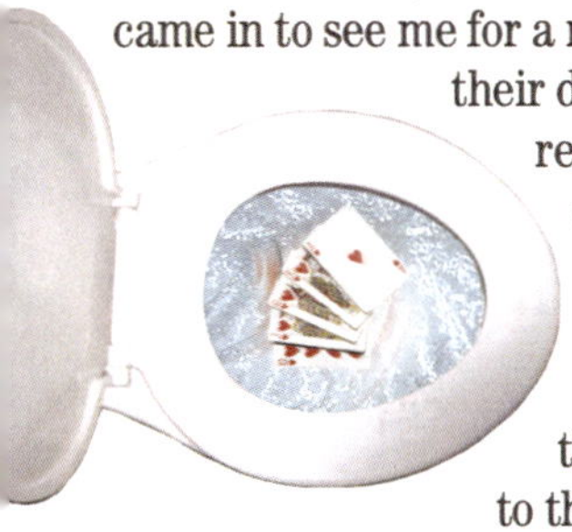

A while back, I had an evening where a middle-aged husband and wife came in to see me for a routine follow up. In between trying to address their diabetes, heart disease, smoking addiction, and reviewing labs, they were busy pointing out the other one's faults and noncompliance. It started to turn in to a mild argument as they each were getting defensive and trying to outdo the other.

The wife then pointed out that one of the things that annoyed her most was that when he goes to the bathroom, he brings in his electronic poker video game and he spends ridiculously long amounts of time in there.

I turned to the husband and asked him about it and he said it was a good stress relief and that he usually could escape there without being bothered. Seeing that this back-and-forth thing could go on all night, I had to intervene with some humor so as to try and break things up.

*I then turned to the wife and said, in his defense, that the reason he was in there so long was that he was working on a "Royal Flush."*

Both he and his wife couldn't stop laughing and they were back on friendly terms. *Dr. Phil, eat your heart out.* ✚

# WHAT???

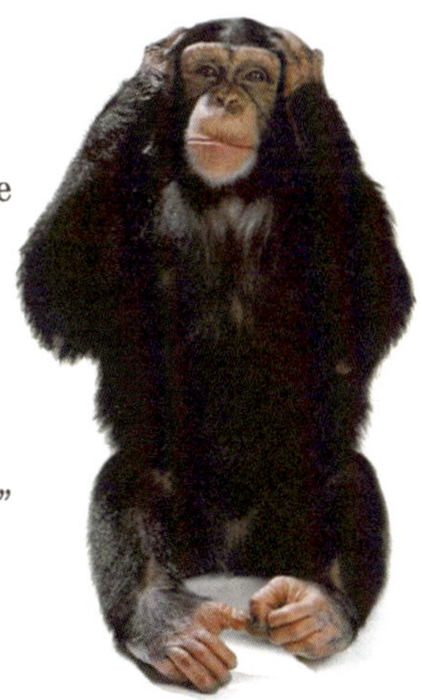

The other day I saw a new patient who had a multitude of problems. I am used to that, doing what I do for a living (pain management). I sat there through the litany of complaints, did my exam, looked at the data, etc. and then discussed treatment options.

The patient looked at me and said, *"I appreciate how much time you've spent with me. I can't imagine how you can sit here day after day and listen to all these problems."*

To which I replied, *"Who listens?"*

I really need to get my meds adjusted. The truth is leaking out. ✚

# AWFUL LONG TIME

As an intern in my second month of training in Nashville, TN, I showed up for my first day on the ward service at the VA. Never having worked at a VA before, I was ill-prepared for the steep learning curve of not only patient care, but also the mastering of the elephant that is the VA system. I met my senior resident for the month: Sister Harris. *Yes, a nun.* No, I'm not making this up. This woman was and is a saint, put through medical school by her convent and planned to return there to provide free primary care for her sisters and community. Myself, a redneck foul-mouthed heathen from south Alabama, felt mildly paranoid at all times the whole month.

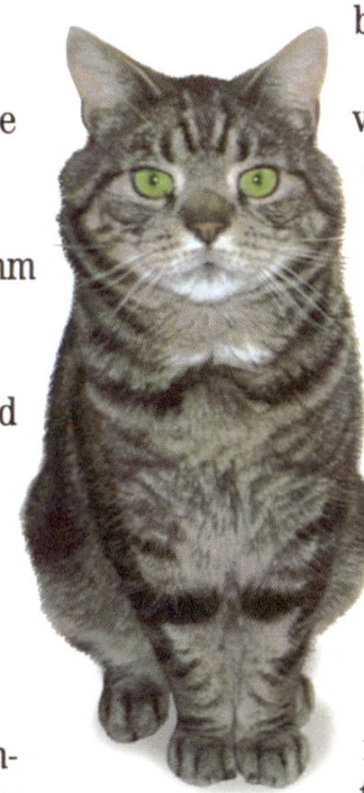

After the first few days I got into the rhythm of the VA-spa, and enjoyed the old-timer patients that frequented the place. My favorite was Harry, admitted with community acquired pneumonia. At 93 years old, he had actually run a blood transfusion tent for General Patton. He had some great stories. Every morning during my pre-rounds, he would gush about how impressive it was to see a young female as a physician, how proud my parents must be, etc. etc.

After the third day, I realized that Harry really liked the ladies. In fact, he was on his fourth marriage, this time to a 32-year-old blond bombshell. I realized his soft spot for young women on the morning Harry was to be discharged. I was rounding with Sister Harris, in her full habit and wimple, as usual. We got to Harry's room, and I informed him and his bombshell wife that he had been afebrile for 24 hours on oral antibiotics and was free to go.

I asked, in my naïve intern's voice, *"Is there anything you need? Anything I can get you to make you more comfortable at home?"*

His reply: *"Well honey, it has been an awfully long time since I saw any pussy!"*

You can imagine Sister Harris' reaction. Harry went home, and we prayed for him for the rest of the month. And I still love to tell this story. ✚

31st Annual

**North American Pathology Conference**

*presents*

# The PATH to Boredom

January 1 to 3, 2008

***Connect with the Zany Leaders in the Field of Cytopathology!***

Located this year at the hot spot of Lancaster, Pennsylvania.
*Who can forget the wild time we had in 1984?*

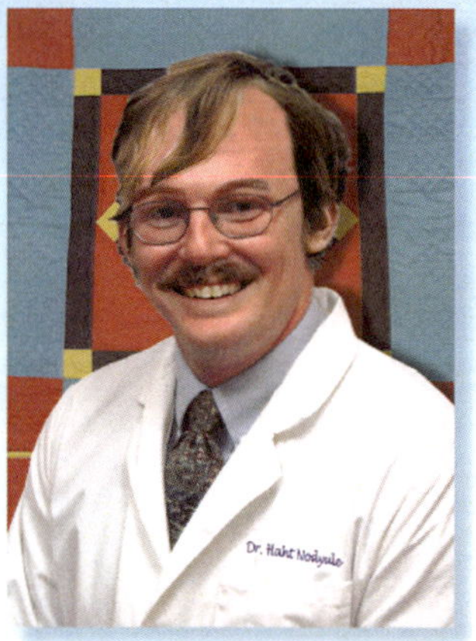

This event will feature cutting-edge lectures, workshops, and a keynote lecture presented by

## Haht Nodyule, MD

Distinguished recipient of the *2007 Hottest Single Pathologist Award*.

Come see his talk entitled:
**Microscopes, Moh's and Malignant Markers: More Fun Than A Family Doctor Trying To Decipher What An RDW Means.**

**Cryo Schmyo:**
How To Get Your Local Docs To Excise EVERYTHING
*by Dyson Toomer, MD*

**Understanding Social Norms IV:**
Ordering A Pizza On The Phone
*by Angelsteen Flankowitz, DO*

**Patient Contact:**
Four New Frightening Reasons To Avoid It
*by Nestor Candlewax, MD*

**Consulting With Peers:**
Using Jargon They Haven't Heard In Decades
*by Slyson Byopsiez, MD*

**Taking CYA to the Bank:**
Why To Always Need More Tissue & Additional Tests (What We've Learned From The Radiologists)
*by Soh Shelly Awkward, MD*

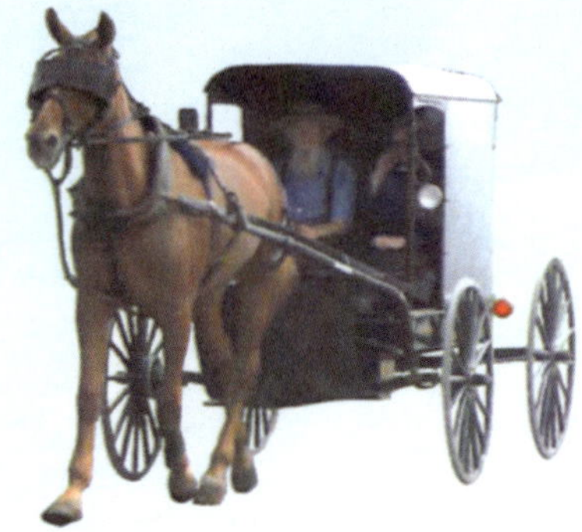

**Atypical Lymphocytes And Criteria For Action Following Automated CBC And WBC Differential Analysis.**
(This one is going to be nuts!)
*by Schlomo Blaristen MD*

We will again have a full area of corporate exhibits, working lunch meetings, and think tanks.

***Don't Miss It!***

**Party each night at the local tavern and watch the Dutch Amish let their hair down. This year's hard rockin' evening entertainment will be the hottest new local band called *Boyz to Mennonites***

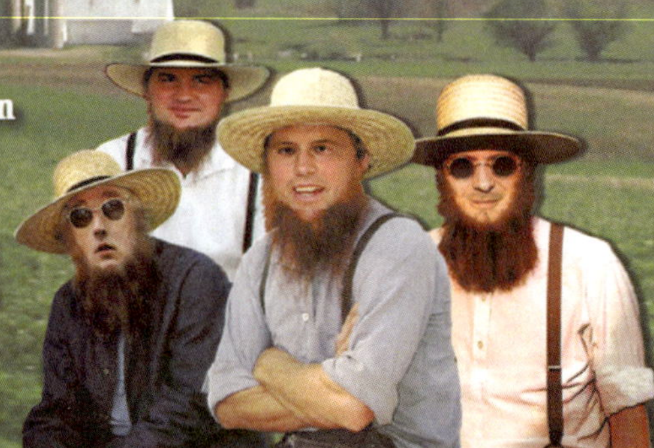

**Don't forget our**

## Annual Casual Social Gathering

**offering opportunities for networking and further exchange with other pathologists.**

**Reserve your space now as last year seven physicians showed.**

**Call 1-555-HOT-PATH Now.**

**Approved for 14 CMME Credits**

## Realistic Perceived Exertion Chart
for Treadmill Stress Tests

**1** **Okay to go!**
"I feel pretty good. This isn't so bad."

**2** **Very, very light intensity**
"This exercise thing isn't so hard. I can do this every day."

**3** **Very light intensity**
"Okay, this is getting a little tougher. But I'm tough, too."

**4** **Light intensity**
"Are my joints supposed to hurt so much? Not so fun anymore."

**5** **Moderate intensity**
"You need to slow this treadmill down. Seriously."

**6** **Moderate to intense**
"Hello, having some trouble breathing. Why are you speeding this thing up?"

**7** **Intense**
"My heart is beating like a rabbit. Why are you smiling you sadistic bastard?"

**8** **Very intense**
"I am sucking wind, I have chest pains and I want to kill you. Stop the f#cking treadmill!"

**9** **Very, very intense**
"Can't breathe. If I live after this I promise to hunt you and your family down unless you stop the treadmill now!"

**10** **Maximum intensity**
"I am going to die. These will be my last words, *'Got a cigarette?'*"

# THOSE DARN NARC SEEKERS

***or . . . You don't get it yet? I'm not getting you high today.***

## True Story #1

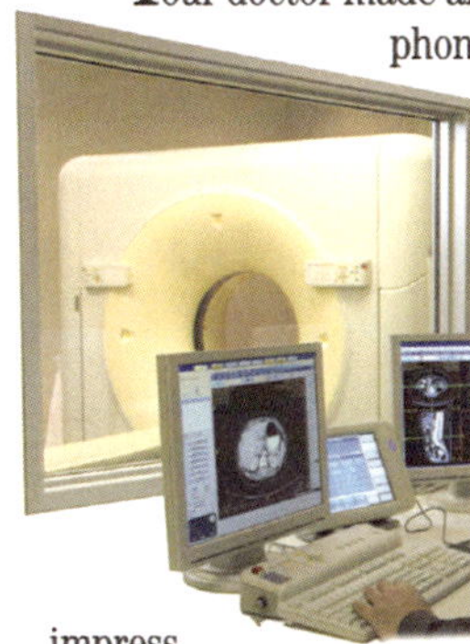

Your doctor made an unprovoked phone call to tell me she thinks you're a malingerer who sticks your finger down your throat to induce vomiting so you can impress us that your pain is so bad you've been vomiting.

You couldn't remember which hospital in Orlando you were at five days ago so I couldn't get your records, but your doctor told me she has them. You used a fake name there. You forgot to tell me you had an identical visit to the ER two miles away two days ago.

You've had so many unnecessary CT scans that you're going to have to sue yourself for malpractice when you get radiation-induced cancer in 20 years. After I spoke to your doctor I cancelled your CT scan.

I wasn't reassured when you told me you've only used a fake name ONCE. Your arms are covered with needle marks from all your ER visits and you haven't washed off the adhesive from your many cardiac monitoring stickers. Every one of your blood tests was completely normal. When I ordered *Toradol* you asked the nurse for *Dilaudid.*

Repeatedly demanding to speak with me after that was a nice touch, but I'm not budging. I was especially amused when you demanded to speak with the senior doctor. *That would be me.* I appreciated it that you had bad aim when you threw something at me on your way out. I made a note of that in your record.

## True Story #2

This is your eighth visit this year for back pain. All my partners give you *Vikes* because you tell them you have a herniated disc, yet you don't have a doctor to care for your chronic pain. You told me you don't have a doctor because you recently moved. One town over.

You elegantly sauntered into the ER in hooker boots and fell sound asleep in the 20 minutes it took me to get to you. I had to do a sternal rub to wake you up. You had no pain that I could observe or reproduce, and when I asked you to sit up you moved as nimbly as a gymnast. My nurse also had to wake you up ten minutes later to offer you NSAIDs and muscle relaxants.

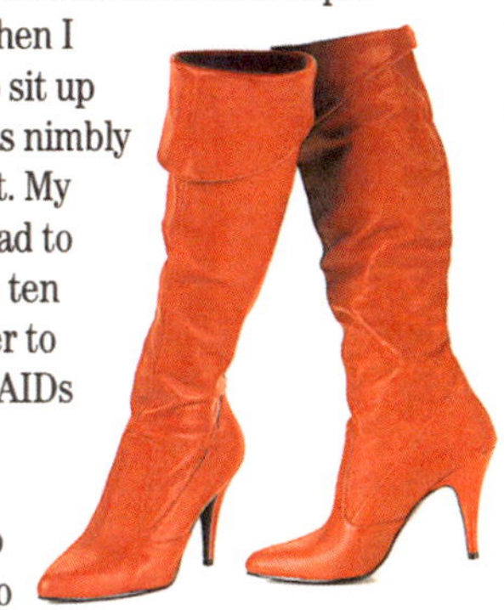

You also demanded to speak with me when the nurse didn't give you what you were expecting. *You can't just sashay in and order off the menu.* We are all out of Oxycontiin tonight, sorry. *Why should I get you high when you already are?* ✚

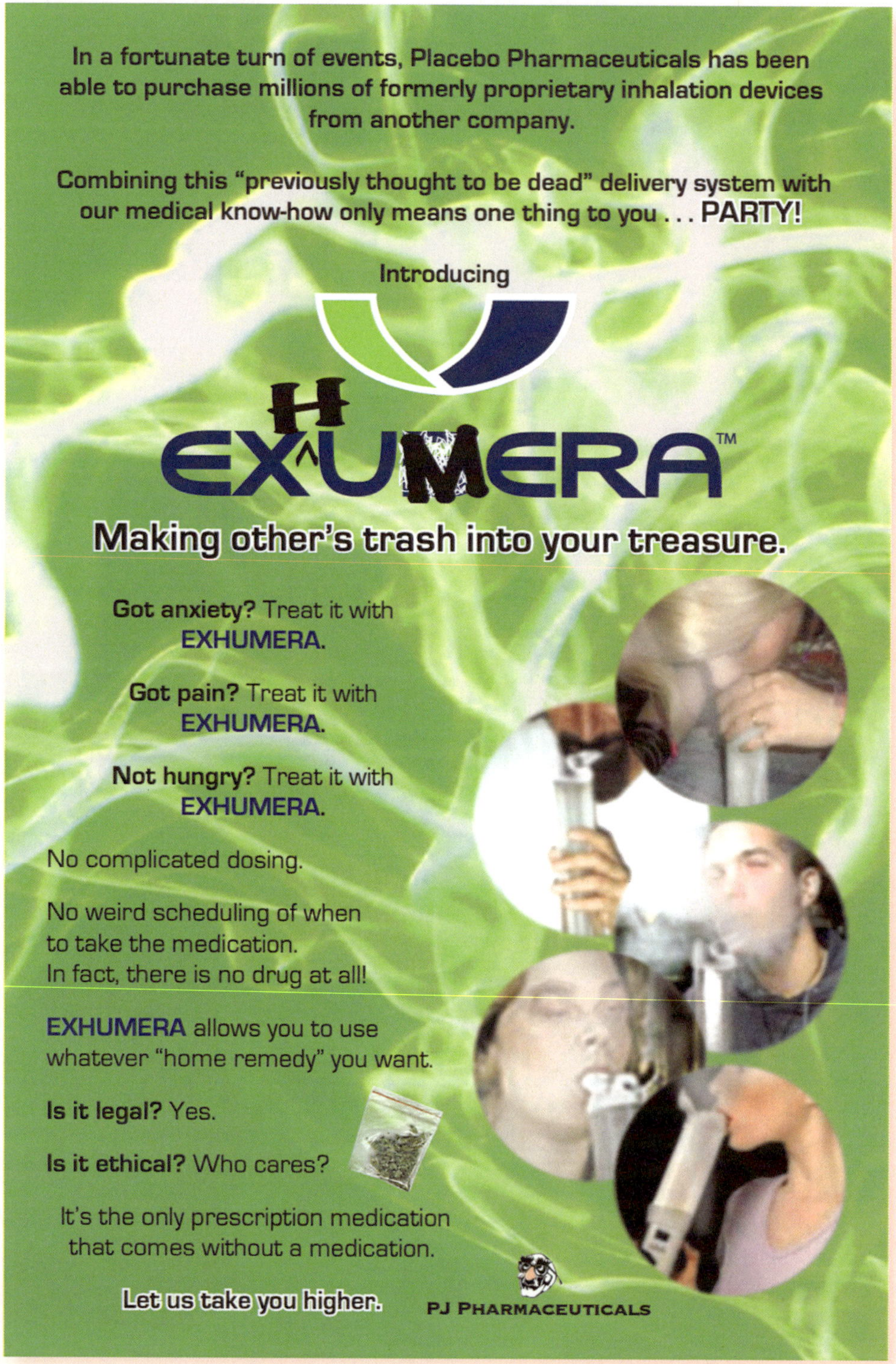


# MORE TRUE STORIES OF MEDICINE

## SIMPLE VOCAB

I recall my first day of medical school when it was explained to us that by the end of our second year our vocabulary would increase by several thousand words. While this was definitely true, it still did not completely prepare me for some of the terminology that I would be expected to know in order to practice successfully in eastern Tennessee.

One of my first patients was an elderly black man who came into the office for follow-up of his hypertension. When I asked how he was doing, he responded with, ***"My nature don't work."***

I looked at him and said, *"Your nature doesn't work?"*

He repeated more emphatically, ***"My NATURE don't work."***

I once again said, *"Your nature doesn't work?"*

He then pointed to his groin area and said, ***"I told you my nature don't work!"***

Finally a light blinked on in my mind and I said, *"Oh, your nature doesn't work,"* and switched him from his beta blocker to another antihypertensive (the former causes erectile dysfunction).

While working in the ER, a young but rather well-worn looking woman came in complaining that, ***"My monkey is sick."*** Being totally confused, I excused myself form the exam room and inquired of the nurses as to how to treat a *"sick monkey?"* After a good laugh, they informed me that *"monkey"* was one of the backwoods expressions used for a woman's vagina.

With my new found information, I was now able to go back and examine this patient and make a diagnosis of Simian Trichomoniasis.

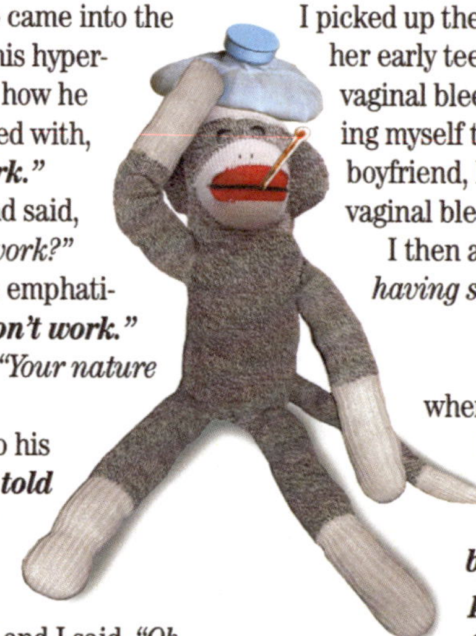

Fifteen years later, again in the ER, I picked up the chart of a woman in her early teens with a complaint of vaginal bleeding. After introducing myself to the patient and her boyfriend, I asked if she was having vaginal bleeding. She denied this.

I then asked, *"Are you not having some bleeding?"*

She replied, *"Yes."*

When I inquired as to where she was bleeding, her boyfriend cleared up the confusion by stating, ***"She is bleeding from that place where a man sticks his thing in."***

I simply replied, *"Oh, I see,"* and after her exam, made a diagnosis of a menstrual period.

Sometimes, however, the patient will make it easy for you. I recently had a fifteen-year-old girl come into the office stating, ***"It feels like the last time I had trichomoniasis."***

Well she was close, this time it was Chlamydia. ✚

# SWEET GRANDPA

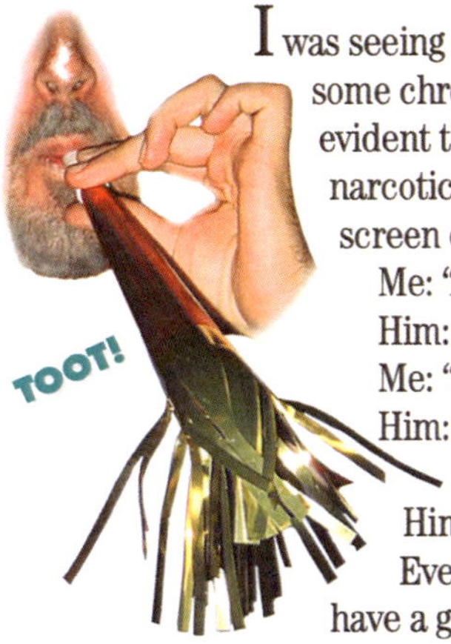


I was seeing a colleague's patient, about 40 years old, with some chronic pain du jour. In my colleague's notes it was evident that he was considering putting the patient on a narcotic contract. I told him we were going to do a drug screen on him. The following conversation ensued:

Me: *"Are we going to see any drugs in your urine?"*

Him: *"No."*

Me: *"So there won't be any drugs in it?"*

Him: *"No, except I did some coke a couple of days ago."*

Me: [clarifying] *"You did some cocaine?"*

Him: *"Well, it was my grandson's birthday party."*

Even in my patient population, a 40-year-old couldn't have a grandson more than an eight years old. But apparently a child's birthday party was a perfectly reasonable excuse to take a toot.

*"Hey Grandpa! Looks like you got some white icing on your nose!"* +

# POOL PLAY

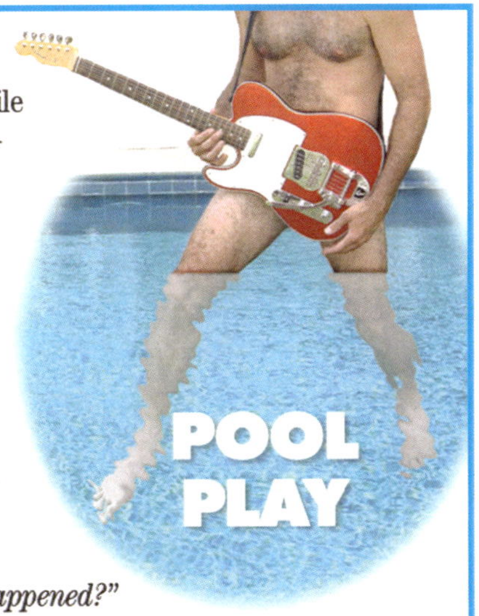

I spent some years doing medicine in juvenile halls. It can be hard sometimes to keep your professional composure when dealing with these kids. Have to bite your lip a lot. One day this young man took off his shirt for an admitting physical exam and right in the middle of his abdomen was this bright, greatly raised, shiny and perfectly round ten centimeter scar. I asked how he got that.

*"I was playing my guitar,"* he said.

*"Well a lot of people play guitars but I have never seen a scar like that before."*

*"It was an electric guitar."*

*"A lot of people play electric gitars. What happened?"*

*"I was playing it."*

*"I don't get it. How did you end up with that scar?"*

***"I was standing in the pool..."*** +

# COCK FIGHTS

I was working a summer holiday evening shift on the trauma end of a busy ED in the deep south. The charge nurse and a registration clerk came wheeling this 20-something, bubba-lookin', very drunk guy down the hall towards our trauma room in a wheel chair. He was yelling, *"I bin' shot! I bin' shot!"*

So I asked him, *"Where were you shot?"*

He responds, *"I don't know, but I bin' shot!"*

So we wheeled him into the trauma room, stripped him, and sure enough, there was a bullet hole in his right groin just to the right of his penis, with another hole in his right buttock. His vitals were stable, he was neurovascularly intact with minimal bleeding, so I asked him what happened.

He dodged the question a few times, then finally admitted, *"Well, ya' see, my uncle and I had got to drinkin', and after six or seven beers we decided to have a contest to see whose penis was bigger, so we pulled 'em out, and I won, and I guess he got mad about that, because he said,*

*'If you keep waving that thing around at me, I'm gonna' shoot it off,'*

*and I guess I kept waving it at him, because he took out his .357 and shot at me!"*

**We thought it couldn't get any classier than this.** We got him back from CT, which was largely normal except that the bullet track went right by his sigmoid colon.

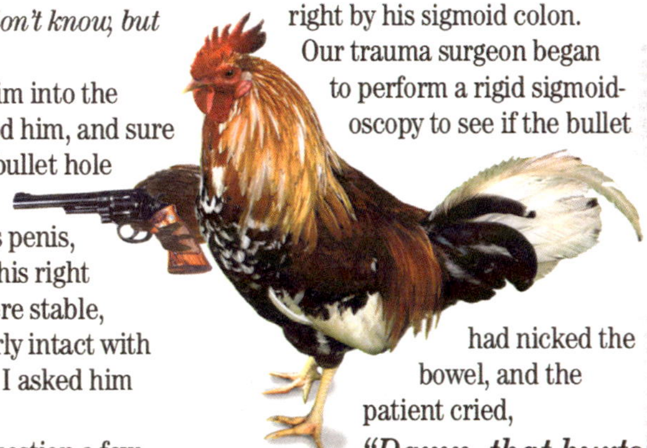

Our trauma surgeon began to perform a rigid sigmoidoscopy to see if the bullet had nicked the bowel, and the patient cried,

*"Damn, that hurts! I don't know how my wife can stand that, but she kinda' likes it!"*

The bowel was normal and the patient did well, so we bandaged him up, sent him home, and have been laughing about it ever since. +

The Placebo Journal Home Business Guide

# HOW TO MAKE A DIET PILL

**You too can make millions in the nutraceutical industry. *No ethics required!* Don't know any science? *Not a problem!* Actually, the less science you know the more successful you can be!**

**STEP ONE** **Combine one word in Column 1 with a word in Column 2 to get your product name.**

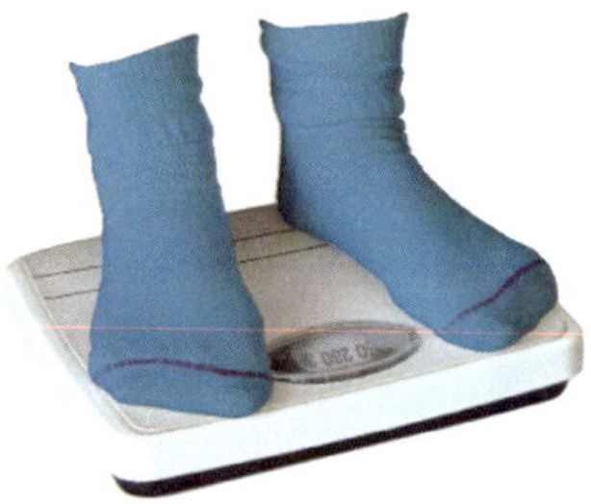

| | |
|---|---|
| Dexa | Fast |
| Ultra | Clear |
| Mega | Slim |
| Carbo | Trim |
| Lipo | Kwik |

**STEP TWO** **Select ingredients.**

- caffeine
- chromium picolinate
- pyruvate
- Hoodia
- psyllium
- chitosan
- yerba maté
- contents of vacuum cleaner bag
- hydroxymethylbutyrate
- guarana
- garcinia cambogia
- citrus curantium
- 7-Keto-DHEA
- conjugated linoleic acid
- grass clippings

**STEP THREE** **Formulate claims. Choose from examples below.**

Today, there exists a safe, all-natural, bio-active weight loss compound so powerful, so effective, so relentless in its awesome attack on bulging, fatty deposits that it has virtually eliminated the need to diet.

*"I lost 30 pounds in 30 days even though I ate all my favorite foods."*

**Lose up to two pounds daily without diet or exercise.**

*"I lost 15 pounds in 30 days without having to change my eating habits or lifestyle in any way."*

**Go from a size 12 to a size 6! Lose inches QUICKLY. Take it off! And keep it off!**

Thousands of dieters are already using it and losing weight faster than they have before – and keeping the weight off. Slim down for good for the rest of your life.

**Tired of yo-yo diets without success?**

Blocks fat before your body absorbs it; the pounds will melt away effortlessly.

Inhibits fats, sugars, and starches from being absorbed in the intestines and turning into excess weight, so that you can lose pounds and inches easily.

**An 'all-natural ingredient' designed to attract and absorb excess calories and transport them out of your system.**

**STEP FOUR** **Before & after photos.**

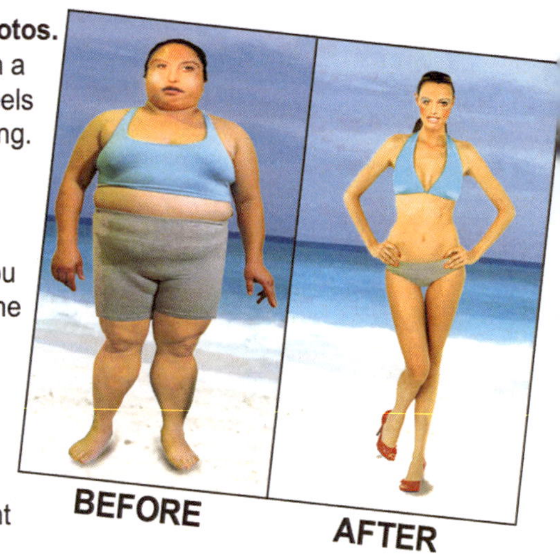


1. Take a photo of a thin woman with a killer body with full makeup and high heels wearing a bikini. Make sure she is smiling. Label this "**AFTER.**"

2. If you can, get the woman seven months pregnant before you shoot the next photo. If she won't cooperate or you have time constraints, take a photo of the same woman without makeup or high heels, make sure she looks unhappy, and run it through *Photoshop* to create a fat person. Add some wrinkles. Label this "**BEFORE.**"

3. Place the photos in an ad and print one of the following underneath:

***"The way our miraculous weight loss cure works is so ingeniously complex, your doctor won't even understand it, and might be skeptical!"***

***"At this rate of weight loss, I'll be out of my overalls in less than a year!"***

***"I had sex!"*** ***"It also cures cancer!"*** +

## A TRUE STORY OF MEDICINE

# A Novel Use for a Vacuum Extractor

A 58-year-old white male presented acutely to our rural emergency room with a foreign body in his rectum. Approximately two hours prior to presentation, he had inserted the ball and had been unable to pass it. Exam revealed a foreign body in the rectal vault; a hard circular object measuring approximately 7 cm in diameter. There was some bruising at the rectum and linear laceration dorsally.

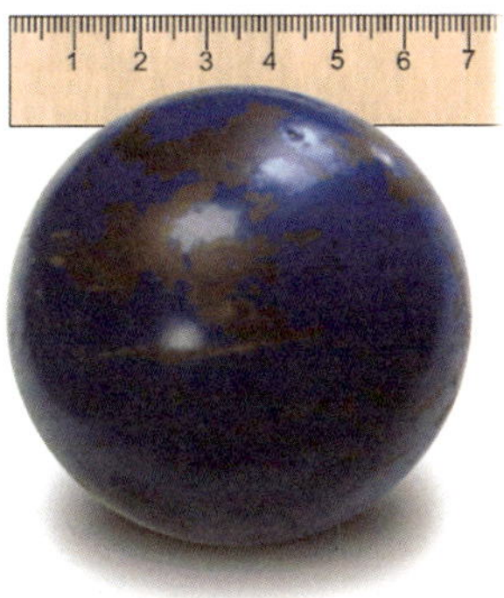

First, I attempted to remove the foreign body digitally and manually, but was unsuccessful. I then unsuccessfully attempted to place ring forceps around it. Finally, I tried a *Kiwi* vacuum extractor. ***Oh, the sweet smell of success.***

After removal and cleaning, the object turned out to be a blue croquet ball. The rectum was inspected following removal of the ball and showed minimal bleeding. This was the only time I have ever used a vacuum extractor and been unconcerned when the delivered entity was blue.

After an extensive literature search, I was unaware of any other documented case of a vacuum extractor used for a found rectal foreign object.

Little did I know I would get a second chance to use this technique for a rectal foreign body, not even three weeks later! This time, a guy came to the ER with an apple in his rectum. I started straightaway with the vacuum extractor, but it didn't work. We had to use a ring forceps to break it up. ***After that I will never eat another caramel apple!***

How I became my small town's magnet for rectal foreign bodies I will never know, but to this day the nurses harass me, saying that every time I am on call people just go around thinking,

***"Gee, what can I put up my ass tonight?"*** +

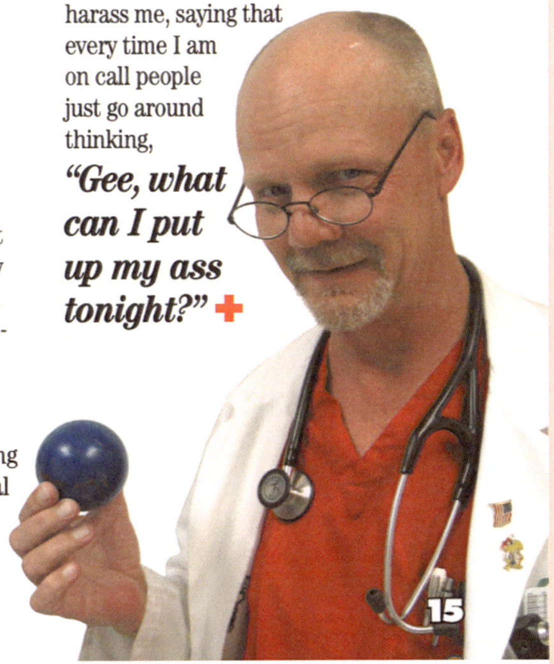


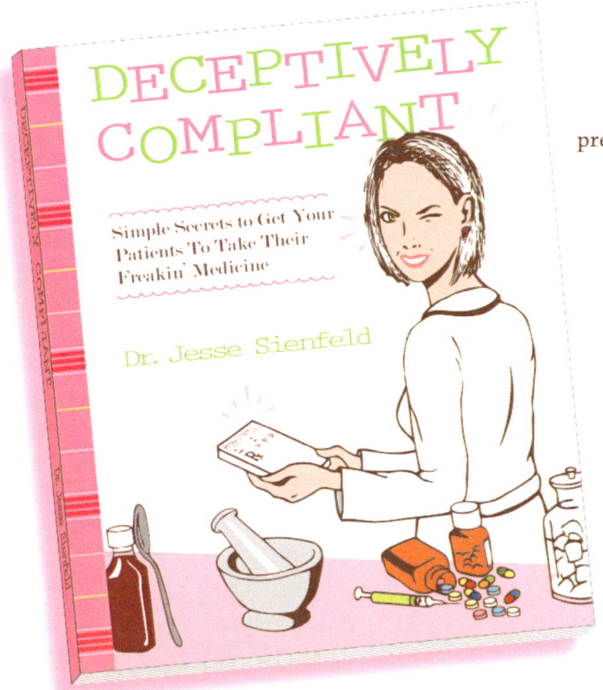


Study after study shows that half the time patients don't use the prescription you give them. Complaints such as *"I forgot", "It made me nauseous,"* or *"It made my muscles ache,"* are all too common. The truth is that most patients simply refuse to listen to your advice.

How can average doctors ensure their patients are getting the meds they prescribe?

**The answer comes from Dr. Jesse Sienfeld and you need to read this book!**

*Deceptively Compliant* is filled with traditional drugs that patients love, mixed with medications they complain about. The result is that even if they did have any annoying little side effects, they won't care enough to complain about it.

Examples include, let's say, combining lorazepam with a statin drug. Or, how about, methadone and a biphosphonate!

With some revealing and humorous personal anecdotes and tips on how to deal with the police and medical licensing board, this book will make the practice of medicine so much more enjoyable.

Also contains advice on solving practical problems for doctors. Dr. Sienfeld addresses how to confuse your patients into taking their drugs. She shows how to use the art of distraction to ignore their common complaints and move them on their way to the pharmacy and perpetual compliance.

**Dr. Jesse Sienfeld's book is practical, easy–to–read, and a godsend for any doctor who wants their patients to just shut the f#ck up already and take their freakin' medicine.**

*"The combination prescriptions worked like a dream. Unfortunately, a couple of my patients died from them. Is that bad?"*
Susanna Gladden MD, California

*"Hey, this book is the same thing I wrote last year. WTF!?!"*
Prisoner #267549 MD, New York

# PJ Smoker Repellant System

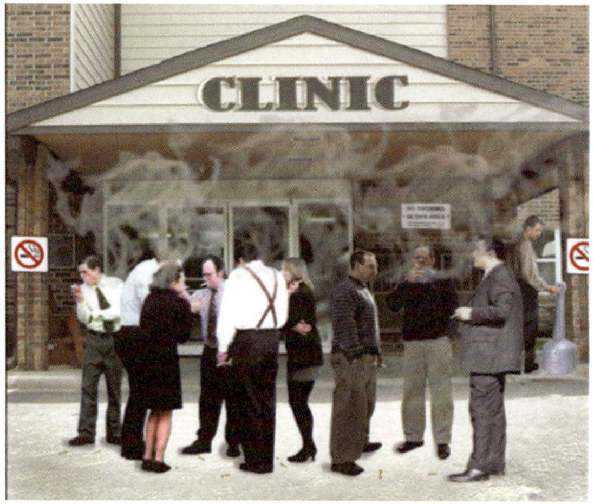

CLINIC


Tired of your patients smoking right outside the front doors of your medical office?

Is using your *No Smoking* sign as both a seat and an ashtray getting you down?

***Well, not anymore with the PJ Smoker Repellant System!***

Cure your most annoying nuisance by deterring flocking smokers from common hang-out sites around your office.

**The PJ Smoker Repellant System is environmentally friendly, does not harm smokers, yet is completely effective after only one application.**

*Trust your problem to the most experienced name in the smoker repellent industry.*

**System includes:**

❶ Our world famous **Smoker-Specific Electronic Sound System** to divert loitering around exits. It features the zany voices of the *Hypoxic Twins* - **Al Veoli** and his sister, **Karcy Noma**!

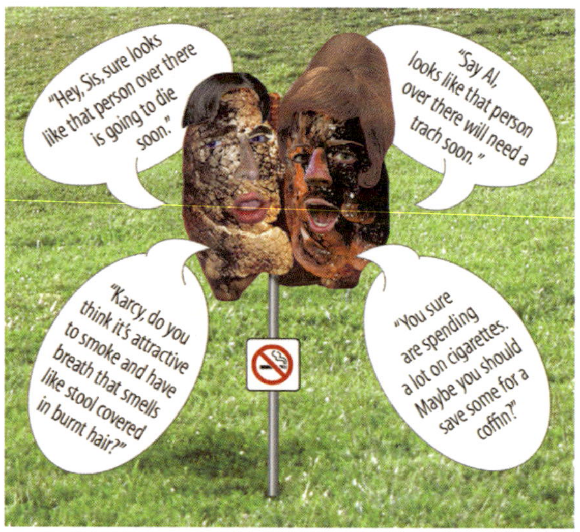

"Hey, Sis, sure looks like that person over there is going to die soon."
"Say Al, looks like that person over there will need a trach soon."
"Karcy, do you think it's attractive to smoke and have breath that smells like stool covered in burnt hair?"
"You sure are spending a lot on cigarettes. Maybe you should save some for a coffin?"


## *We don't hurt them ... just make them leave!*

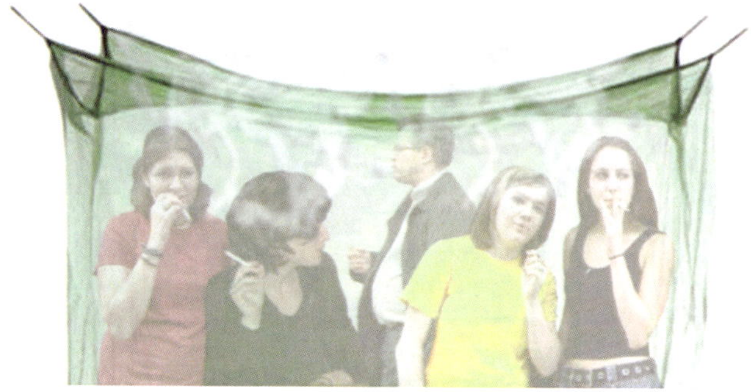

❷ **DRAGNET**, our advanced knotless mist netting for easy capture and release of pest smokers. It can also be used to create an 'invisible' barrier to keep smokers away from their favorite places to roost.

❸ Our patented **PUFFTRACK Electric Shock System** with a 110-volt electric shock generator* for those most resistant smokers who just will not leave.

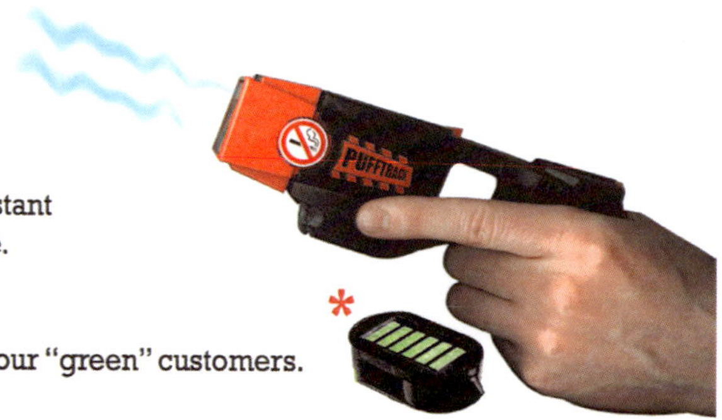

* Solar-powered adapter for our "green" customers.

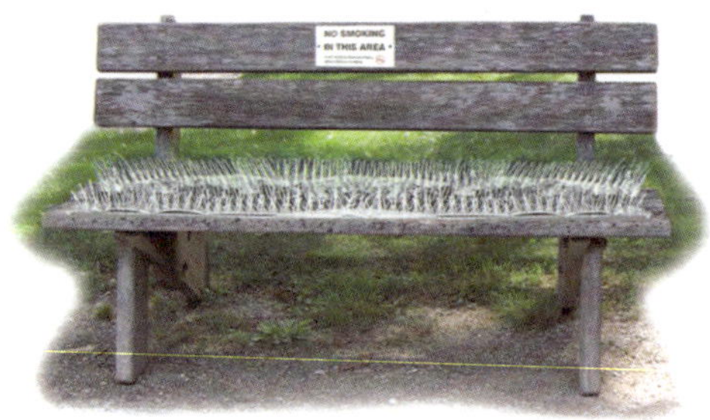

❹ Structural anti-perching and loitering deterrents complete with **Spike Strips** for outside sitting areas and all those hard to get at nooks and crannies around the outside of your medical office.

***Free Installation!***

***Two Year Guarantee!***

All this for only $1999. Order now by calling

**1-555-PUFFOFF**

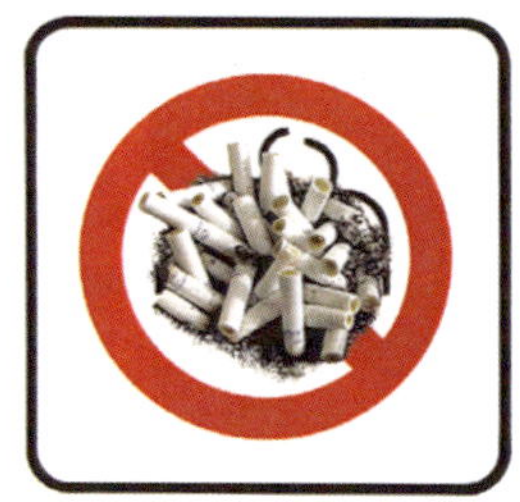

# MY “REALISTIC” 24 HOUR SHIFT IN THE ER

## THE FIRST 12 HOURS

**6:45 a.m.** As I pulled into the parking lot, the doc who I was relieving was already sitting in his car and sped away.

*Not a good sign.*

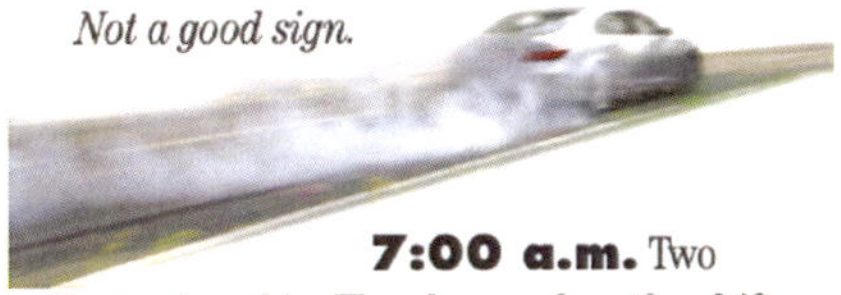

**7:00 a.m.** Two patients signed in. They knew when the shifts changed. The first was hung over and vomiting with abdominal pain.

*"I swear it really does hurt, Doc!!"*

I asked him if he was allergic to anything (besides soap and water) and then I ordered labs. As I walked to the bathroom to put my jacket up, I noticed the doc's bed was untouched in the call room. *Not a good sign.*

**7:03 a.m.** Nurses beeped me out of the restroom. *Damn!*

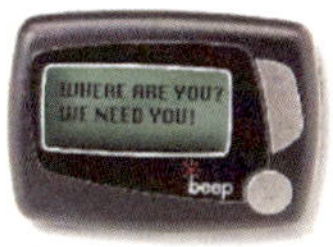


**7:04 a.m.** The second patient who signed in was 28 and claimed he had chest pain for *"three days."* Had to wonder why it was an emergency now? Answer - he's a "spoda." He was spoda be at his parole officer's office for a drug screen.

*"Can I have some morphine for this pain?"* Must have been what he was shooting up for the month or some street equivalent. Now he'd have an excuse for a positive drug screen.

**7:25 a.m.** The first ambulance rolled in with a 94-year-old nursing home patient hollering and screaming at the staff. Turns out that he's always like that and the nursing home dumps him on us when they get tired of it. They stated that he was complaining of chest pain. Even the nurses wondered how he could tell them he had chest pain? The answer was that they knew that a complaint of chest pain would get rid of him for at least a few hours and hopefully overnight.

**7:35 a.m.** First lab came back (already ?,there must be a CLIA inspection today) on our abdominal pain fellow. A white count of 28,000. *Could it be that he really was sick for once?* Ordered the abdominal CT scan.

**7:45 a.m.** "Spoda" had an abnormal EKG. Must be from all the crack and methadone. He was happy about the prospect of spending the night and asking for morphine constantly . . . his idea of heaven.

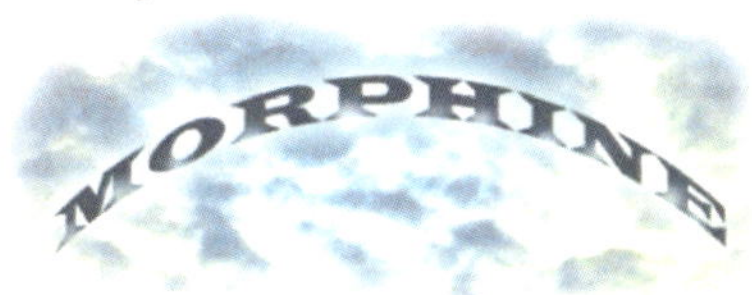


**8:00 a.m.** More ambulances. The nurses were yawning. No one actually needed the ride.

**8:10 a.m.** The first public health department clinic patients started showing up. Their clinic was already full and they send all of their overflow to us for "liability reasons," in case someone was actually sick.

**8:20 a.m.** Pediatric clinic was full and started sending us their overflow for "liability reasons." I couldn't help but notice that they never sent over anyone with insurance. Plus, I had to listen to the pediatricians gripe later about the Minute Clinic in town, and how it upsets the "continuity of care1" Yet, there are pedi patients I have seen 10-15 times a year whom have never once been able to get in to see an actual pediatrician. *No, I'm not flattered when these kids call me "Daddy?"*

**8:35 a.m.** VA clinic starts sending us their overflow for . . . Well, you guessed it.

**8:40 - 9:00 a.m.** Sorted out who was ill, sick, or really sick.

**9:10 a.m.** "Spoda's" CKMB and Troponin were up slightly. *Did he forget to mention his dad died of a heart attack when he was 25?*

**9:25 a.m.** After talking with the on-call internist and cardiologist, I got the orders written for telemetry and got ready to send him up. Patient decided, *"No way! I got things to do today,"* and tried to leave AMA. He stayed after I threatened to call his parole officer.

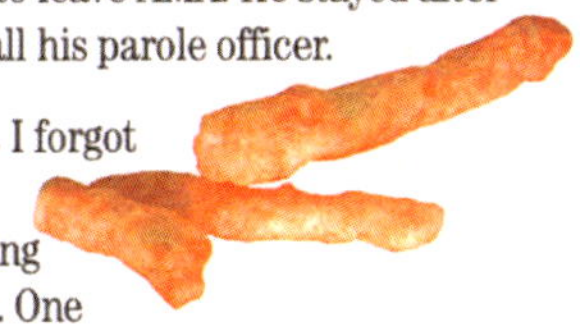

**10:00 a.m.** I forgot it was Monday. Everyone was trying to get out of work. One mom brought her child in for "vomicking." The child was sitting on the bed munching on *Cheetos*, the world famous cure for all vomiting. Turned out the kid had an appointment with his doctor in one hour but, *"he's too sick to wait."* Mom wanted a work excuse for herself.

**10:10 a.m.** Truck driver with a blood pressure of 210/120 and a heart rate of 140. *"I don't know why!"* and denied any drug use. Urine drug screen shows methamphetamine, of course, and the patient acted indignant that I would *"even check him for that !"*

**10:20 a.m.** Tried again to go to the bathroom. *Yup!* The nurses beeped me out again. I will talk to them about "separation anxiety" right after I try to explain to my urologist why I can crack walnuts with my urinary sphincter muscles.

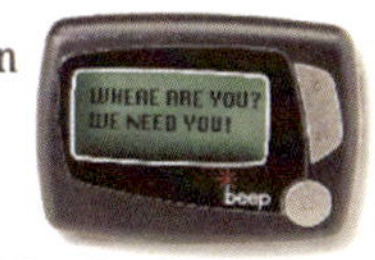


**10:22 a.m.** Radiologist started calling with x-ray "discrepancies" from yesterday. Why don't they read them when they're done, especially when they make more for reading the x-ray the next day than I get paid for seeing and treating the patient after reading his x-ray myself? Now we also had to hunt down all the charts and call these people.

**10:30 a.m.** "Spoda" had his abdominal CT done. The preliminary report read like one of Hillary and Bill's testimony transcripts. Full of "could bes, maybes, cannot rule outs . . ." *Does he have *%@#$ appendicitis or not?* The clinical exam was useless as he groaned to palpation of his abdomen, skin, hair, and even shoes. Asked the radiologist to call it to the surgeon as it was always fun to do that. I can usually hear the bellowing clean across the hospital!

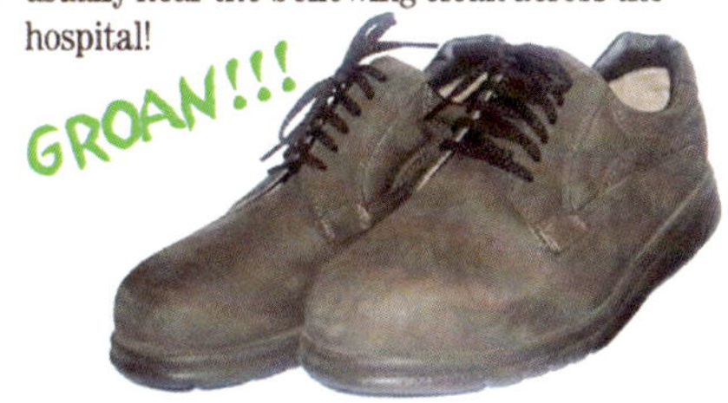


**10:45 a.m.** Wondered if I could charge by the pound for pelvic exams?

**10:45 a.m.** Had already asked seven patients to hang up their cell phones and pointed to the big signs in the room. One was a family member taking cell phone pictures of grandma's ostomy site to send to friends " *'cause it's really cool."*

**10:59 a.m.** Had already seen two toothaches, two back pains, and one "migraine." *Gonna be a bad day.*

**11:18 a.m.** Very obese lady came to the ER because her incision site was dehiscing *(I wonder why?)* Turned out that she had the surgery done in another part of the state and her surgeon insisted that she come here when she called him. Of course, he has made all the money he was gonna get from the DRG so there was no use in seeing her again.

**11:29 a.m.** Wrote memo to myself to write a letter to the governor to see if he could make vicodin an over-the-counter drug. *It would sure help.*

**11:35 a.m.** Two ambulances arrived from the same nursing home. One patient had very low blood pressure and high

*continued on next page*

## MY "REALISTIC" 24 HOUR SHIFT IN THE ER *continues . . .*

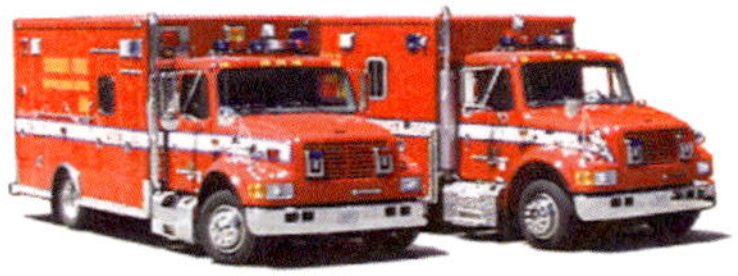

glucose and the other had an altered level of consciousness with a blood sugar of 20 and a BP of 190/100. Checked out my hunch and yes, they were roommates at the nursing home. Apparently the diabetic one got the other patients BP med and the hypertensive patient got the oral hypoglycemic agent.

**Noon** The lunch rush. Odd how people tend to have emergencies at meal time and when they get off work.

**12:15 p.m.** The telemetry unit called. Our chest pain parole violator had left AMA and they wanted to know if we had seen him.

**12:20 p.m.** X-ray department called. They couldn't find the little old, demented man who they were X-raying on the table. They wanted to know if we had seen him.

**12:30 p.m.** X-ray called back. They found him. He had rolled off the x-ray table onto the floor behind the table. They asked if I could come over and examine him and order a CT scan of the head. I told them to have the radiologist do it as it was his turf. *"He's gone to lunch and won't be back for an hour,"* is the response I got. So I used my lunch "break" to do his job.

**12:40 p.m.** I'm getting mighty fluent in Spanish lately. I've had some dreams in Spanish, but I'm not sure why it's the duck speaking it.

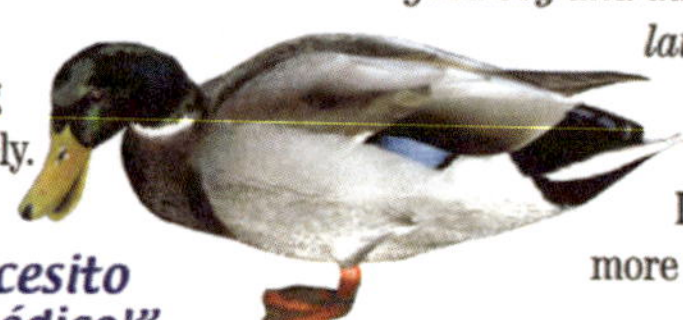


**12:45 p.m.** Snuck down to the doctors' lounge to grab lunch while I could. Most of the staff docs tried not to stare at me as I gulped down my lunch in two minutes. The GI guy told me, *"You know that's not good for you."* I grunted in agreement as I grabbed everything I could to take back with me to eat later that night. Of course, I ran into one of the numerous little old ladies on her way to x-ray and she eyed the food I was carrying stating, *"That's where you've been while I've been suffering! Feeding your face!"* I just smiled at her and noted mental odds that everyone of her tests would be absolutely normal, yet demand to be admitted anyway.
*Of course I was right.*

**1:00 p.m.** Every patient I saw today had been hurt or sick for "three days." I wondered what the hell happened three days ago. I thought about staying inside and hiding every three days.

**1:15 p.m.** One of our very frequent flyers arrived by EMS and said, *"this time, I'm really gonna kill myself! I mean it!"* Her only answer was the unit clerk's gum popping and the ER nurse saying, *"Oh, promises, promises! Why do you get our hopes up like that? If you want, I'll help you do it if you really mean it. I mean, we have WAYS of killing you that no one can detect. That way your family gets the life insurance money !"* The patient demanded to be taken to another hospital where "they understand me better." Two points for the nurse as it almost worked. But EMS refused to move her.

**1:45 p.m.** Received a transfer patient the on-call doc had accepted from another hospital. Despite hospital by-laws that HE had to see them and admit them from the ER, he called and asked the nurses to see if I *"would be a good boy and admit her for me and I'll see her later. I'm awfully packed at the office!"* I looked at our packed waiting room and sighed. Later that night, he did it three more times.

**2:00 p.m.** Code on the floor in the long-term care wing. I never understood before what the term "Chinese fire drill" meant but now I did. God bless the ER nurses; at least they knew what Epi was! Not that it mattered. The patient had obviously been dead for some time and someone just now noticed it. I also realized that at every code, there was always the same hugely obese nurse/therapist that showed up, but no one knew who she was. And I swore I'd seen her at other hospitals too. Even during my residency, the upper level residents pointed her out. *Weird.* No one ever had the nerve to ask who she was.

**2:40 p.m.** Two MVA's arrived by ambulance; both from the same wreck but not in the same car. Despite my warning her not to, the charge nurse put them next to each other. Instant dueling symptoms and both tried to out-moan the other. Family started to show up and the yelling quickly escalated to threats and fists. Someone paged security and when the 85- year-old guard finally arrived, we had to put him on a monitor for chest pain.

**3:15 p.m.** Realized that the urologist was out of the country on vacation when all of his patients started showing up with kidney stones and acute urinary retention. The covering urologist was in another town. *Scchhwing!!*

**3:40 p.m.** Nurse handed me the phone; a pregnant lady who was due the next day wanted to come in for "a checkup" today. It seemed that she hadn't seen her OB/GYN doc in four months since *"we got into a fight."* The nurses were laughing at me as they watched me try to explain to the lady what the facts of life were. Did I previously say, *"God bless the ER nurses?"*

**3:55 p.m.** EMS brought in a toothache by ambulance. The patient was upset that he came by ambulance and was being put into the waiting room! *"I thought you had to see me right away if I came by ambulance!"* he shouted.

**4:00 p.m.** School has now let out. *Let the games begin!*

**4:15 p.m.** EMS called with CPR in progress on a 95-year-old nursing home patient. I asked the obvious, *"Ummm, what's the patient's code status?"* No one knew. When the patient arrived, there in the stack of paperwork was her Do Not Resuscitate orders. The code ended, EMS was mad and the nurses called the nursing home to chew them out.

**4:25 p.m.** During our "code," one of the frequent flyers with back pain walked into the room as we were doing CPR and wanted to know *"when the hell someone's gonna see me !"* I told him that if his heart stopped, we'd move him to the front of the line.

**4:55 p.m.** Tried to use the restroom again. I got smart this time and used the nurse's restroom; they couldn't find me.

**5:30 p.m.** A 12-year-old boy who fell off of a fence with an obviously broken arm. His mid-forearm was angulated up at 45 degrees! Now I had to call the after-hours on-call orthopedist. Unfortunately, it was Dr. "Need to Retire" who told me to splint him and he'd see him tomorrow at the office. I spent several minutes telling him how that would not be a good idea but he hung up on me. By a small miracle, another orthopedist happened to walk by and I hugged his shoes begging him to see the kid. He did, set the arm and I offered to give him my first born in gratitude.

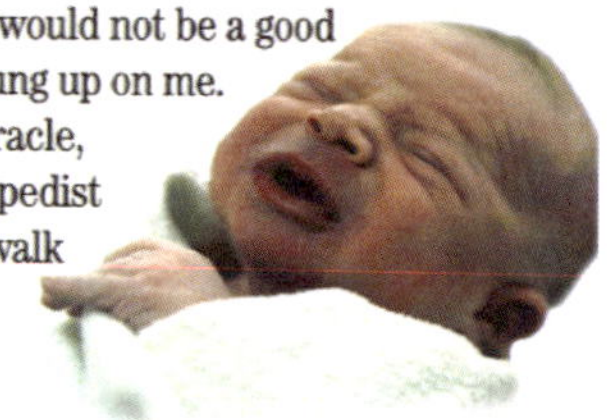

**6:12 p.m.** Hospital operator called a Code Blue for the ER waiting room!? Everyone rushed there to find no one in any distress! It seemed the operator was not taking her schizophrenia meds and was hallucinating. Then the administrator showed up wanting to know why we had patients in serious condition sitting in the waiting room!

**6:40 p.m.** 80-year-old, little old lady came in with chest pain; actually a delightful patient who downplayed her symptoms. I was worried because she was nice! Of course, 30 minutes later, we were cardioverting her. Fortunately she did okay and ended up in the unit. Isn't there a law about the chance of a patient surviving being inversely proportional to their value to society?

**7:00 p.m.** *Halftime!!* I was halfway thru my shift – only twelve more hours to go. +

***The rest of the 24-hour shift will continue in our February issue.***

## MORE TRUE STORIES OF MEDICINE

# THANK GOODNESS IT HAD A WIDE BRIM

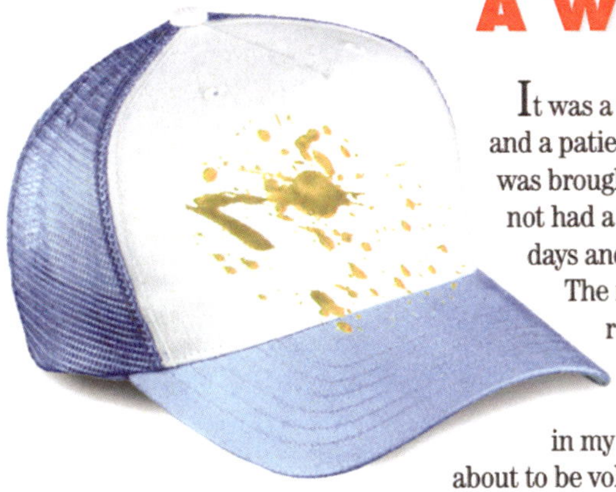

It was a typical day at the walk-in clinic and a patient from the local nursing home was brought in for abdominal pain. He had not had a bowel movement for several days and had a history of constipation. The nursing staff had tried the usual routine of laxatives, softeners, enemas, etc. with no results. I got the usual quiver and cramp in my stomach knowing my finger was about to be volunteered to relieve this gentleman. Thank God I attended 20+ years of school to qualify myself for the job.

Luckily, the gentleman was accompanied by his son who generously helped in getting him undressed for the "procedure." After several minutes the *pooecotomy* was complete and the patient was feeling much better. I asked him to get dressed and noted his hat had taken some *shrapnel* and asked the son not to put his hat on.

Just before they departed I went to check on the gentleman and he was already proudly wearing the poo-stained cap. At this point his dignity and mine were tarnished enough, so I shook his hand and sent him on his way.

I am sure the nurse who undressed him at bedtime raised an eyebrow wondering just what happened at the office!! +

# EYE-OPENER

I was getting set for minor eye surgery – removal of some granulomae from my eyelid. While scheduling with the surgeon/ophthalmologist, he said my surgery would be at about 11 a.m., and that I'd be his seventh surgery that morning.

*"Wow,"* I said, *"aren't you going to be pretty tired by then?"* (I wanted a surgeon who was fresh and perky).

He answered, ***"Hell no, by then I'll just be sobering up!"*** +

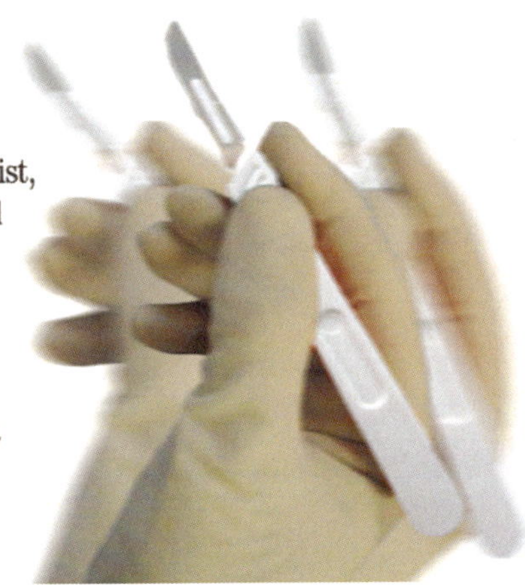

**While they chose "Strong Medicine for America," the *American Academy of Family Physicians* had a lot of rejected slogans:**

***Family Practice – It's What's for Medicine!***

***I Can't Believe They're Not Specialists!***

***Family Doctors: You Know They Care. Otherwise They'd Be Radiologists.***

***Strong – Yet Surprisingly Soft***

***The Other White Doctors***

***Do You Really Want A Doctor Who Drives A Nicer Car Than You?***

***Low Prices, Low Morale – Always***

***We May Not Be Specialists But Damn It We're Still Special Too.***

***McMedicine – I'm Lovin' It!***

***Family Doctors: Speaking English For Over 200 Years!***

***(And maybe a few more.)***

## PLACEBO JOURNAL MEDICAL ALGORITHM OF REALITY

# "It's Personal."

Patient will not state his complaints to your staff, but instead tells them, ***"It's personal."***

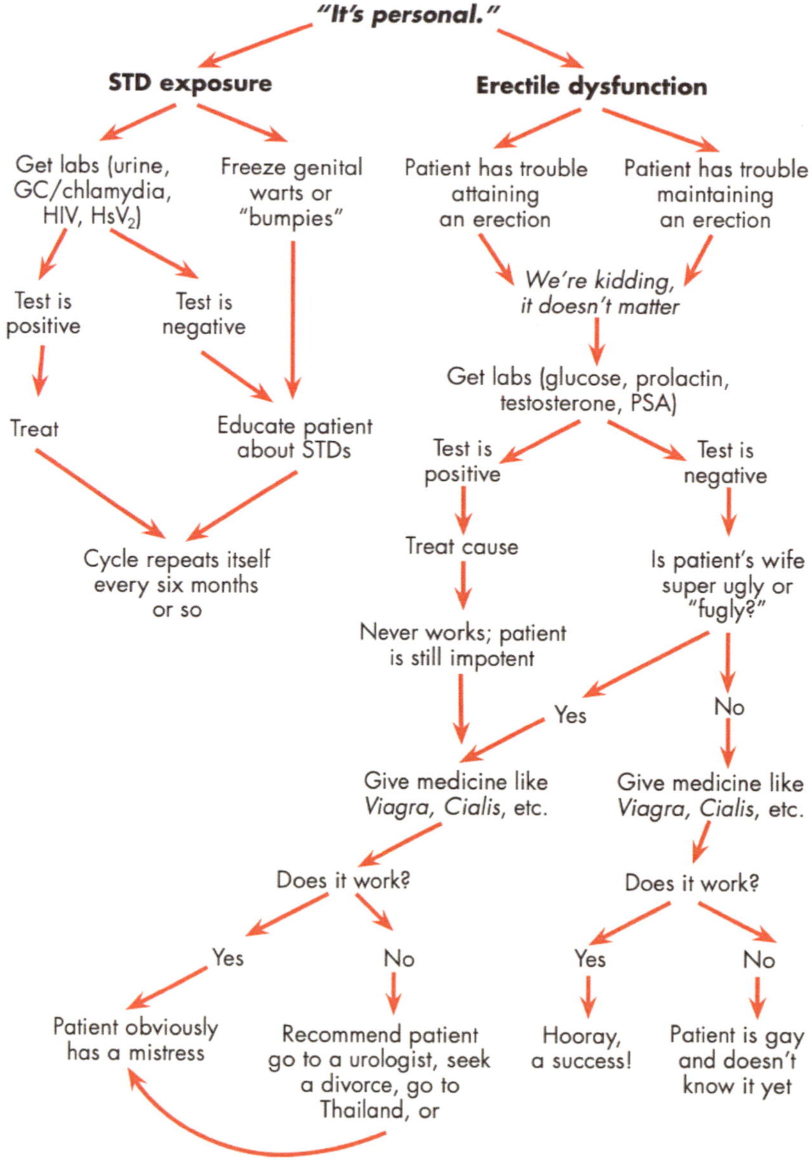


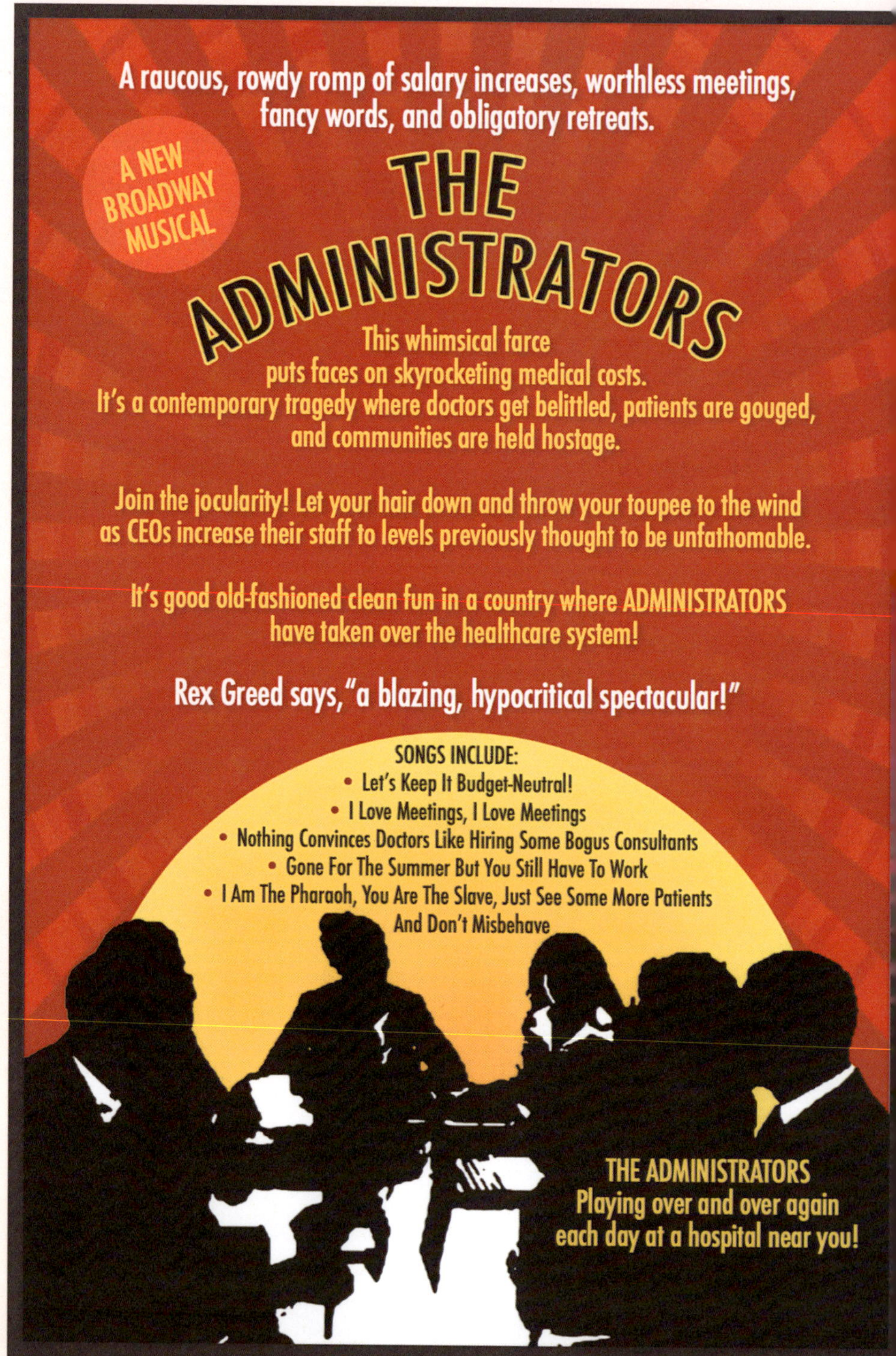

A raucous, rowdy romp of salary increases, worthless meetings, fancy words, and obligatory retreats.
A NEW BROADWAY MUSICAL
THE ADMINISTRATORS
This whimsical farce puts faces on skyrocketing medical costs.
It's a contemporary tragedy where doctors get belittled, patients are gouged, and communities are held hostage.
Join the jocularity! Let your hair down and throw your toupee to the wind as CEOs increase their staff to levels previously thought to be unfathomable.
It's good old-fashioned clean fun in a country where ADMINISTRATORS have taken over the healthcare system!
Rex Greed says, "a blazing, hypocritical spectacular!"
SONGS INCLUDE:
• Let's Keep It Budget-Neutral!
• I Love Meetings, I Love Meetings
• Nothing Convinces Doctors Like Hiring Some Bogus Consultants
• Gone For The Summer But You Still Have To Work
• I Am The Pharaoh, You Are The Slave, Just See Some More Patients And Don't Misbehave
THE ADMINISTRATORS
Playing over and over again each day at a hospital near you!

# HOPEFULLY NOT!

A couple days ago I had a pleasant visit with a mid 30-year-old man who had a bump on his leg which was worrisome to him. He'd hit his knee playing with one of his children about a week ago and was concerned about possibly having a blood clot. After examining him and reassuring him it that was just a hematoma, I told him it would most likely resolve on its own.

Upon leaving he thanked me and said, ***"We'll be seeing you."***

I paused a minute and then said, *"I think I'd find a different phrase to use at the end of the conversation, considering your occupation."*

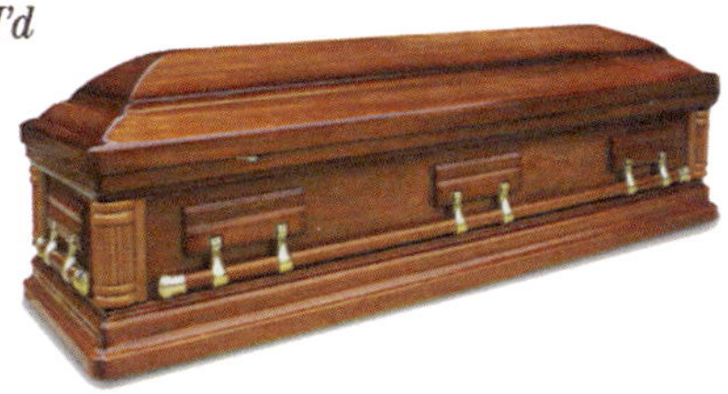

He thought about it and started laughing . . . he is our town's mortician. ✚

# WHAT WERE WE THINKING?

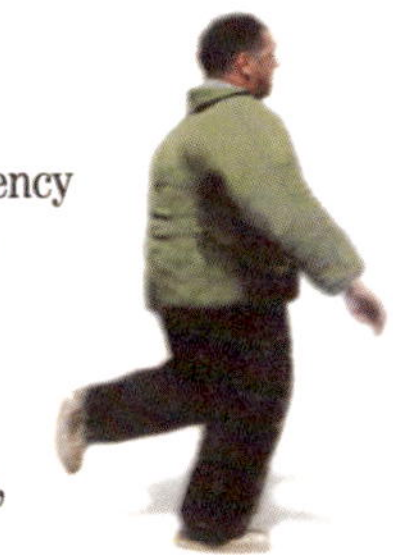

Back in 1987, I was in the third year of my psychiatric residency and was doing a rotation at a large urban ER. One of the patients I was attending to was a LARGE, ANGRY man who was not only acutely psychotic but he was high on crack as well. He was also well known to the staff for prior episodes of aggression.

While I was out of the room consulting with a fellow resident, this LARGE, ANGRY, PSYCHOTIC, HOPPED-UP patient eloped from the ER. The other resident and I promptly began to chase him and ran outside after him. As he got further away from us, we both stopped for a moment and reflected on the situation. I turned to my fellow resident and said, ***"Wait a minute, what are we going to do if we catch him?"***

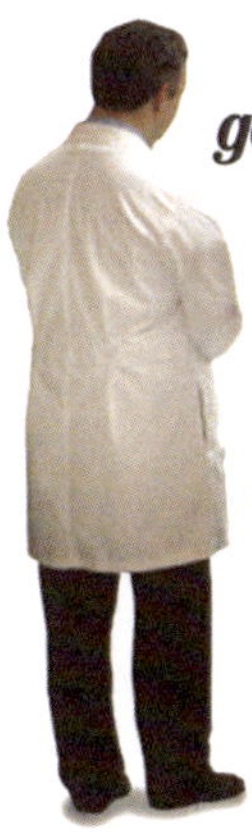

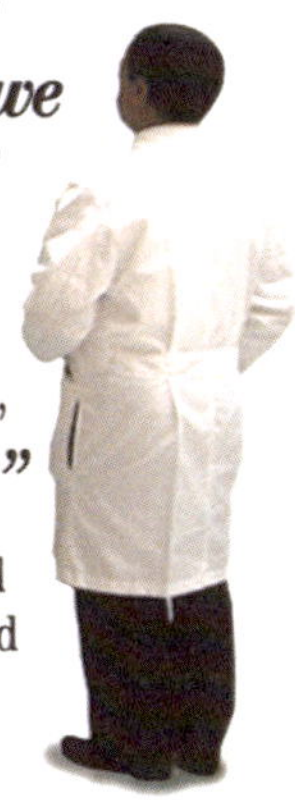

He looked at me, shrugged his shoulders, and said, ***"You're right."*** and we both turned around and returned to the ER.

NOTE: Police were notified and the patient was apprehended shortly thereafter and returned to the ER. Needless to say, he was placed in a secure room and I am alive today to tell this tale. ✚



# GETTING STUCK

I am a medical intern in a program where a lot of our patients are native Spanish speakers, and I, in the local vernacular, am an east coast *"gringa."* Sure, I took Spanish in college but never became more fluent than such useful phrases as, *"Que lastima mi computadora es descompuesta!"* (How sad my computer has malfunctioned) and *"Donde esta los banos?"* (Where are the bathrooms?) The latter actually being quite useful.

In July we had a month long down and dirty medical Spanish class for the new interns to get us up to speed and I was feeling pretty good about the whole thing. Seeing patents as a real MD and what not and hable en espanol tambien.

Not long after my first month I meet this gentleman who cut his hand jumping over a certain fence covered in razor wire and he needed a few stitches in his hand before going back. I gathered my supplies and thoughtfully explained, all in Spanish, to the gentleman what was about to happen during the procedure, including how many stitches he was about to get.

*"Ha tenido puntas?"* (You need stitches?), I asked.

Strange look from the patient. He nodded no.

*"Usted nessicita siete or ocho puntas."* (You need 7 or 8 stitches), I repeat.

*"Verdad? Aqui?"* (Really, here?), he replied with an even stranger and now hopeful look from the patient.

I heard the snicker from the border patrol agent behind me as he told me,

***"Puntadas ma'am, not puntas. Puntas are whores."***

Oh well, our patient was a lot less happy about getting stuck then, well, doing the sticking himself. I was happy not to be taken in for solicitation as I'm sure that's not the first time I made that mistake. ✚

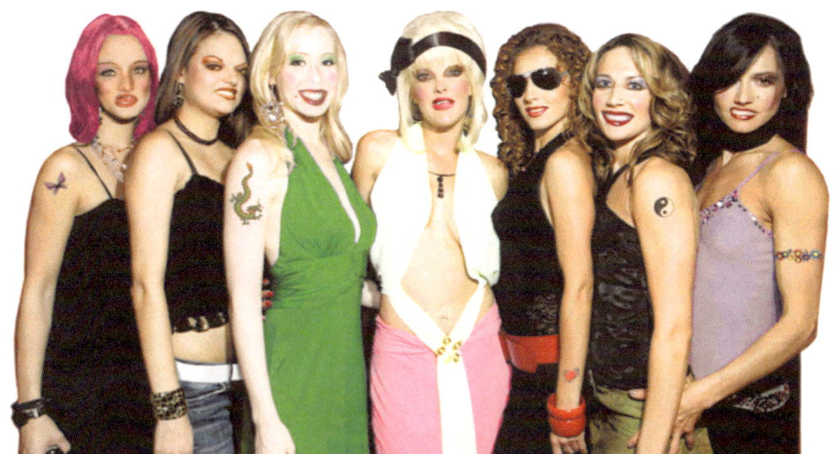

# COTTAGE CHEESE

Every once in a while, something happens to you that changes the way you think, feel, and eat for the rest of your life. My life-changing event took place when I worked for a private ambulance company. My partner and I were called to a nursing home to pick up a cute little old lady and take her to the hospital for some tests.

We stopped at the nurses' station, grabbed the patient's paperwork and headed down the hallway, weaving our gurney around wheelchairs filled with slumped over sleeping old people.

When we arrived at the room, our little old lady was just finishing her lunch. I walked up to the side of her bed just as she was pushing a huge spoonful of cottage cheese into her mouth.

I waved and said loudly, *"Hello."*

She looked over at the empty space next to me, so I made a big giant wave, like I was in a parade and she saw me. I think.

*"Are you ready to go to the hospital?"*

She didn't seem to notice and looked back down at her cottage cheese.

A tiny little nurse came in the room and announced, *"She doesn't hear too well."*

She stood on her tiptoes next to our patient and in a voice that would make an Army drill sergeant proud yelled, *"THESE BOYS ARE TAKING YOU TO THE HOSPITAL."*

I jumped back covering my ears and yelled, *"Good God Almighty!"*

Her voice was so loud I heard it echo down the hall, *"take . . . take . . . hospital . . . hospital . . . hospital."*

The sweet little old lady didn't look up but just nodded. She was intent on getting that last spoonful of cottage cheese in her mouth.

Nurse Bullhorn opened her mouth to say something and I covered my ears again. But in her normal voice said, *"She's all yours,"* and left the room.

The next twenty minutes were spent yelling at the top of our lungs and jumping around like clowns trying to coax this little old lady to slide onto our gurney so we could leave. She, on the other hand was more interested in finding the large curds of cottage cheese she had spilled on her shirt and getting each one in her mouth.

On the way to the hospital I couldn't help but notice that she seemed to be having trouble with something in her mouth Something was stuck in a tooth or behind her dentures and she couldn't get it dislodged with her tongue. Her mouth was in perpetual motion.

I was going to ask her if she would like to rinse out her mouth, but my voice was hoarse and my throat was sore from yelling at her earlier so I just continued doing my paperwork.

When we arrived at the hospital emergency room entrance, Larry and I pulled the gurney out of the back of the ambulance and set it on the ground. I bent over and asked in a normal voice, *"How are you doing?"*

Then I remembered who we were dealing with and I put my face directly in front of her face. Taking a deep breath and opening my mouth up wide I began to yell, *"HOW . . ."*

**That's as far as I got.**

At times like this you have to marvel at what an amazing organ the brain is. Sensing imminent danger, my brain went into emergency mode. Time and space was now an ultra slow motion movie. In that split second of time, I saw her mouth suddenly stop moving. Whatever she had been hunting for with her tongue, she had found it. I saw the tip of her tongue protrude just a little bit between her dry, cracked lips. Her cheeks puffed out from the increase of air pressure in her mouth. She looked up at the empty space next to my head and then a huge curd of cottage cheese exploded from her mouth. In slow motion the curd came at me, like a huge asteroid tumbling through space, throwing off little balls of spit in all directions . . . slowly, tumbling, towards my open mouth.

I could hear my brain trying to warn me. In a deep, slurred, drug-induced dream like voice it said, ***"Sheee hawked a looogey. Miiiike cloooose yourrrrrr mouuuuth! Ohhhh NOOOOO! Close youurrrr mouuuth!"*** Time raced back to normal as the cottage cheese asteroid entered my mouth's atmosphere, became a cottage cheese meteor, and slammed directly into the back of my throat.

I immediately made the international sign for choking. Clutching my hands around my neck, I stumbled backwards and dropped to my knees, gagging and coughing, trying to dislodge the curd from the back of my throat. There are seven different types of shock. I was in five of them. This was the grossest thing that had ever happened to me in my entire life.

My partner had witnessed the whole thing and he turned white as a ghost. His hands instinctively made the international sign for choking around his neck and he too began gagging. This is known as 'sympathetic choking.'

I was now rolling around on the ground about to lose consciousness, not from lack of oxygen but from the realization of the enormity of the grossness of what just happened to me. I tried giving myself the *Heimlich Maneuver* by throwing myself against the side of the gurney. That dislodged the curd from the back of my throat and moved it into my mouth. I could feel with my tongue the texture of the cottage cheese curd.

This was the second grossest thing that had ever happened to me in my entire life. I wasted no time in spitting every molecule of moisture out of my mouth, but not before I reminded myself that this curd of cottage cheese had just been in that lady's 90-year-old mouth.

**I began to dry heave.**

My partner saw this, rolled around the side of the ambulance and also started dry heaving. That is known as 'sympathetic heaving.'

A crowd was now forming around us. Doctors and nurses wondered why these two highly trained medics had abandoned such a sweet little old lady and were lying on the ground heaving their guts up.

One of the nurses came over to me and asked, *"Are you okay?"*

In between heaves I sputtered, *"Everything's fine, show's over, move along."*

Getting to my feet, I tried to pretend nothing had happened. It was difficult to pull it off since I was retching every few seconds. I wanted to rinse out my mouth with gasoline.

I looked at Grandma Spitty-Poo. She was oblivious to the near death experience she had just caused. She just laid there on the gurney searching the front of her shirt for more of her lunch.

I haven't eaten cottage cheese in over five years now. It took me two years and a lot of therapy before I would even walk down the dairy aisle at the supermarket. I used to like cottage cheese. I used to like a lot of things: drinking milk, spitting watermelon seeds, talking to people without flinching and keeping my hand over my mouth, eating white chocolate-covered raisins, and meeting little old ladies. ✚

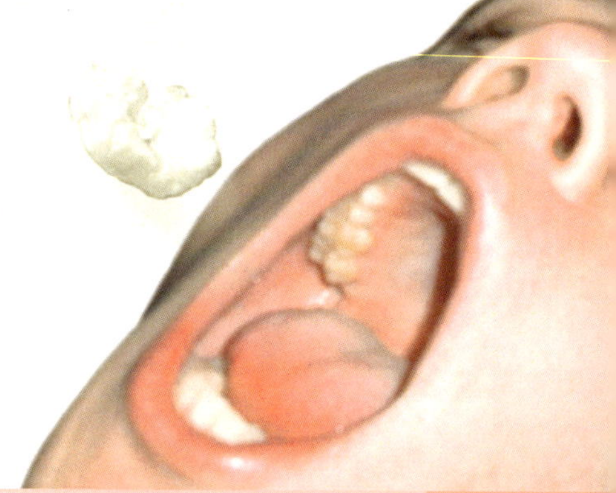

*What if there was an online service for physicians only, where you could meet other single physicians?*

*And what if the site had the technology to scientifically and cytologically match you with the perfect physician?*

**NOW THERE IS! INTRODUCING:**

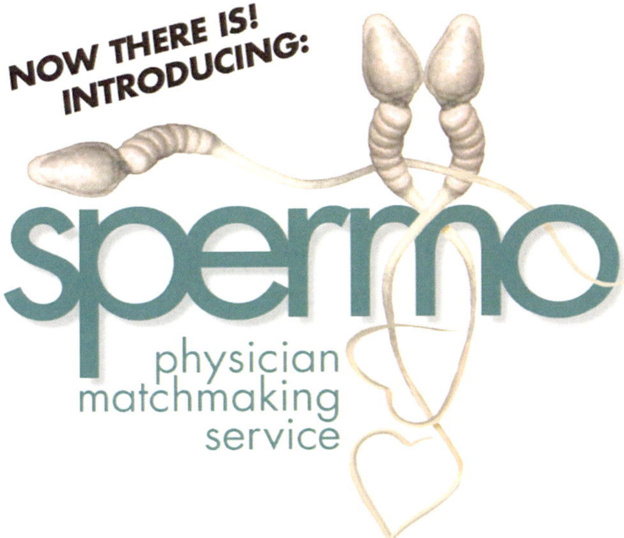

spermo™

physician matchmaking service

***THE PHYSICIAN-ONLY IN-VITRO MATCHMAKING SERVICE!***

Staffed by world-renowned experts, ***SPERMO*** will match you to your physician mate using TWO scientifically proven methods; the Common Sense Approach and the Cellular Compatibility Technology Approach.

Log on to ***www.SPERMO.com*** today and find that special doctor who understands that you are more than just you. *You're a doctor too!*

***SPERMO:*** *Because only doctors truly understand (and want to mate with) other doctors.*

**SENILOQUEL** is an antipsychotic drug that you can trust to help calm **aggressive behavior** and **agitation.**

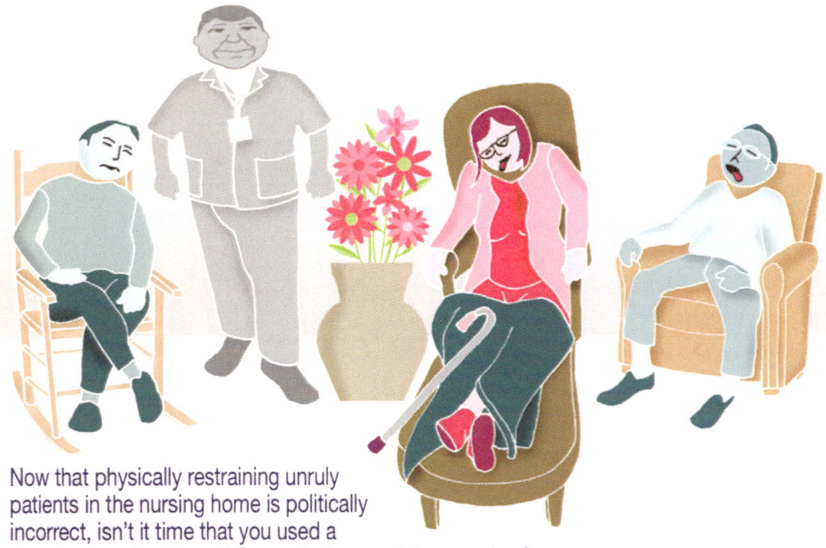

Now that physically restraining unruly patients in the nursing home is politically incorrect, isn't it time that you used a chemical handcuff in order to make it run a little smoother?

**SENILOQUEL** makes your patients calm down without the annoying need for human touch or compassion.

**SENILOQUEL** stabilizes the moods of nursing home patients and it is effective in making many residents sit, stay, and even roll over. In fact, we guarantee to put Grandpa to sleep.

Why hire extra staff when it is easier to get reimbursed for giving patients extra pills?

There are some Alzheimer's patients for whom nonpharmacological approaches simply don't work. For those patients, there's **SENILOQUEL**!

**SENILOQUEL is not approved for dementia-related psychosis but it sure does work!*

**IMPORTANT SAFETY INFORMATION:**
SENILOQUEL does have some mood-stabilizing properties. It also causes Neuroleptic Malignant Syndrome (NMS), tardive dyskinesia (TD), hyperglycemia, and a whole host of blood disorders but who really is going to know if SENILOQUEL is the culprit? SENILOQUEL is not approved by the FDA for, well, anything.

Seniloquel®
quityapping fumerate

**PJ PHARMACEUTICALS**
*The Realistic Drug Company*

# NOW THAT'S SERVICE

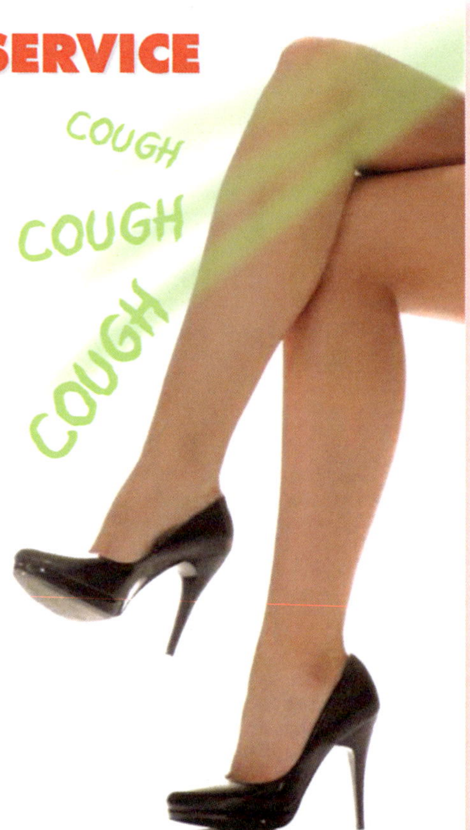


Years ago I went to see my doctor one morning on my way in to work. I had been sick with a nagging cough for about three weeks. So, I broke down, got an early appointment, and dressed for work. My doctor's office had two waiting areas. After you were "promoted" from the mass waiting area, you went to a smaller area with a sofa and a couple of seats. I got my "promotion" and was sad to see that when I got to the next level there were three other sickly souls in front of me. They all looked ill, while I was looking fairly good for someone with a annoying cough.

The doctor's office door opened, and there he was . . . my doctor. *"Hallelujah,"* I thought, *"he is here, and he's going to start seeing us."*

He took one look at the sea of sickly patients, and amongst that sea was me – young, blonde, and in a suit with high heels. He took one look at me, smiled, and motioned me in. *OH, THE LUCK!* (I did feel guilty, but hey, I had to get to work – these poor souls were just going to go home and crawl back in to bed – which is where I really wanted to be).

I went in to his office and sat down across from him at his desk. Suddenly it dawned on me, we weren't in the examining room. We were in his office, a place I had never been before. Still not catching on, I thought, *"Hmmm . . . this must be a new approach he is trying. Interview the patient in the office, then send her into the adjoining exam room."*

He leaned back in his chair, smiled flirtatiously at me, and very casually asked me how I'd been. Then it hit me . . . ***. . . he thought I was a drug rep!***

Not knowing what to do, I started in with a discussion of my disgusting, nagging cough and how long it had been hanging around. You should have seen the look on his face when he put it all together. *I know he had to be thankful for the adjoining exam room!*

I was nice and pretended like everything was normal. I decided not to embarrass him any further by asking him if he always made the less attractive, sickly patients wait while he chatted it up with the drug reps. We went into the exam room where he quickly listened to my cough and wrote me a script. ✚

## PJ MEDICAL ALGORITHM OF REALITY

# Childhood ADHD & Autism Spectrum Disorder

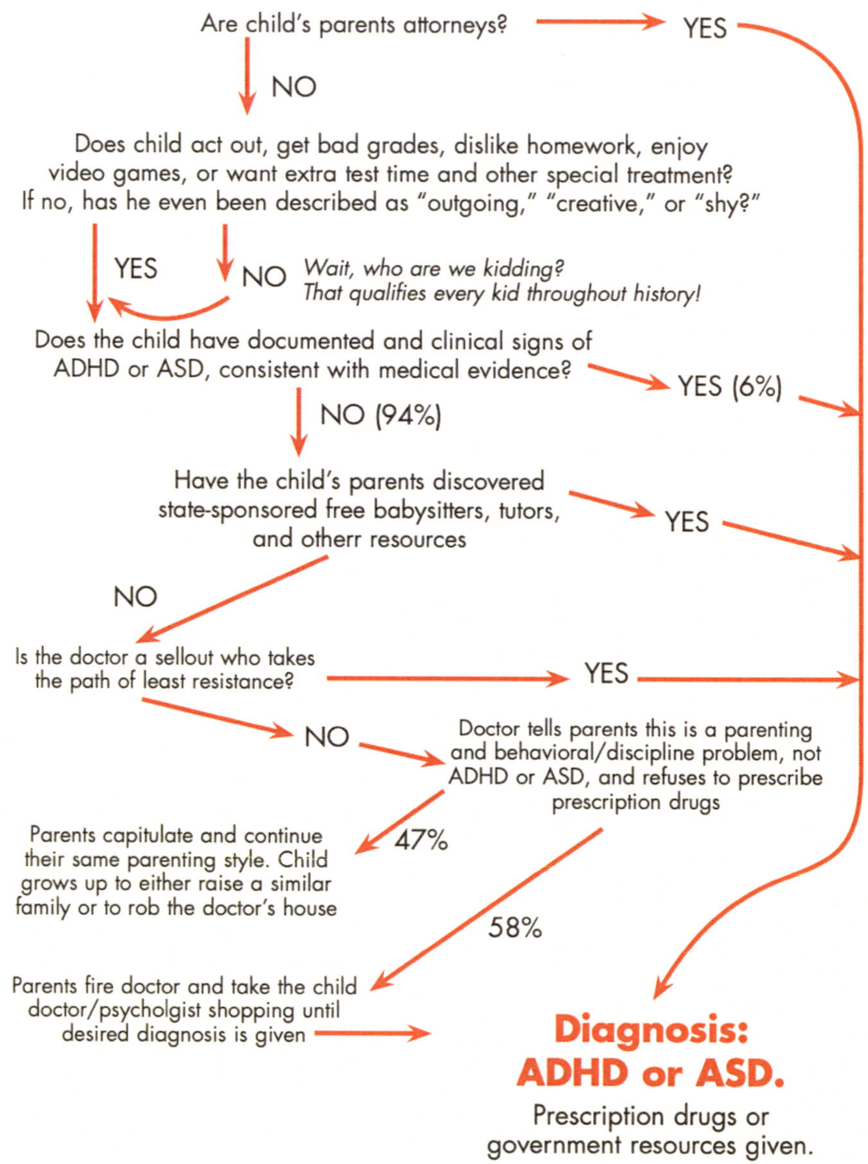

## TRUE STORIES OF MEDICINE

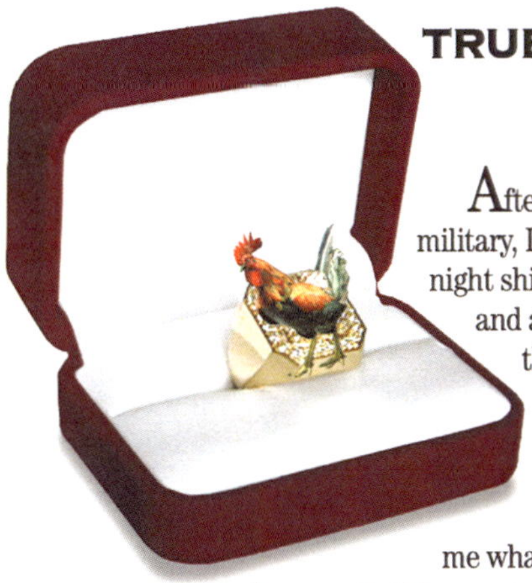

## CUTTER

After almost 20 years as an ER nurse in the military, I thought I had seen everything. During the night shift, a young soldier approached the triage desk and asked to see the doctor. I questioned him as to the nature of his problem, and the young man turned red and mumbled about something being "stuck." Curious, I took him to a room, handed him a gown and asked him to disrobe. After I returned, I asked him to show me what was stuck and where.

Apparently this young man had bought a "cock ring" and placed it on his member. The problem was that it was too small and would not come off, cutting into the flesh and causing it to become dusky in color. Non-plussed I stated, *"No problem I can fix that,"* and I removed the ring cutter from the drawer. I told him, *"I will just cut it off."*

Apparently this poor kid thought I was intending to cut off his penis and not the ring because he got extremely pale and then passed out falling off the gurney. He subsequently sustained a two-inch head laceration that required a head CT and sutures! ✚

## PBM FELONY

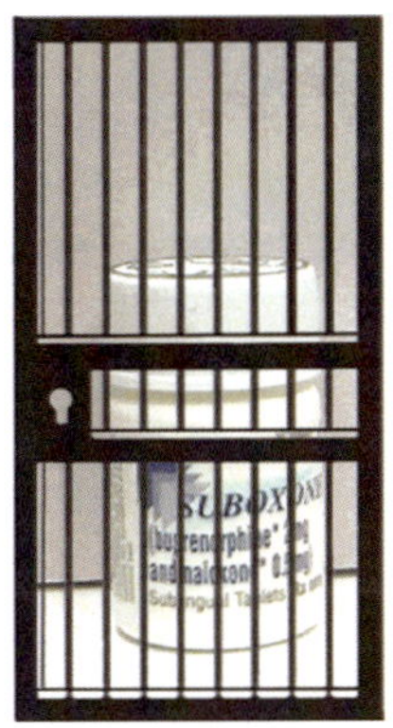

I am licensed to prescribe *Suboxone*. This is a narcotic used to treat opioid dependency. It requires a special course for non-addiction specialists. The idea is to reduce the use of methadone as well as methadone clinics and allow more freedom. *Suboxone* is a Class III opiate while *Methadone* is a Class II.

I received a call from a PBM (pharmacy benefit manager). They challenged the use of *Suboxone* and insisted that *Methadone* was the preferred drug. I explained, as above, why I wanted *Suboxone*. The lady at the other end insisted it was not going to be approved. Rather, they would authorize my prescribing *Methadone* for the patient's addiction. I asked her for her name, address and phone number. She asked why. I explained she had asked me to commit a federal felony and I thought that itself was a felony. She said she had not. I explained that I am licensed for treatment of opiate addiction with *Suboxone*. The use of methadone for treatment of addiction requires a different license and certification as an addiction specialist. Not having these credentials, my writing for *Methadone* for addiction is a federal felony. She hung up.

I received approval for *Suboxone* treatment a few minutes later. ✚

## Find out how our AccuSham Holter Monitor can benefit your practice.

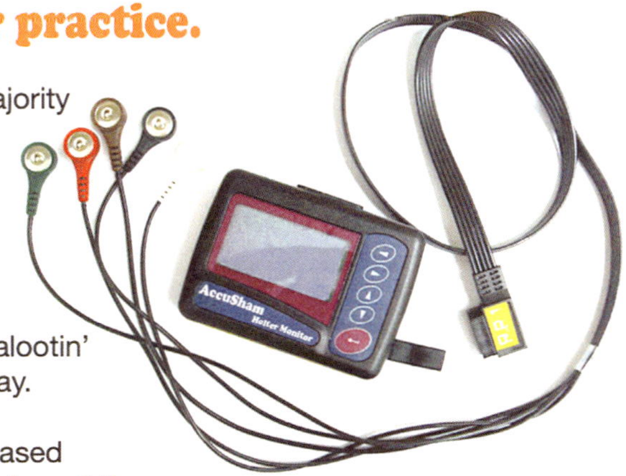


The overwhelming majority of patients who claim to have palpitations really have no cause. Heck, we all know that. In fact, most of them never have anything that even gets picked up on those high falootin' real Holter monitors anyway.

Our faux digital, PC based AccuSham Holter Monitor has all the wires, leads, bells, and whistles of the real thing but never records a thing!

**ONLY $24.95**

Compare to the real ones that cost almost $5000!

***Is it cost-effective for your practice?* You betcha!**
***Is it time-consuming?* Not anymore.**

The AccuSham Holter Monitor comes with:

- A fancy looking shell from discarded and outdated real Holter monitors.
- Five new leads (green, red, brown, black, and white) that look extremely professional.
- A printed event report that easily can be reproduced and placed in any patient's chart or EMR (CD ROM extra).

Our motto:

**Why go to extremes when it's all from caffeine?**

The AccSham Holter Monitor is so cheap you can place it on any patient and still claim your $200 reimbursement with CPT code 93230*

**This is fraud and we really don't recommend doing this.*

**Placebo Device Depot**

Toll Free 1-555-ARRHYTHMIA

www.placebodevicedepot.com

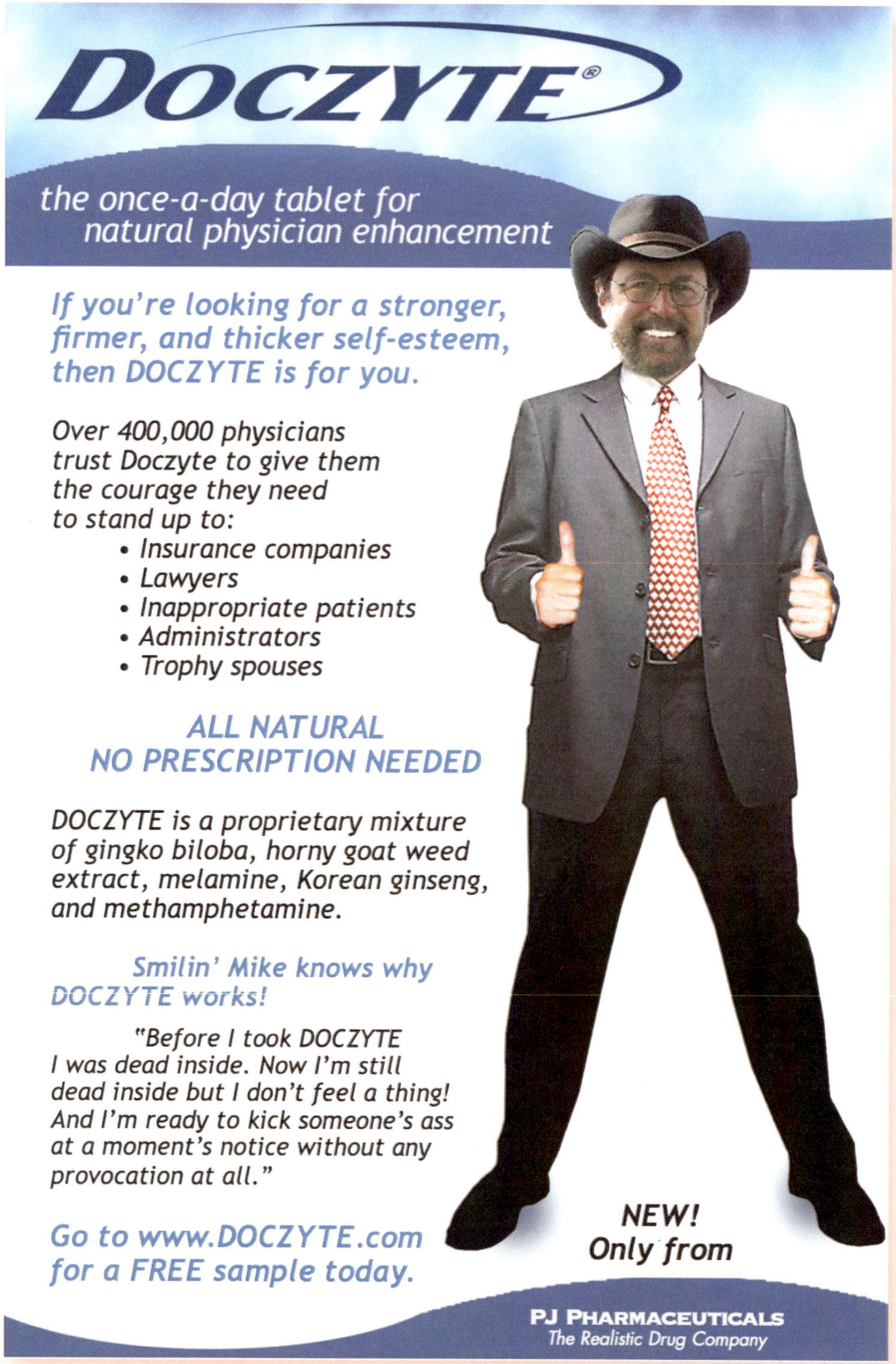
DOCZYTE®
the once-a-day tablet for
natural physician enhancement
If you're looking for a stronger, firmer, and thicker self-esteem, then DOCZYTE is for you.
Over 400,000 physicians trust Doczyte to give them the courage they need to stand up to:
• Insurance companies
• Lawyers
• Inappropriate patients
• Administrators
• Trophy spouses
ALL NATURAL
NO PRESCRIPTION NEEDED
DOCZYTE is a proprietary mixture of gingko biloba, horny goat weed extract, melamine, Korean ginseng, and methamphetamine.
Smilin' Mike knows why DOCZYTE works!
"Before I took DOCZYTE I was dead inside. Now I'm still dead inside but I don't feel a thing! And I'm ready to kick someone's ass at a moment's notice without any provocation at all."
Go to www.DOCZYTE.com for a FREE sample today.
NEW!
Only from
PJ PHARMACEUTICALS
The Realistic Drug Company

# SOUR GRAPES

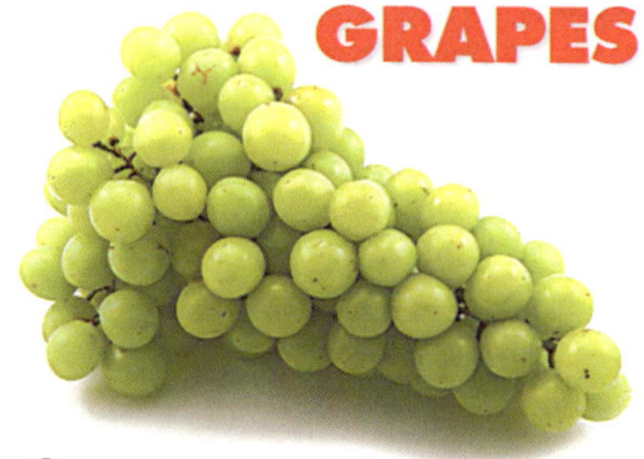

Several years ago, I received a small segment of bowel from an obstruction release and segmental resection. I am a pathologist.

When I opened it, it was full of beautiful intact California green grapes. Uncharacteristically, I actually went up and talked to a live patient.

I told her the situation and asked her what she'd been eating.

*"Raisin bran."*

I then noticed she had dentures.

*"Did you have your dentures in when you ate the raisin bran?"*

*"No, I let it get soft in the milk and then ate it."*

The unchewed raisins apparently had re-hydrated in the small bowel.

The patient did fine and promised to always chew up her raisin bran in the future. ✚

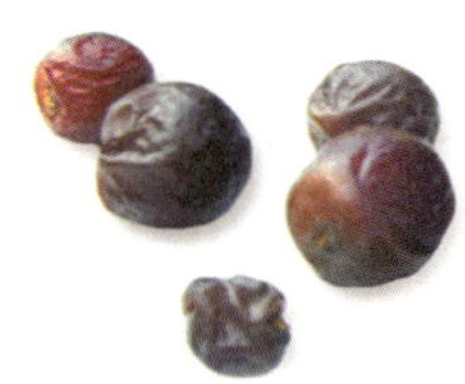

## TRUE STORY

# AND OFF HE WENT TO THE GOLF COURSE

After completing a hip pinning, Orthopod Dr. DeChuck *(not his real name)* took the patient to the Recovery Room and then retired to the surgeons' locker room to change. At this point, the patient regurgitated the eggs, bacon, orange juice, coffee, and grits that he neglected to tell DeChuck that he had for breakfast. This prompted the usual drill of suction, reintubation, and attention to cardiac issues that frequently accompany these events. Dr. DeChuck returned to the RR and observed all these efforts for a good three or four minutes before pronouncing, ***"Well, the leg is straight,"*** and then headed off to the golf course.

Epilogue:

Fast-forward many years later and I'm having a cup of coffee in the surgeons' lounge and commenting to no one in particular about the economy, the Middle East, terrorism, and the *Rangers* losing the *World Series*, when an old friend and long-time colleague put down the *WSJ* and observed, ***"At least the leg is straight."***

This has become the comforting comment in situations when things head south. ✚

# The Second Annual North American Allergy Conference *and Singles Cruise from Oregon to Alaska*

## Join us this August 5th to 9th for the hypoallergenic ride of a lifetime.

AGENDA:

**Sneeze or Sniffle: You Be the Judge**
by Ryan Phima, MD

**Anaphylactic Reactions in the Office – How to Call 911**
by Artie Caria, MD

**Dust Mites – Why We Can't Blame Everything on Them Anymore**
by Urshio L. Skratchin, MD

**Angioedema – That Ain't a Good Thing**
by Jennifer Hymenoptera, MD

**Why Calling Ourselves Immunologists Makes Us Sound Really Smart**
by Cletus Dummhead, MD

**Dermatographism – How to Really Make Some Cool Designs**
by X. Cory Ashun, MD

**RAST Testing – Is there anyone you shouldn't be doing it on? And other stupid questions**
by Polly Posis, MD

**Asthma – Stealing the Thunder from the Pulmonologists**
by Lee Aktiv Rundizeez, MD

**Food Allergies – Why We Still Have No Idea What We Are Doing With This One**
by Noah Glootins, MD

**Environmental Controls – Why No Patient Ever Follows Our Advice**
by Franc Legionaiire, MD

**Eosinophils – Should This Take Over As Our New Cellular Mascot?**
by Khan Tak Durm Ititus, MD

**Peanuts – The Ultimate Evil!**
by Al Lergan, MD

**Venom Immunotherapy – The Newest Techniques** with our special guest speaker and esteemed Voodoo Priest Mr. Abdah Bosuti

**Rhinosinusitis – What Rhino? Where's the Rhino? But, seriously folks, we can treat this**
by Eosin Philbin, MD

**How to Convince Patients You Are A Real Doctor Or At Least Get A Date With One Of Them**
by Keynote Dinner Speaker Doug Farrago, MD

### AFTER THE LEARNIN' COMES THE PARTYIN'

Dance your booty off with our special cover band made up entirely of fellow allergists:

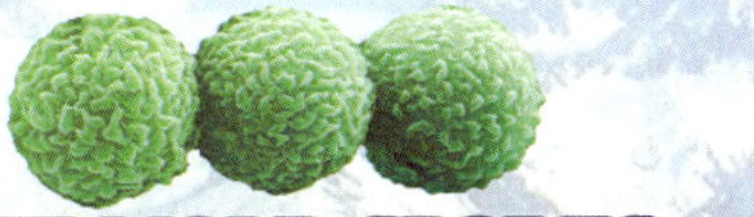

### THE MOLD SPORES

singing songs by such groups as *Weezer* and *Kansas* (including "Dust in the Wind")

Don't forget the other activities on the cruise which include such great games as:

**Guess The Pollen Levels**

**Spin the Epipen**

**Zinc Oxide Face Painting**

**Photomicrograph Triva Game with Slides!**

**I, Spy Molds, Grass, Trees and Weeds**

Cost for members only $1495

Call our offices today at 1-555-ALL-ERGY to book yourself a ticket*. You just might get lucky on this trip – *lucky enough to get some great CME credits, that is!*

** Free plastic dust mite bed cover sheets for the first 100 who ask!*

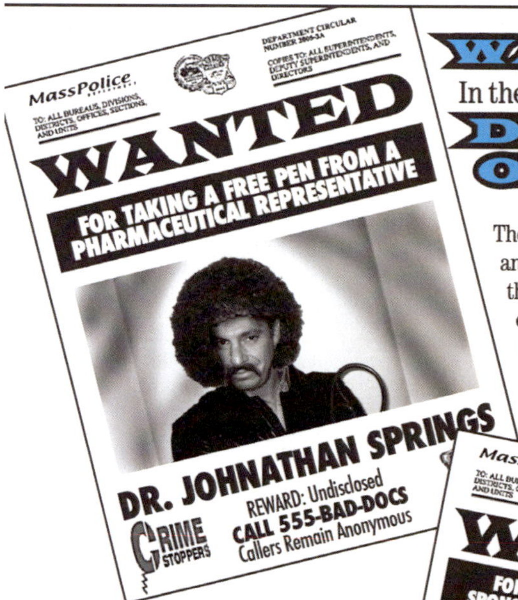


# WANTED

In the state of Massachusetts

# DEAD OR ALIVE

These physicians remain at large and need to be apprehended for their perceived conflict of interest, embellished crimes against humanity, and concocted notion that they are the cause for the increased cost of healthcare.

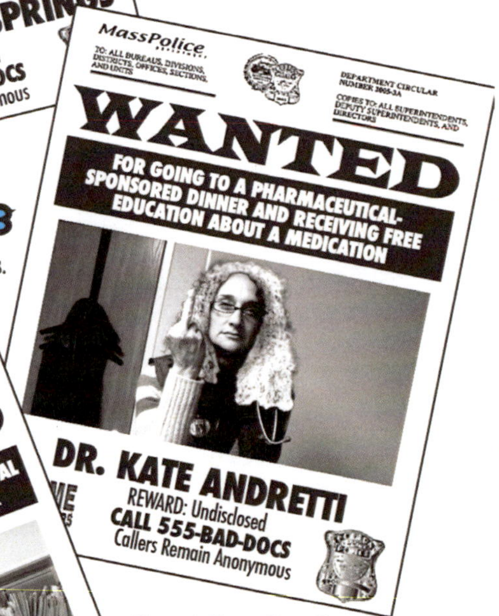


# WARNING:

These criminals are highly dangerous. Do not apprehend on your own.

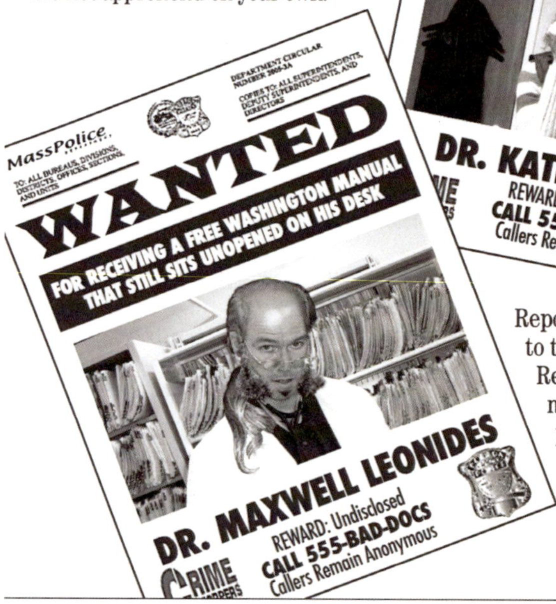


Report them directly to the Governor or State Representative so they may use these doctors for propaganda and their own political gain.

**REWARD: Undisclosed**
**CALL 555-BAD-DOCS**
**Callers Remain Anonymous**

PANNIVIA, the all-new, pro-biotic yogurt sensation that's taking health food stores by storm!

PANNIVIA, is an all-natural yogurt that's proven by pseudoscience (even better than regular science!) to help restore the natural balance of bacteria and fungal elements to the colon! Other yogurts boast that their overpriced probiotic yogurts have active bacterial cultures. But where do they get their bacteria? Who knows!

With our overpriced product, you are guaranteed 100% pure human-pannus-grown bacterial cultures, AND the yeasty goodness that only a morbidly obese and extremely sedentary human pannus can provide!

That's right! Not only are you restoring the delicate balance of nature to your colon, you're providing work for thousands of morbidly obese and home-bound Americans who before PANNIVIA were considered disabled!

**PANNIVIA! SCRAPE SOME!**

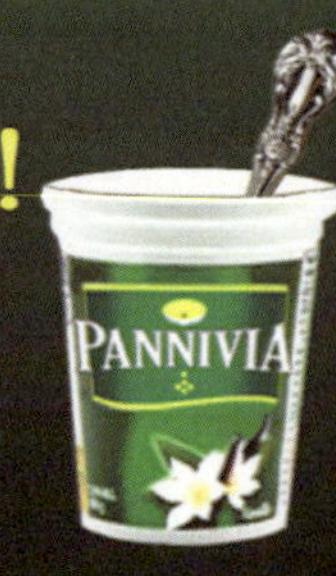


Coming soon from PJ Herbal Pharmaceuticals:
**PANNUSBOCK**
All-natural pannus-borne lager!

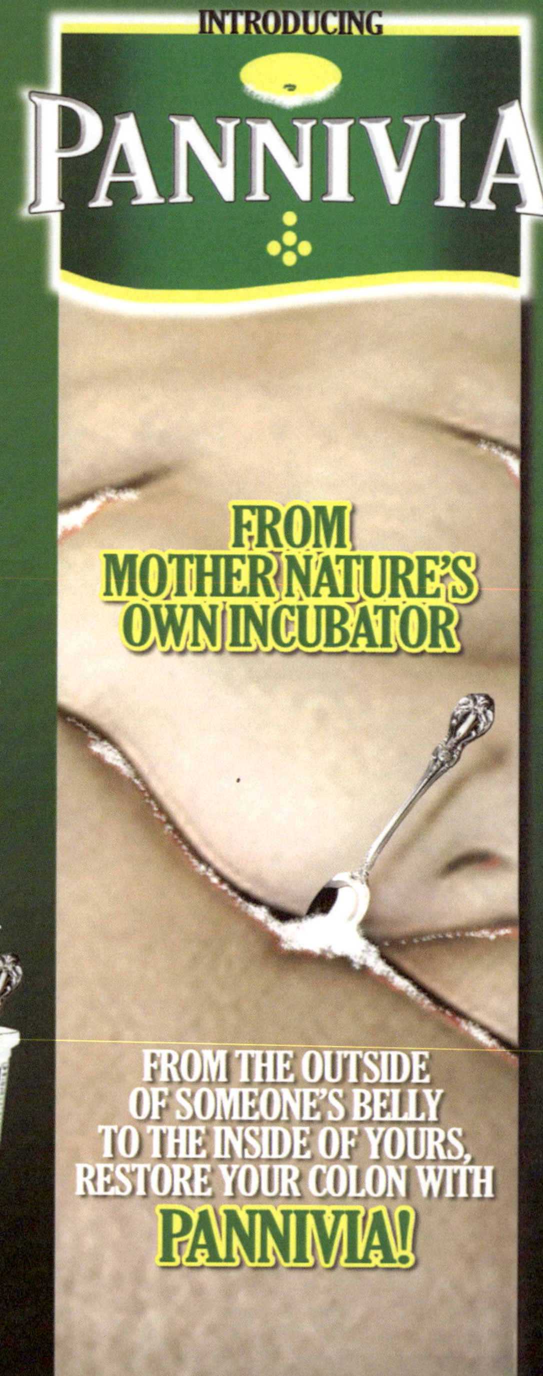

# Reinventing Your Carreer After Being A Physician

**AIR TRAFFIC CONTROLLER**
*What do you think being on call is all about?*

**DRUG DEALER**
*Well, this one is obvious.*

**DATA PROCESSOR**
*You can thank the EMR for this one.*

**LAWYER**
*You have been trained in defensive medicine for years. How about putting it to good use? Besides, you know which doctors suck in your hospital. Start handing out your cards right outside their offices.*

**CONSULTANT**
*This is just a made up job anyway. And you have seen all the other idiots who do it.*

**SURGEON GENERAL**
*I mean really, what do they do anyway?*

**ADMINISTRATOR**
*If you can't beat 'em, join 'em. You'll need to lose some IQ points first, though.*

**POLITICIAN**
*They even do less than the administrators but it is a better way to pass around your half-naked pictures on* Facebook.

**PHARMACEUTICALS**
*There are so many choices here to make a living while losing all credibility as a physician. Jump right in!*

**FAST FOOD RESTAURANT**
*No one takes more orders and juggles more items at the same time than you. Besides, you may make more money than being a doctor.*

**CHEF**
*Heck, medicine is now a cookbook job anyway. It can't be much different than whipping up some créme brulé.*

**NEWSPAPER DELIVERY PERSON**
*You've been giving news to patients every day of your life so why not continue doing the same.You still have to get up early but you can now go to bed early and once again, you may get paid more.*

**HAIRSTYLIST/MANICURIST**
*How many nails have you treated or cut off? How many backs have you shaved to do a procedure? Now you can do it in a nicer atmosphere.* +

A TRUE STORY OF MEDICINE

# REMEMBER, DRINK THE GOOD STUFF

There is much to recommend modern medicine over "the good old days" of cod liver oil, leeches, and hot iron cauterization, and I do not seek to return to those times. That said, we all hear the occasional anecdote to make us envious of the doctors of yore. Last night at supper, I was listening to a long-time family friend tell tales of old Apalachicola and the "Forgotten Coast." They have always done a little drinkin' down here (accounting for most of the snake bites) and between the tales of oysters and shrimping, our friend recalled an old local man from more than fifty years back who always kept a big glass jar of clear liquid on the floor by his side, and sipped from it liberally whenever he went by. One day the local went to see the (only) town doctor, to complain about a recent, progressive numbness in his legs that had begun to concern him greatly.

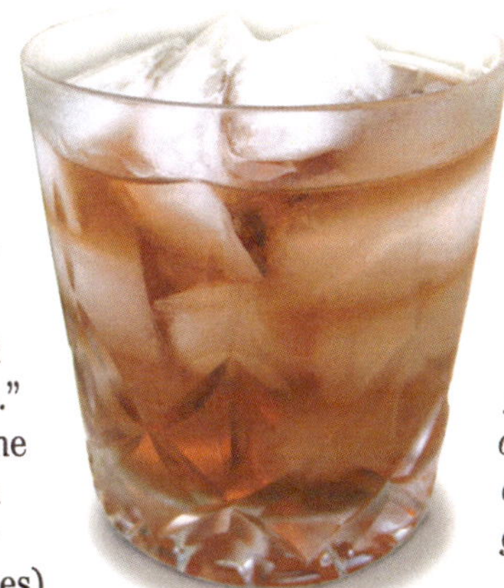

The old doc was said to have stared hard at the glass jar and asked the patient what he was used to drinking.

*"Shine!"* replied the patient proudly ("Moonshine" whiskey, for you suburban types).

*"Well,"* replied the old physician, *"You've got to cut that "shine" out for good! From now on, all you can drink is good bonded whiskey."*

The patient thanked him, threw away the home brew, and started drinking only store-bought liquor. A couple weeks later he saw the old doctor, reported the numbness gone, and it never did return.

It must have been fun to be a doctor able to recommend drinking the good stuff as a path to better living. +

YOUR GOVERNMENT NEEDS YOUR HELP TO SPREAD THE WORD ABOUT

# MEANINGFUL USE.

The country doesn't understand what this simple concept means. Please go to www.wearewayoverourheadonthis.com to get a bumper sticker for your vehicle. Only doctors like you can make our healthcare system run better. All you need is for us to tell you what to do.

Just go on the site, click on the free bumper sticker logo and sign up by giving your full name, birth date, address, social security number, license number, DEA number, complete a short essay on why you want to help the government, a small test to see if you're competent and provide three different secure electronic signatures. From there you can download a full application to be filled out and notarized and then sent in to us. *It's that simple!*

## PICK ONE OF THESE GREAT BUMPER STICKERS FOR FREE:

15,000 Hours Will Get You 15% With **MEANINGFUL USE** . . . *okay 1.5%*

**MEANINGFUL USE:** *Trust us, we're the government.*

**Meaningful Use:** *The Other White Noise*

**MEANINGFUL USE:** From the same people who brought us OBAMACARE!

**MEANINGFUL USE:** *Even We Don't Know What It Means*

**MEANINGFUL USE:** *THE BEST THING SINCE LEECHES AND BLOODLETTING*

**I've Got Your Meaningful Use Right Here!**

**Meaningful Use:** *Don't think this means you're not going to get screwed in the end!*

Allow 8-19 weeks for delivery.

**MEANINGFUL USE =** How to be used, meaningfully.

**Support your country, support your patients, support healthcare reform and support change . . . all with a simple bumper sticker.***

*Not all applicants will get a bumper sticker. Some will actually be audited by our *Medicare* claims bounty hunters. What can we say, shit happens. ✚

**Are you a Urologist tired of spending your days digitally examining people who usually forget to wipe?**

***Urology just isn't as sexy as it used to be . . . until now.***

## Get back in the OR with *PJ Surgical's* new organ harvesting technology!

# CADAVER-JECT

***Corpus Cavernosum Allograft* Technology**

With our patented method of corpus cavernosum tissue collection, now you can loiter confidently in the doctor's lounge, knowing that no longer are you the sadistic laughing boy of surgery. *Gone are the days when only orthopods perform bone transplants!* Not only is our penile tissue transplantation technology guaranteed to enhance those refractory ED cases, it also will enhance your pocketbook and your long-damaged self esteem!

***Return to the basic tenets of your Urology training: 1) Giving old guys a boner 2) Getting rich doing it!***

Still need a new *Ferrari* and one more trophy girlfriend? Procure an additional windfall by offering your patients

**CADAVER-JECT *CELEB!***

With CADAVER-JECT *CELEB* you can tap into the DNA of the most famous members in the world. Your patients can choose DNA from:
• *Karl Hungus* • *Long Duck Dong* • *Dirk Diggler* • *Mister Ed*

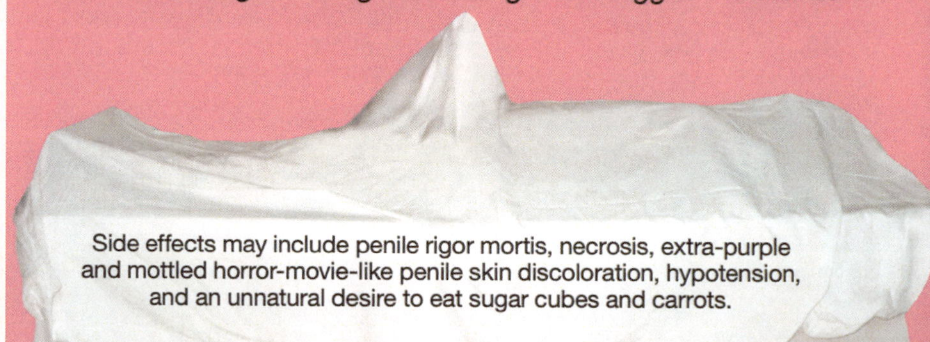

Side effects may include penile rigor mortis, necrosis, extra-purple and mottled horror-movie-like penile skin discoloration, hypotension, and an unnatural desire to eat sugar cubes and carrots.

Who are you going to call when your clinical day is just too overwhelming?
We have your answer in two words.

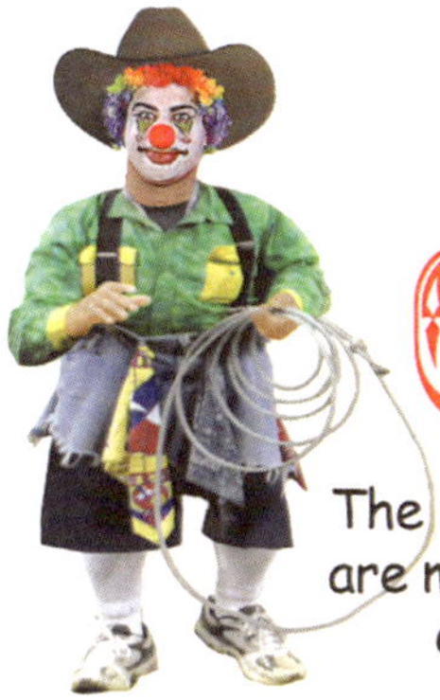

# RODEO CLOWNS

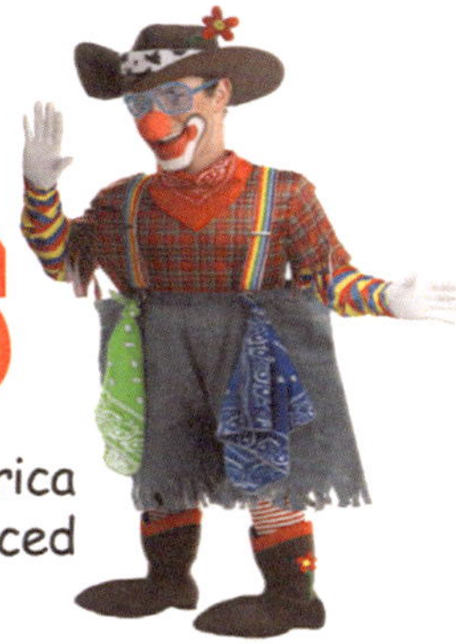

The Midget Rodeo Clowns of America are made up of the most experienced entertainers in the business.

No other team of professionals will be able to distract your toughest patients like the members of the MRCA.

The MRCA are now available for your medical office – in any part of this great country.

- An obese patient complaints they can't lose weight? Bring in a midget rodeo clown.
- A fibromyalgia patient is still in pain and all your medications are exhausted? Bring in a midget rodeo clown.
- An elderly patient has a list a mile long? Bring in a midget rodeo clown.

Each MRCA member is trained to distract, protect and provide an alternative target for your patients. By blending the perfect complement of facial paint and diminutive size, you are guaranteed a reprieve from even your toughest of patients.

When your
**STEPD™**
Shiny Thing Easy Patient Distracter
no longer works
then we have your answer.

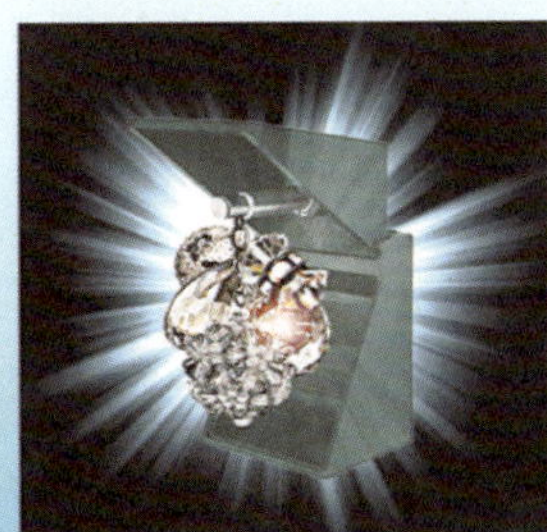

Prices are negotiable.
Call 1-555-GOT-MRCA now.

# TOP 10 Things Our Patients Say That Are Always Wrong

**10.** *"I am allergic to Benadryl."*

**9.** *"The cold is moving into my chest."*

**8.** *"My cough is from an infection, not my smoking."*

**7.** *"My normal temperature is 96, so 98.9 is a high-grade fever for me."*

**6.** *"My wife made me come in, but there is nothing wrong with me."*

**5.** *"My bowels haven't moved for a day and a half, so I know I'm constipated."*

**4.** *"I know this is Lyme disease, I found it on the internet."*

**3.** *"My weight has to be a gland problem – I eat like a bird."*

**2.** *"I think I got it off a toilet seat."*

**1.** *"I have a high pain tolerance."*

## Oh, what the heck, here's a few more

**6.** *"I don't like to take pills."*

**5.** *"I don't really like going to the doctor."* (but your chart is larger than the PDR)

**4.** *"I have chest pain but I know it's not my heart."*

**3.** *"I have chest pain and I know it's my heart."*

**2.** *"I don't have anything wrong with me except my work comp injury."*

**1.** *"I don't believe in medicine."* (then WTF are you doing here?)

TRUE STORIES OF MEDICINE

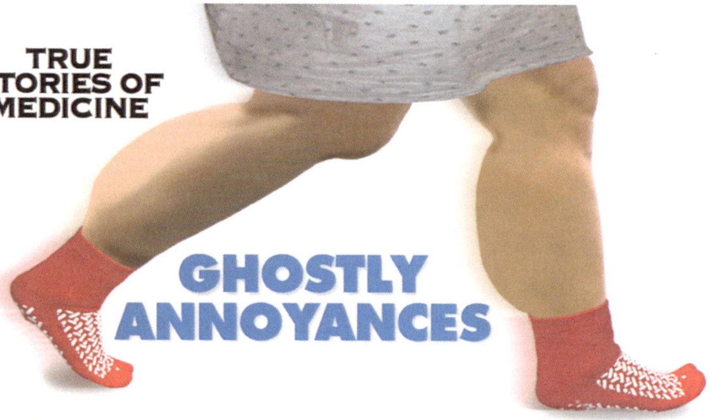

# GHOSTLY ANNOYANCES

Bariatric surgery has been around for decades, but sometimes outcomes are less than desired. As an ICU nurse at a large teaching hospital I took care of an unfortunate lady who lingered for about six months before passing off this earth. She had become an institution in the ICU, having taken up residence there and becoming known by all the staff. After she passed away the bed was filled next by a gentleman with a myocardial infarction.

After his first night, when asked how he slept, he responded that he had a weird dream about being chased around by an obese lady who was demanding that he get out of her room. ✚

# REAL PHONE MESSAGE

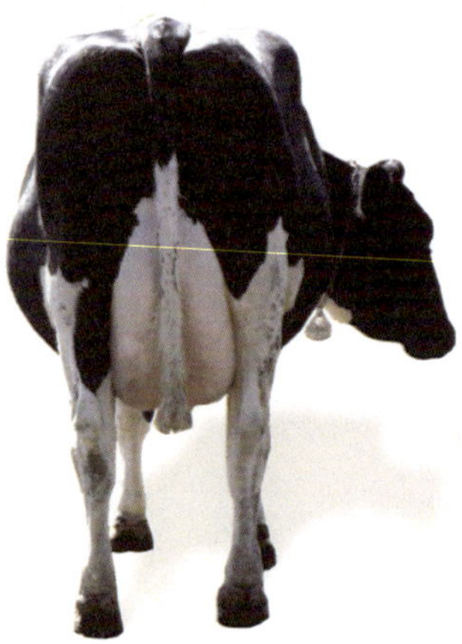

The story is not that interesting, but the phone message itself is hysterical . . .

***"patient states he was standing by the fence and got ran over by a cow one week ago, very painful."***

Suggest patient yeild to cow?

*Welcome to primary care in Oklahoma!* ✚

*Introducing Placebo Pharmaceuticals' newest weapon in the war against ED!*

# LAZARUS

## A Revolutionary New Treatment for Erectile Dysfunction

- Are prescription ED drugs too expensive?
- Did your last Internet-purchased "Canadian *Viagra*" turn out to be *Smarties*?
- Do you nearly die from hypotension every time you have sex due to the synergy between the nitro you just took for your sex-induced MI and your favorite prescription ED drug?
- Do vacuum pumps scare you or embarrass your partner?
- Does a *Gumby*-like penis implant creep you out?

EASY TO USE!

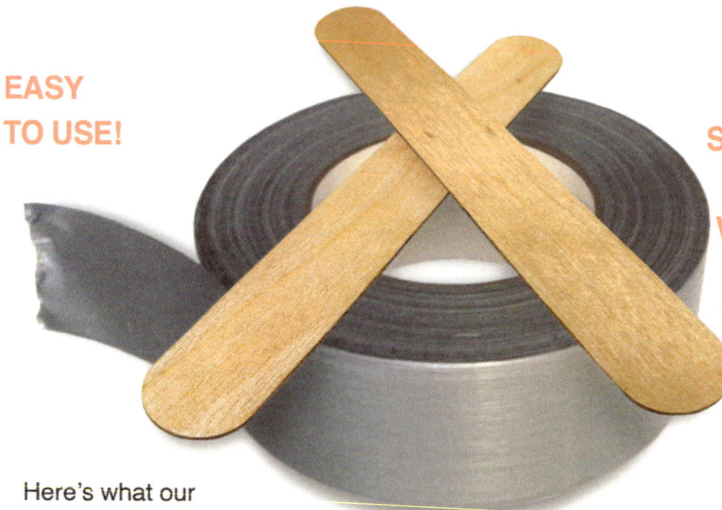

JUST STRAP IT AND WRAP IT AND YOU'RE GOOD TO GO!

Here's what our satisfied customers have to say about our amazing breakthrough device . . .

*"Holy mother of God, this product had me going 'til eternity!"*

*"My 20-year-old girlfriend kept screaming 'Jesus Christ' and I didn't have the heart to remind her that my name was Bill."*

*"Now I know how Abraham fathered a child at age 180."*

*"My penis has grown to biblical proportions."*

**PJ PHARMACEUTICALS**
*The Realistic Drug Company*

# TOP 15 Ways to Cheaply Boost Staff Morale

**15.** Have all providers go bottomless for the day.

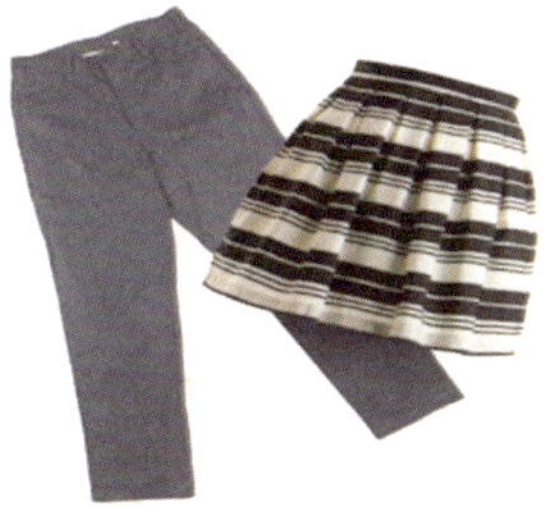

**14.** Dress as your favorite patient; extra points for mimicking the correct smell.

**13.** Pretend you are an administrator for the day and do no work.

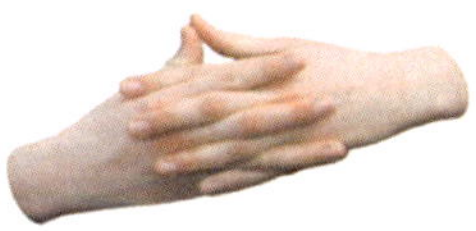

**12.** Hide your favorite demented patient and play hide-and-go-seek.

**11.** Go on an outing to your favorite cemetery and see who can locate the most patients . . . er, ex-patients.

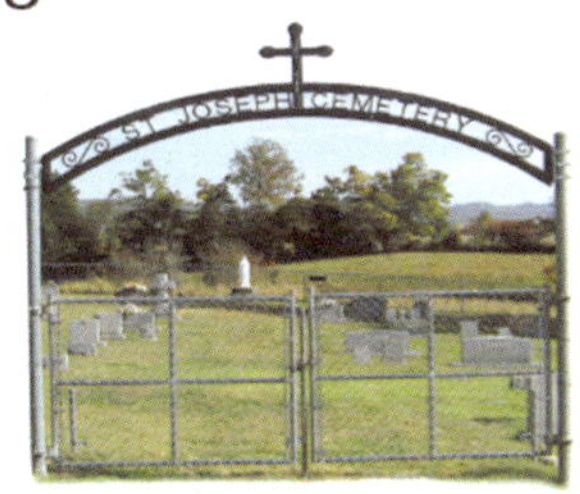


**10.** Play the insulin game. Each staff member takes 30 u of regular insulin and see who passes out first. Have plenty of candy or glucagon around.

**9.** Grease the hallway with *Vaseline* and see who can slide the farthest. This can also be left on the floor for the rest of the day to see how many patients fall (a cruel but hysterical game).

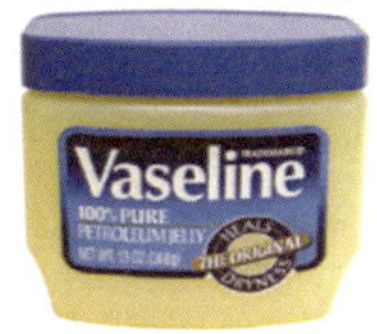


**8.** Play Russian roulette with urine containers. Save enough samples of urine and place some apple juice in other ones. See who makes the most mistakes with a taste-testing contest.

**7.** Have a creative cookie swap with treats that look like different stool samples you have collected over the years.

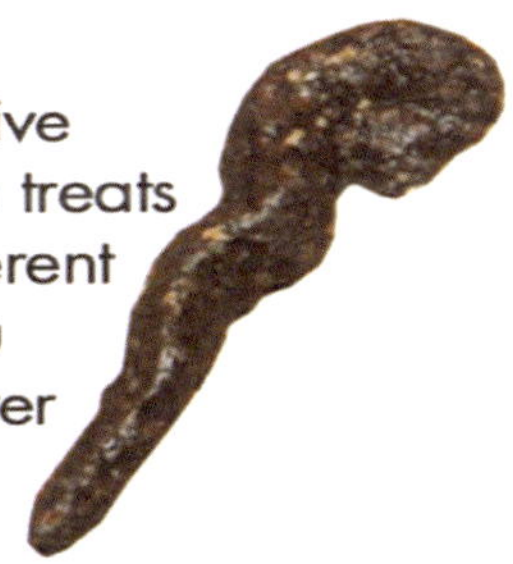

**6.** Decorate the office like a morgue and see how many patients it creeps out.

**5.** Have a Cinco de Pendo Day and have everyone wear adult diapers for the day.

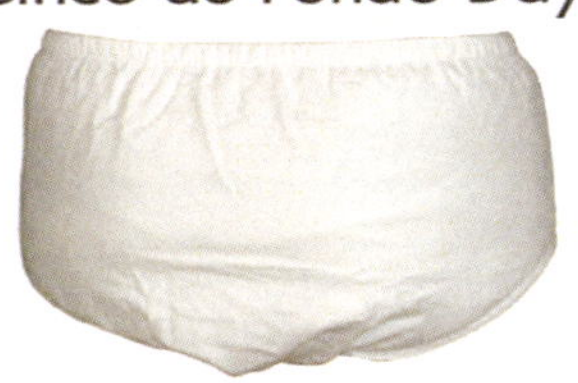

Then lock the bathroom door and see who uses them.

**4.** Give each staff member a list of five annoying patients and have them call their place of work with meaningless questions or angry demands.

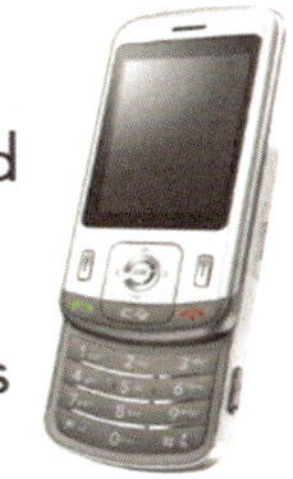

**3.** Have your staff bring their children to work for a day and then set up a fake code to scare them *(into never going into the medical field).*

**2.** Invite the hottest drug reps to come in at the same time to compete for your business. This does nothing for your staff but you will love it and your staff can be happy vicariously through you.

**1.** Hold a monthly potluck day where one member brings in a homemade dish that contains medical marijuana. +

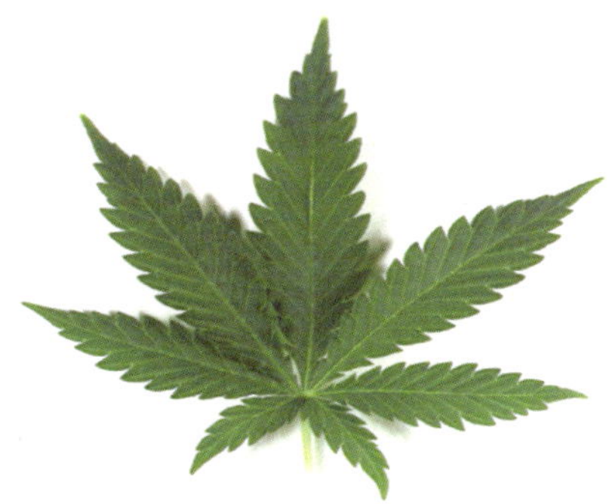

You've agreed to make rounds on a few patients this weekend, or maybe you're taking over an inpatient team from a partner. That list the other doctor gave you has some notations by patients' names that are intended to bring you up to date. They look pretty reassuring . . . but are they really? Here is a short guide to . . .

# Interpreting the "Comments" Section of Your Hospital List

| What the doctor says: | What is really going on: |
|---|---|
| Family very involved | Member constantly at bedside taking notes and criticizing everyone from the cleaning lady to the chief of surgery |
| Recent mental status changes | Alcohol withdrawal seizures followed by DTs |
| Needs help accepting diagnosis | Insists his lung mets can be cured by antibiotics/herbal supplements/acupuncture/pyramid power |
| Has difficulty with invasive procedures | Terrified of needles; requires mega-doses of *Ativan* for blood draws |
| May need extra TLC | Soul-sucking emotional leech – allow 45 minutes for each visit |
| Some problems with symptom control | Demands ever-increasing doses of IV narcotics |
| Has strong views on tx plan | Control freak who demands name & dose of every med and refuses it unless indication was previously explained at length |
| Good understanding of healthcare system | Patient is not only an RN but related to hospital CEO ✚ |

Prevent fibrosis and restenosis while sporting a medical piece of elegance.

# Fashion Stents

***Sure you have fashion sense but do you have Fashion Stents?***

You're mature. You've made it in life.
You've done it all and had your first or even second heart attack already. But you feel something is still missing.

***New from PJ Biopharmaceuticals comes our newest drug eluding stents with a little extra pizzazz.***

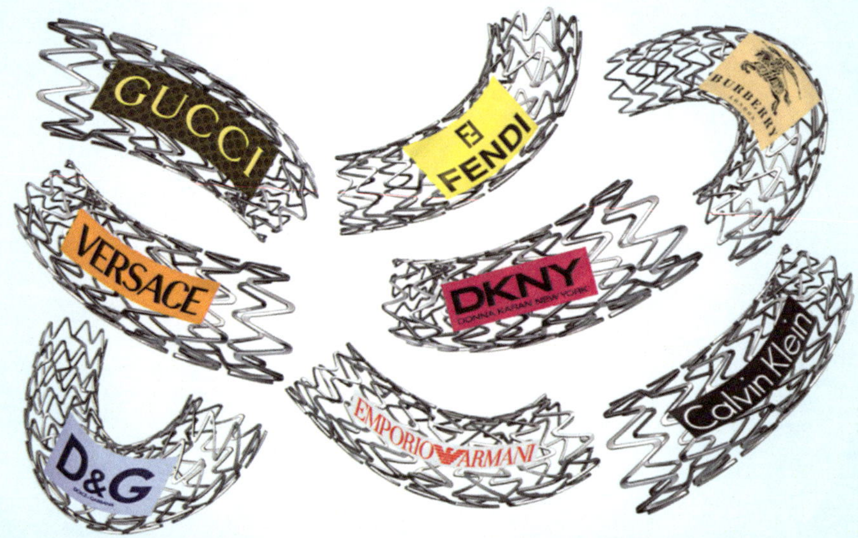


Each Fashion Stent allows you to have your interventional cardiologist to deploy a piece of hardware with a famous design or logo. Options include:
•*Armani* •*Burberry* •*Calvin Klein* •*Dolce and Gabbana* •*Donna Karen* •*Fendi* •*Gucci* •*Versace* •*and many more!*

Does it matter that no one will ever see it?
No, because you know what's in your heart (literally).
And class doesn't need to boast.

## Get Your Fashion Stents Today!

Coming soon in gold and silver. ✚

## MORE TRUE STORIES OF MEDICINE

# Jamaican Me Crazy

My Jamaicans-with-vaginitis month began with a chief complaint of a "bump on my poom-poom," which sadly for her revealed itself to be "herp-herp."

Patient number two actually had no vaginitis. The intake history proceeded thusly:

Me: *"Are you sexually active?"*

Patient: *"Oh, you know I'm Jamaican, mon. We love dat thing."*

Me (working to hold a straight face): *"Great. Do you have one partner? More than one partner?"*

Patient: *"Well I'm not lettin' just anyone in m'kitty."*

Me: *"Excellent plan."*

I had treated patient number three two months previously for trichomoniasis. She came back with similar symptoms stating that her fiancé was, *"with another girl on the side."* I explained reinfection to her as she railed against the injustice of it all.

*"Dat pisses me off! I keep myself clean down there and now I get this naasteeness all again. I cleaned myself good this morning. I knew you'd be down there and I knew you didn't wanna see no nasteeness!"*

I shrugged understandingly and silently thanked her for doing so and proceeded to get her comfortable for the exam to exclude any other infections. As I began helping her lay back on the table, she speed dialed her cell phone.

*"You sonofabeech! I can't believe you give me that naasteeness agin! I'll be havin' no more relations wit you now. The doctor here gonna tell you!"*

By now she is fully settled into both stirrups and is proffering her cell phone towards my free hand. I wave the phone away with a *Surgilube* slathered speculum and, biting my cheeks tell her, *"Just tell him to come in and get treated."*

Laying back again she finished, *"Even the doctor don't be wantin' nutting to do wit you!"* as she snapped the phone shut. ✚

# *You just want to save lives . . .*

. . . but people are constantly after you to sign this, discuss that, attend a meeting here, or an intervention there. Even when you're in the bathroom, **YOU CONSTANTLY GET STOPPED!** Here at *PJ*, we know that you make use of hallway mirrors, newspapers, and pretend cell phone calls to get where you're going, and usually fail at not getting stopped . . . **UNTIL NOW.**

Introducing the

# GPYes!

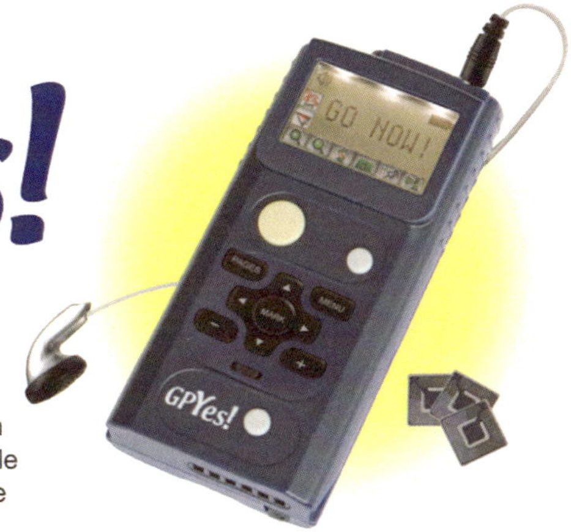


***How it works:***

*1)* You place a small transmitter sticker on the ID badge of every employee you want to avoid. Getting this done generally requires a hug or a "Well done" pat on the chest. (More difficult to employ on female co-workers, but they'll never find you for the harassment inquiry anyway!)

*2)* Upload the blueprints of your clinic or hospital.

*3)* Tell ***GPYes!*** your destination, and through a covert in-ear microphone, the ***GPYes!*** tells you when to walk, when to run, when to crawl; when to stop, and when to turn. You get where you're going while easily avoiding anyone you've marked with a transmitter. *It's that easy!*

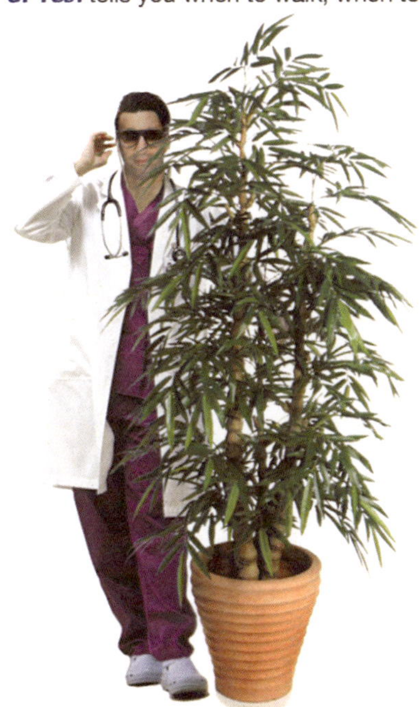

***And the GPYes! also works in reverse!***

You can track the movements of the tagged employees, and catch them red-handed! Imagine the joy of giving the hospital board pictures of:

- Administrators playing golf during the day
- Utilization Review schmucks buying smack from a dealer in the alley
- Anti-physician board members getting it on with ER-frequenting crack whores in the janitor's closet.

***Getting rid of time and money-wasting employees has never been easier!***

***ORDER YOURS TODAY!***

***Exclusively from PJ Covert Electronics***

# WEBINAR on SEPTEMBER 15th, 2011

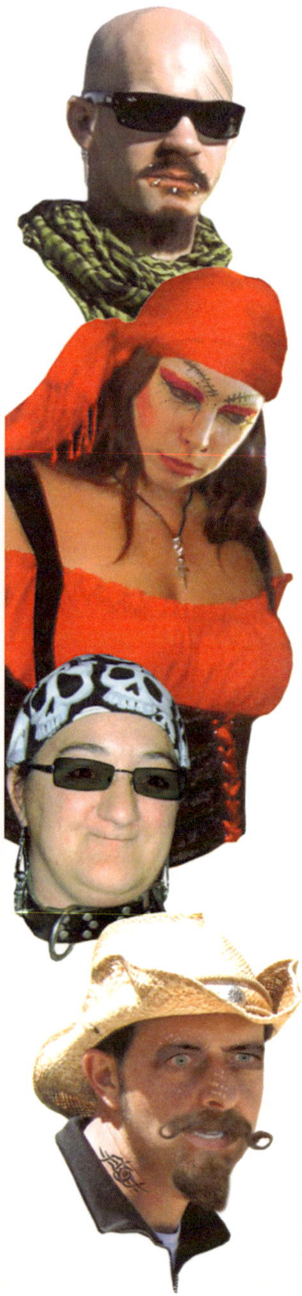

### The newest business phenomenon sweeping the country fairs is coming to a hospital webcast near you.

PJ Consulting brings your system the magic of "carnies" and blends them with your administrative skills to build the optimal hospital management team.

**Join our large, live, on-demand, secure video webcast to learn how to run your "joint," manage "the kitty," and make your doctors truly work for their "scratch."**

We have harnessed the power of the carnie and unearthed their secrets only to reveal them to you. Much of which, by the way, you have already been doing!

- Learn from the experts on how to really bait and switch.
- Improve your performance in fooling doctors into believing they are special.
- Hottest trends in stringing the medical staff along while having your plans already made.
- Master the art of showmanship and creativity while still accomplishing nothing.

***We have developed the most robust, scalable, interactive webcasting platform in the industry to allow you to bring the art of grift to your healthcare system.***

Learn the carnie secret language and use its ever-changing form to fool physicians or board members.

### GOALS

As a hospital "agent" you can:

- Use the technique called the "alibi" to fool a physician into thinking he will apparently get his bonus only to invent a further, unforeseeable, condition of the game.
- Put on a "bally" to attract recruited physicians even though the system is "flat" or rigged.
- Confuse specialists with a "call" and become the "butcher" who takes every penny from a "mark" by confusing him and then forcing him to practice anyway.
- Make the system a "gaff" or unwinnable for doctors because the physicians are such a "Hammer-Squash" or dumb or stupid (also called a "Larry").
- Increase your "scratch" in the "kitty" so that your CEO gets a huge bonus.
- Create ways to hide the "oats" or dirty cash from the government to use as "patch money" in order to induce board members to turn a blind eye. Also known as "juice" or "ice."
- Target those "sharpies" who may be experienced doctors who are wise to traditional carny . . .er, administrator scams.
- Hire outside "shills" who are consultants who then pretend to be a casual helper on the doctors' sides only to screw them in the end.
- Create "sugar shack" events for all employees with food, games, and fun in order to make them feel important and forget how little they are really paid.

# HOW TO BECOME A HOSPITAL "CARNISTRATOR"

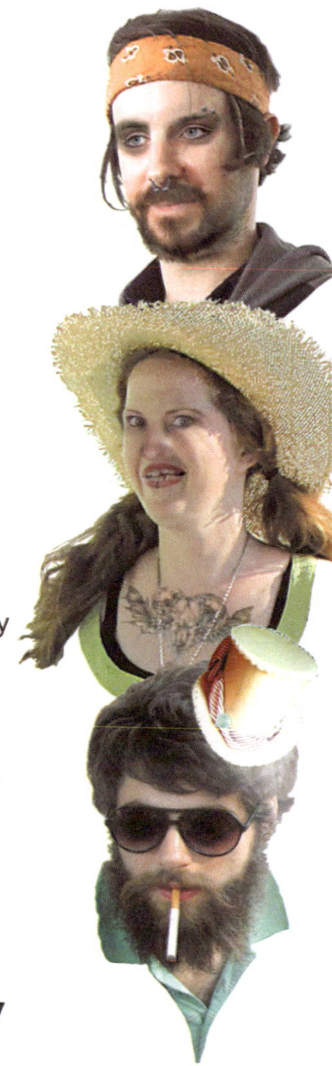

***Order now by going to www.carnistrator.com and bring the power of the side show to your main event!***

BELIEVE IT OR NOT.

# MY "REALISTIC" WEEK IN THE CLC

or Community Living Center (formerly nursing home care unit)

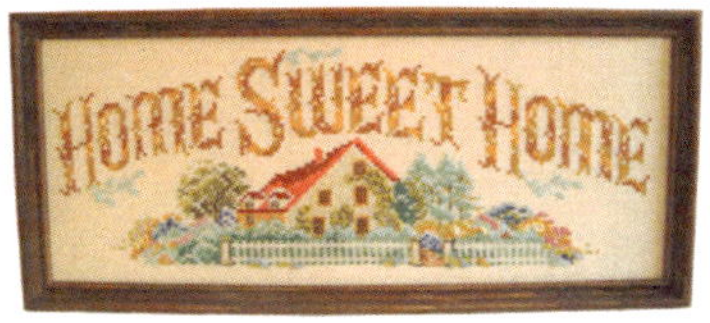


There has been a national push to make these facilities more homelike for the residents, a great idea but difficult to mesh with the other initiatives like discharging people from the hospital much earlier and sicker than before and also establishing a stronger palliative/hospice program. So I guess the unit is homey if you happen to have neighbors who are either terminally ill or dragging an IV pole with a bag of antibiotics trailing behind.

## MONDAY

I met with Len and his family to discuss his upcoming above-the-knee amputation. Len is an ultra light pilot with an amazingly positive outlook on life. At 78 years of age he had taken his 350 pound friend on his first flight over the desert. When the engine conked out his friend panicked and pushed the rudder pedals causing them to smash into a tree. Len's leg and pelvis were broken and his friend fell a distance to the ground.

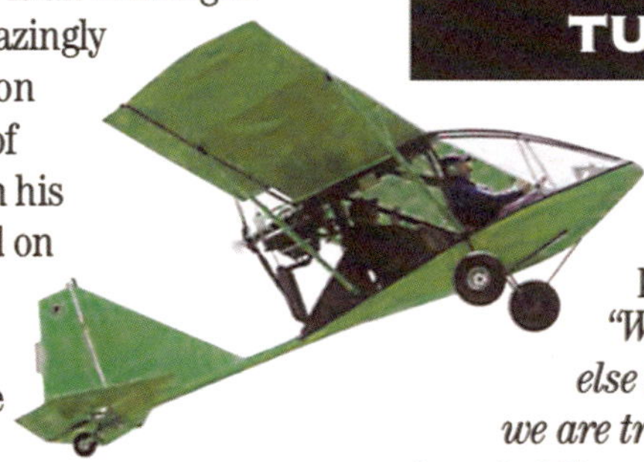

*"That's awful,"* I said.

*"No that was good, I saved my friend's life,"* Len replied. *"You see since he had fallen so far the hospital did a CT of his rather abundant abdomen and discovered an asymptomatic renal cancer. It was removed and he is still alive."*

Anyway, his daughter asked me how amputations were done nowadays and how long it would take. Not missing a beat, Len pulled the starter rope on his imaginary chain saw, making the appropriate *RRRRRRR!!* And with a grand slicing gesture said, *"Fifteen seconds with a* McCullough, *thirty seconds with a* Craftsman.*"*

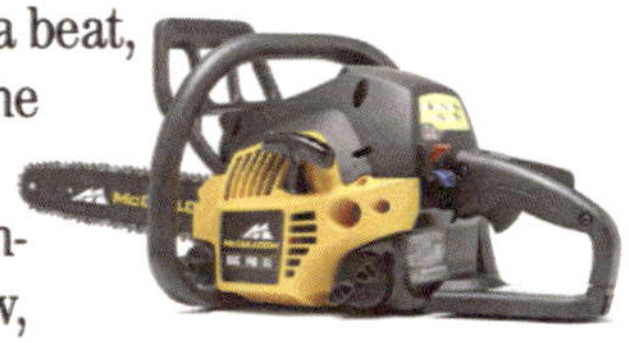

## TUESDAY

Fred, an admission today for "short term rehab" (a hospitalist euphemism for, *"We don't know what else to do for this guy so we are transferring him to you for rehab"*) arrived following a series of disasters. They happened during his six weeks in the hospital after an admission from the ER for "not feeling right." It is less than reassuring to review the record to find that the sitter that he "no longer needs" was still at his bedside all last night due to his confusion and attempts to escape! Oh, and by some miracle he also still needs the 6L/min of oxygen to keep his sats in the mid 80s. Yeah, he's ready for rehab . . . *not.*

## WEDNESDAY

Wayne was admitted for ongoing radiation therapy for throat cancer, one of the many poorly publicized benefits of smoking. He has already had a PEG tube inserted because he can't swallow without aspirating and also a trach to protect his airway. As I enter his room this morning he is standing at the toilet, holding his PEG tube over the bowl apparently thinking it was his penis, the growing puddle at his feet and his wet pajama bottoms at least were reassuring that he isn't in urinary retention and we probably don't need to fret about benign prostatic hypertrophy.

## THURSDAY

Tony has been encephalopathic intermittently due to bathing his hepatitis C infected liver in alcohol for years. This afternoon as I pass his room I can hear a hollow clunking sound coming from inside as well as mumbled profanity. Upon entering to investigate I find him walking around the bed looking for his other "shoe." On his left foot he has managed to wedge his plastic urinal around it and he is looking for the matching "shoe" for the right.

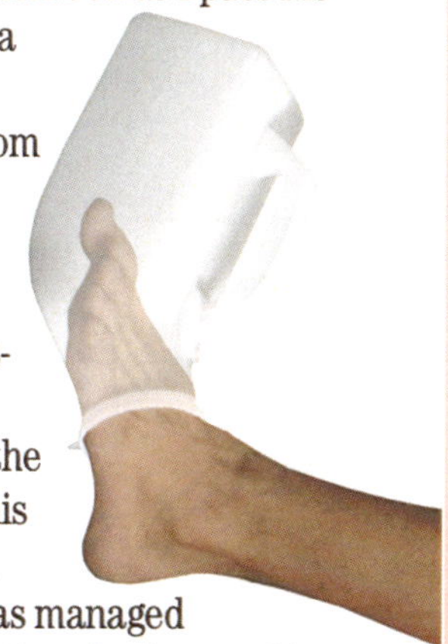

## FRIDAY

Our youngest resident, in her 30s with multiple sclerosis, has lost much of her social inhibitions due to the progression of her disease. She pretty much says whatever comes to mind and explains that it is her MS talking if anyone is offended. She was having a conversation with another resident who had stopped in his wheelchair to say hello. When she discovered that he was a Muslim she peered with concern at his shoes. *"You aren't going to try to light those and blow us up are you?"* she asked. ✚

# CAN I GET A . . .

As a medical student, I spent a month rotating at a hospital whose house staff consisted primarily of foreign medical graduates. One day our neurology attending asked us (a group of five residents and me) if we knew the best way to differentiate between seizures and syncope. I knew it must be a trick question so I stayed quiet. The residents looked at one another sheepishly until one brave Nigerian man spoke up, *"The difference is a weakness."*

All the cogs and wheels were turning in our brains trying to figure out why a person lying on the floor from a seizure versus a fainting spell might be weaker than the other one. I imagined trying to pick them off the floor like limp noodles. The attending rolled his eyes.

*"Why would weakness be a distinguishing feature?"*

The resident became more persistent. *"Yes, it's a weakness!"*

*"No it's not!"* shouted the attending.

*"Yes, that's what I say. A weakness, weakness, WEAKNESS!"*

I was astonished at his certainty in the face of something so seemingly irrational.

Then one of the other residents piped up, ***"He's saying 'witness.'"*** ✚

# Sometimes Delerium Is A GOOD Thing!

I work in a nursing home and we received Mr. Nacho from the hospital late in the afternoon one Thursday. In reviewing the hospital notes there was an indication that nights had not been particularly restful for him nor the nursing staff as he was often up and about confused and restless. As a gentleman in his late 70's his prostate had been encroaching on his urethra for some time leading to the amazing discovery of 1600cc of urine in his bladder. He was admitted to the facility some days before and thus when he came to us having failed several voiding trials he now had an indwelling Foley catheter.

The first evening with us he was up and about several times and even wandered away from his bed with the Foley bag still firmly attached to the railing before he was caught by the staff. *Ouch!* In a very unusual turn of events, the balloon did not rupture freeing the catheter. The catheter tubing itself BROKE allowing the trapped distal end to remain in the bladder!

The next morning upon our arrival and before he was off to urology for his emergency cystoscopy to retrieve the retained catheter fragment and drain his bladder of 800cc of urine he commented to his nurse, *"Boy, did I sleep well last night!"*

When she responded, *"That's not what I heard."*

His comeback was, ***"Why, was I snoring?"*** ✚

# MY MOST EMBARRASSING MEDICAL MOMENT

## RECOGNIZE ME?

I am a gastroenterologist and I do hundreds of colonoscopies every year. Some years ago, at Christmastime, I was at the mall shopping when a women came up to me and said, *"Doctor XXXX, how are you doing!"*

It must have been obvious, from the look on my face, that I had no idea who this woman was. She very quickly turned around and shoved her rear bumper in my face saying, *"Oh! Now do you know who I am?"*

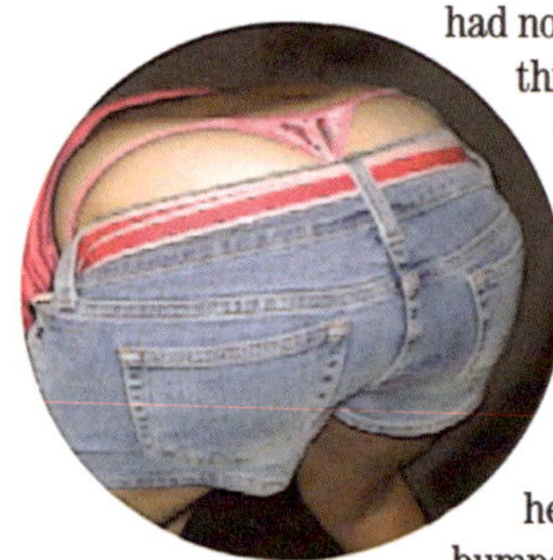

**I was totally mortified!** When I looked around there were several people staring at me with that look . . . *"you pervert!"* I quickly pulled up the hood on my coat and exited the mall. For years I could not go back during the holiday season. I still, to this day, do not know who the woman was. She either never came back to see me for follow-up or has never owned up to her action! ✚

## REACTIVE

As an allergist, I do scratch or prick tests on top of the skin, and intradermal or ID tests at times to increase sensitivity of our testing. One day at the nurses' station, where we also test patients, my nurse and I were discussing the need for an ID skin test for histamine as a control if the prick histamine skin test is reactive enough.

Giving an example, my nurse cocked her head in the direction of the patient, five feet away and said, *"For instance, Mr Smith, who has a HUGE, RED, SWOLLEN PRICK . . ."*

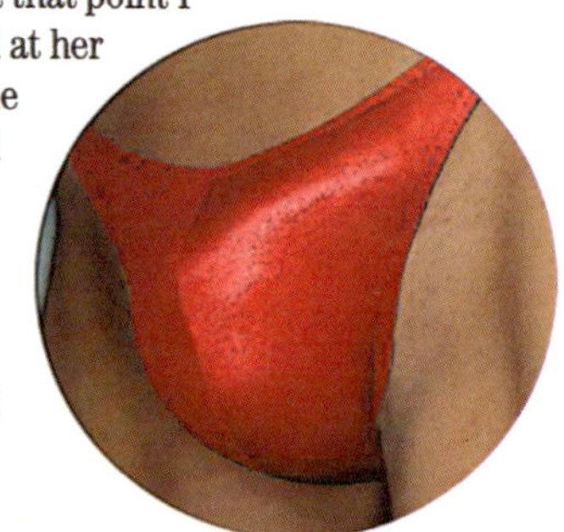

At that point I looked at her and she looked at me with a look conveying the same mixture of, *"I can't believe I just said that/I can't believe you just said that,"* and also, ***"I've gotta run for cover so I can laugh my ass off!"***

We both retreated to my office where we broke down with laughter so hard I nearly wet my pants. It took several long minutes before either of us could compose ourselves enough to be seen in public again, much less face Mr. Smith! ✚

## Try the newest and hottest medical game to hit the virtual world

# ANGRY DOCS

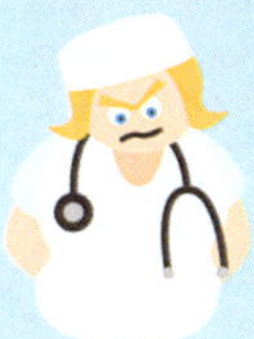

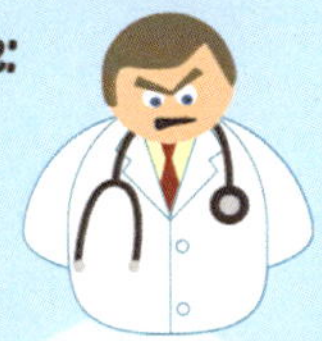

Launch the ANGRY DOCS via slingshot into the:

- Hospital full of administrators
- Trailer full of redneck patients
- Lawyer's office
- Sickna insurance company building

**Watch the ANGRY DOCS that you control attempt to try and retrieve their lost souls that were stolen by the healthcare system.**

RULES: • Hit the evil criminal directly or destroy the building they are in. • Use the special abilities, which some ANGRY DOCS have, to gain an advantage on your enemies. These skills include a thick skin, a sense of humor, or a total sense of helplessness. • Score points as you advance level after level.

**The survival of the ANGRY DOCS is at stake.**

Dish out revenge on the ones who stole their profession.
Play on your iPod, iPad, or EMR between patients or even during the visit!
Use the unique destructive powers of the ANGRY DOCS to lay waste to the fortified buildings.

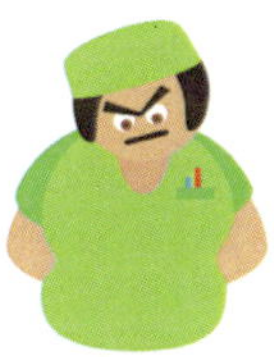

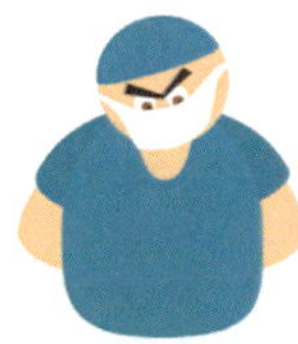

ANGRY DOCS features hours of gameplay, challenging physics-based demolition, and lots of replay value. Each of the 120 levels requires logic, skill, revenge and brute force to crush the enemy.

**You can cry about our broken healthcare system or you can play ANGRY DOCS. Either way nothing will change. But which one is more fun?**

Reviews:

*"Finally a mobile gaming platform that makes me want to hurt someone."*
Roland Goertz, MD and President AAFP

*"If you're dead inside like me than you want to check this out."*
Peter W. Carmel, MD and President AMA



## ARE YOU READY FOR THE NEWEST WAY TO LEARN HOW TO DO A LUMBAR PUNCTURE?

**Now from PJ Toys comes a game suitable for medical students who are ready for that next level of training . . .**

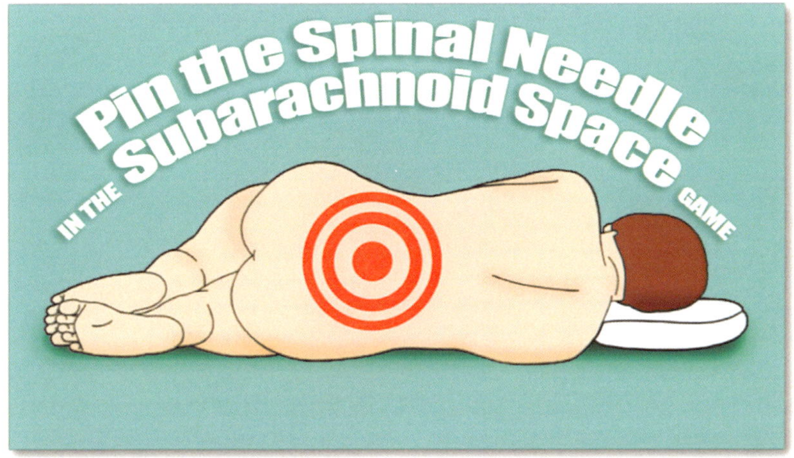


**RULES:**

1. Each student given a real stylet to try and hit the target.
2. The students are spun around until they are disoriented which they pretty much are at this stage of their training anyway.
3. Each blindfolded player aims for an imaginary line between the tops of the iliac crests.
4. The student who pins his needle closest to the area of a successful lumbar puncture (L3-L4 interspace or the L4-L5 inter space) wins.
5. Students who hit the L1-L2 and pierce the conus medullaris get extra scut work to do!

**Make any learning experience more fun with this classic teaching game!**

You can even use this to decide if the student passes by his rotation.

**A GREAT CALL-ROOM DRINKING GAME!**

Not to be used on real patients (except maybe some county hospitals).

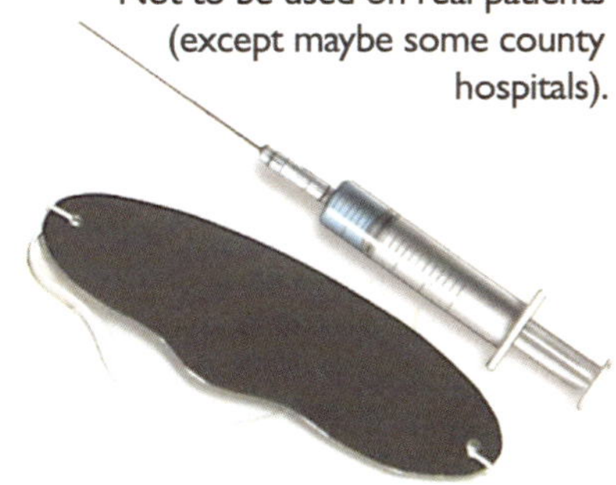

**$19.99** gets you one large poster of a typical late night Gomer. You will have to supply the blindfold and stylet (usually stolen from the hospital).

## BEST ON-CALL PHONE MESSAGES FROM PATIENTS

# CONCEALED

I got a phone call from the police department in a nearby town – seems a patient of mine had been apprehended for possession of methamphetamines. She had confessed and even told them where the contraband was concealed . . . suffice to say it was in a place only a female can hide "stuff." Turns out she told the police that I was the only person she "trusted" to retrieve the hidden package. Both I and my supervising physician declined the "invitation" that I am sure was intended to be a compliment. ✚

**The patient says his pain level is 10.
As a physician you find this hard to believe.**

## NOW FINALLY, THERE ARE TOOLS TO HELP CALIBRATE A PATIENT'S PAIN LEVEL!

***Introducing our newest pain testing tools to help your patient's understand exactly what a 10 actually feels like.***

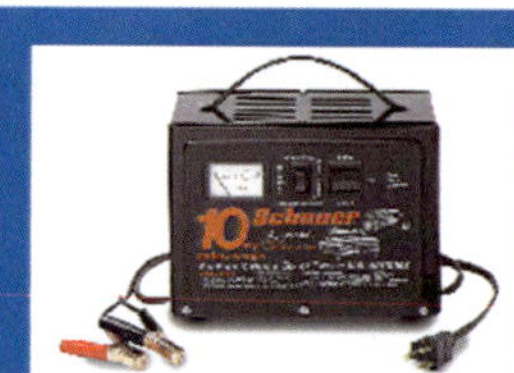

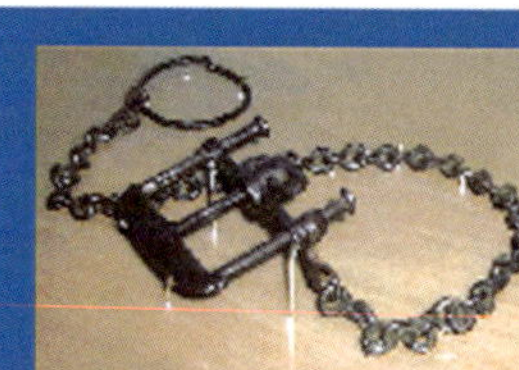

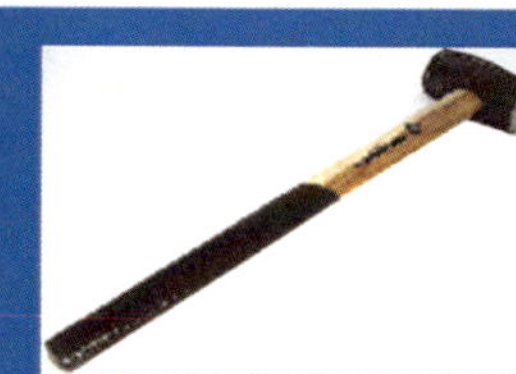

### DELUXE MODEL

Field tested in South American countries

Adjustable voltimeter that readily delivers a charge every time allowing for accurate pain titration

The latest in torture technology

Covered by MediCare and MedicAid

### PORTABLE MODEL

The latest in thumbscrew technology

Simple to operate

Tighten until bone crunches – *now that's a 10!*

Dealer inquiries welcome

### ECONOMY MODEL

BEST SELLER!

Old reliable classic design

Handle is crafted from space age materials

Applies swiftly to toes or fingers – *will register a 10 every time!*

## PJ PAIN MANAGEMENT TOOL COMPANY

**PROVIDING TOOLS FOR THE WORKING PHYSICIAN**

### ANOTHER TRUE STORY OF MEDICINE

# YANKEE DOODLE

I was working the day shift at our big city ER. The complaint said "nasal foreign body." Of course, I was expecting a three-year-old, but it turned out to be a gent in his 60's.

It seemed that he had some elbow macaroni stuck up his nose. Keeping my most professional demeanor (admittedly, a struggle in the best of circumstances), I asked politely how it might have passed that elbow macaroni came to reside in his nose.

With an indignant look, he told me that he puts dry elbow macaroni in his nose at night to cut down on the snoring. The wife's look wasn't indignant, but she certainly thought that this was a very reasonable thing to do. In the morning, when he did the usual elbow macaroni extrication, a piece was MIA.

So I dutifully looked in his nose for the errant macaroni. Not seeing it on first inspection, I got a nasal speculum to get a better look.

No macaroni. *Bummer.*

I then had to report to my pasta patient that I couldn't see the macaroni, and, perhaps, it had come out that night.

*"Well, look again!!!"* he insisted. I was thinking that if he had just waited a couple of hours, we would have the competent crew in and they could have found it.

I looked again. No macaroni.

*"I'm sorry, I'm not seeing any-macaroni. It must have fallen out."*

*"No, I think YOU are too F#ckng STOOPID to see it."* (Wonderful, I thought, like some Presidents before me, I hadn't quite worked out my withdrawal strategy).

*"Perhaps you're right. Let me get one of my colleagues to check."*

*"Fine. Just make sure it isn't that* . . . (at this point he threw in a racial slur about my Korean co-worker, getting his nationality wrong in the process) . . . *out there!!!"*

Time for my exit. I did have trouble explaining to my co-worker what I was talking about. He thought I was kidding.

In the end, the missing macaroni was never found. The patient stormed out en route to the other ER across town where there would be competent help. I didn't ask the wife for a pasta salad recipe. ✚

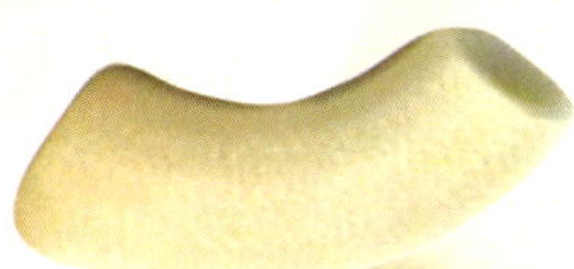

## TRUE QUICK BITS AND MALAPROPISMS

*"How did you fix the constipation?"*
***"I stuck my finger in there and cleaned myself out."***
*"Why?"*
***"I couldn't ask anyone else to pick my ass."***

***"The student squozed the BP cuff too tight."***

*"How do you feel?"*
***"It's better than jury duty!"***

***"This drug releases endogenous orphans."***

***"I'm so fat, I feel obeast."***

***"My sister thinks I have OCCD."***
Is that obsessive Catholicism?

***"That medicine you gave me really opened up my vagina and I am going to the bathroom a lot now!"***

***"I never smoked because I couldn't figure out how to inhale."***

***"The sores on the top of my mouth hurt when I gargle with salt water. Should I stop?"***

***"I'm inhaling and exhaling so my breathing doesn't become confused."***

Female patient was on oral contraceptives. She grew tired of taking them and gave them to her boyfriend, so ***"someone was taking them."*** She became pregnant.

A female patient was being seen for Morton's Neuroma, a painful condition wherein the nerves between the bones of the feet become tortuous and quite sensitive to pressure. We had changed her medication from *Oxycodone* to *Oxymorphone* when the former lost its ability to control the pain. Two days later she called stating that after discussing the condition with her trainer, she was found to have ***tied her shoes too tight!*** ✚

# MEDICAL T-SHIRTS WE'D LIKE TO SEE

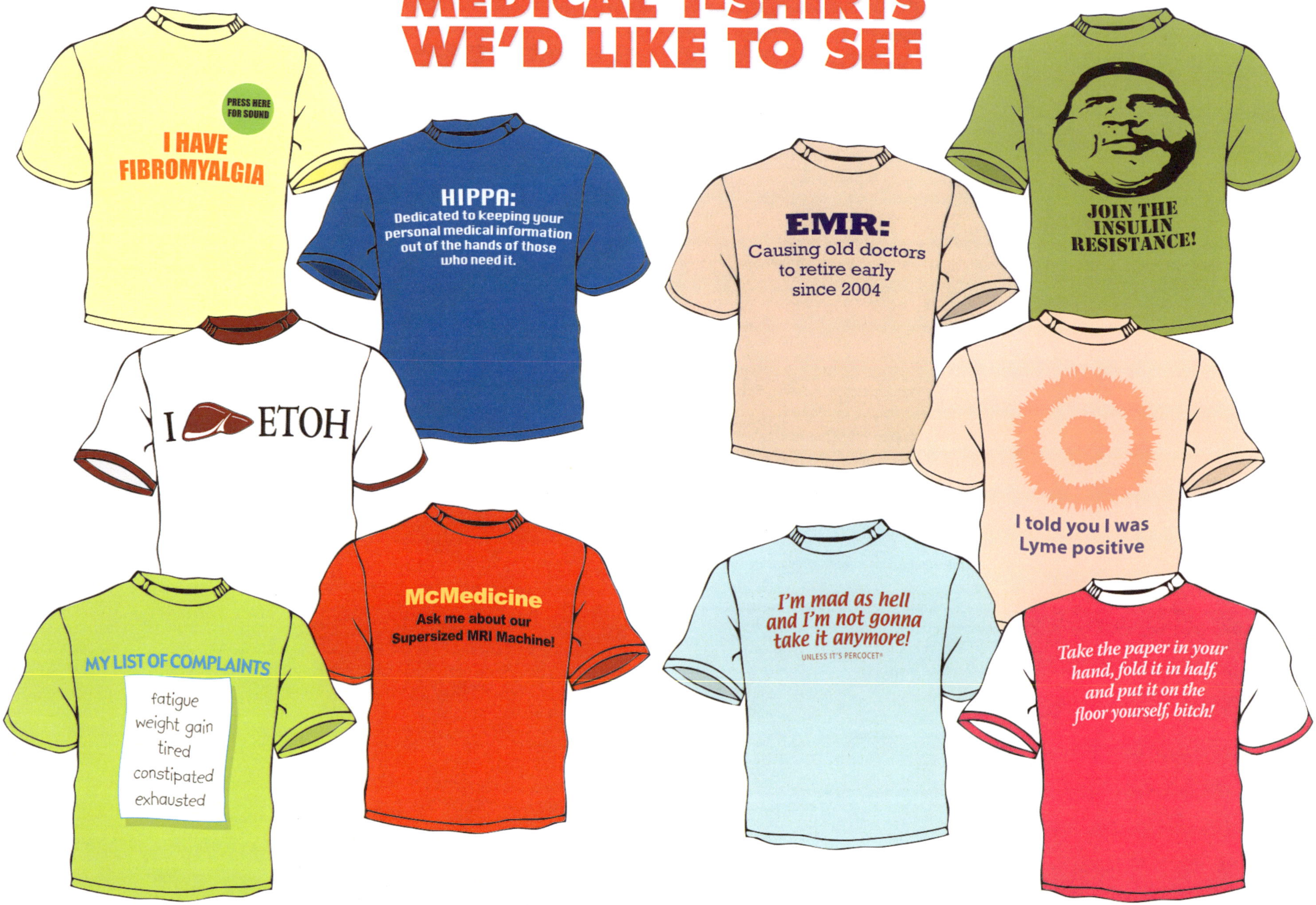
PRESS HERE FOR SOUND
I HAVE FIBROMYALGIA
HIPPA:
Dedicated to keeping your personal medical information out of the hands of those who need it.
EMR:
Causing old doctors to retire early since 2004
JOIN THE INSULIN RESISTANCE!
I ETOH
I told you I was Lyme positive
MY LIST OF COMPLAINTS
fatigue
weight gain
tired
constipated
exhausted
McMedicine
Ask me about our Supersized MRI Machine!
I'm mad as hell and I'm not gonna take it anymore!
UNLESS IT'S PERCOCET®
Take the paper in your hand, fold it in half, and put it on the floor yourself, bitch!

**SEND US YOUR IDEAS . . . WWW.PLACEBOJOURNAL.COM**

# THOSE DARN NARC SEEKERS

## THE NOTE

Okay, so Billy wasn't a pure narc seeker but the story runs the same course, as you will soon see. Billy had ADD and came to me when he transferred from another physician. I have a few patients on stimulants for adult ADD but to be honest, I am really not sure what to do with these people. This is a restricted class of drugs that is often sold on the street due to the huge black market demand. Billy's paperwork showed he was tested by a PhD and was found to be diagnosed correctly and therefore could benefit from the meds. Heck, I read the whole exam to make sure and I had no cause to deny him this treatment plan.

Billy was also seeing the chronic pain people and they were taking care of those medications. It made me more suspicious of Billy but I knew that they were testing him regularly so he would be caught if he was doing anything mischievous. And that is how it went for about a year until I saw the scanned note in my EMR. Billy got himself fired from the chronic pain doctor's office for not showing up regularly. *Uh oh.*

It was then that I decided to test Billy's urine. The results did not show narcotics in his system so he wasn't getting any off the street. *That was a good thing.* It didn't show any stimulants so he wasn't taking of my meds either. *Hmmmm.* Oh, but it did show a lot of cocaine.

My nurse told Billy that he was no longer getting any more *Ritalin* from me and he was not happy. Though he was not being fired from my practice, his ADD would not be treated with stimulants by me anymore. A few weeks later he called from the lab asking to have his urine tested again. I saw no reason to do that and he was alerted to that fact. I saw him in the office a few days later. The lab, in their infinite wisdom, did the test without my order and it was clean. Billy had proof, he thought, that he could now get his stimulants. I explained to him that it didn't work that way. It was a done deal. Again not happy, he sat and thought for a while and hit me with another request.

*"I've had this problem with stealing lately,"* he said.

*"Really? How much of a problem,"* I responded.

*"Not too bad but my lawyer wanted me to ask for a note."*

*"If it wasn't too much of a problem then why do you have a lawyer?"*

*"Well, I have been in and out of jail the last few months."*

*"Good to know. Well, what kind of note does your lawyer want?"* I said, knowing the answer all along.

*"Well, since you weren't treating my ADD then he wants you to say that this caused me to steal."*

*"Yeeeaaaahhhhh . . . uh, no."*

Dead silence.

*"Okay, so I can't get my ADD meds now?"*

*"Let me summarize this for you. No ADD meds. No notes allowing you to steal. In fact, that raps this visit up."*

And off he went. Probably to steal again. And I guess somehow that will be my fault too. ✚

# A TRUE STORY OF MEDICINE

## PICC HUMOR

A woman with a PICC line (peripherally inserted central catheter) kept coming to the emergency room because it kept getting infected. When the staff asked her how she cared for the line, she admitted that her cat liked to play with the connections (the ends that comes out of the skin and where IV is hooked up to - sorry I don't know the technical term for them, maybe they are called ports?) and the cats would lick them and bat them around. When she was told that having the cat play with the PICC line was not a good idea and was causing her infections, all she could say was, *"But Pussy enjoys playing with them so much!"* ✚

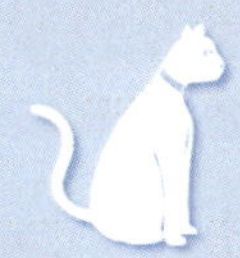

## THE TICK?

At my hospice meeting yesterday, the previous night's on-call nurse related this story.

*"I was woken up by a call from so-and-so's wife at 11pm. She found a tick on his scrotum; what should she do?*

I told her to use alcohol, it would help it detatch and 'shrivel it up.'

So, to clarify, she asks, *"the TICK?"*

The nurse went on to say that he put it in a jar so she could see it when she got there the next day . . . to which, of course, I replied, *"the TICK?"* ✚

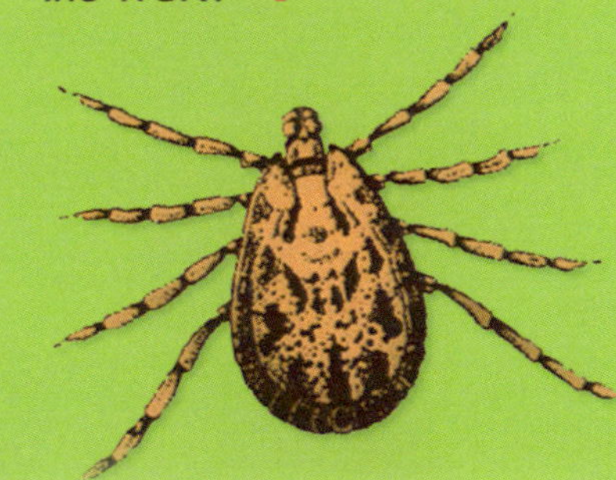

# RIDES at a Medical-Themed Amusement Park

**With all the insurance company profits, we only feel it is fair they should be mandated to invest some of their billions into something . . . Get ready for summer!**

The Centrifuge

The Trainwreck

The Swiss Family Robinson Meth Lab

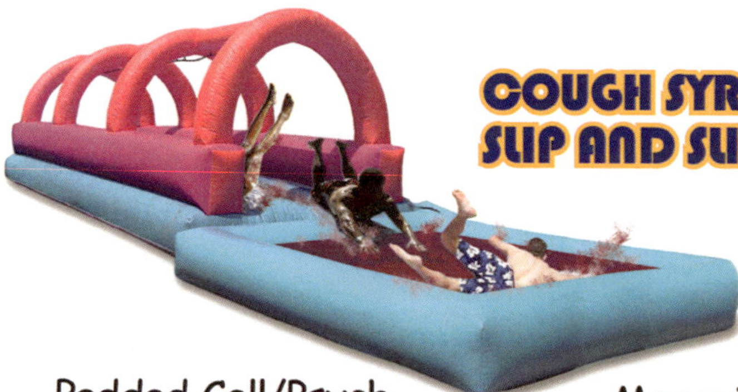

**COUGH SYRUP SLIP AND SLIDE**

Padded Cell/Psych Ward Fun House

The Clinical Care Roller Coaster

Haunted Forensic Ward

Tower of Rectal Pressure

It's A Narc World

Meconium Splash Mountain

Ho White's Scary Medical Adventures

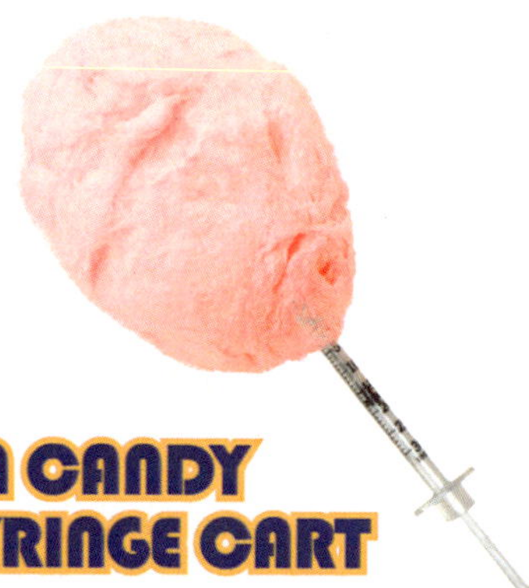

**THE COTTON CANDY ON AN INSULIN SYRINGE CART**

The Psychiatrist's House of Revolving Doors

The Slot Machine Arcade

The Towering Hemorrhoid Inferno

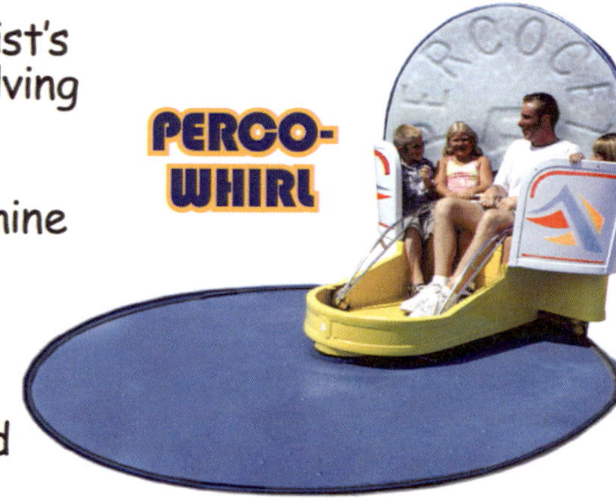

**PERCO-WHIRL**

The Administrator's Midway of Expensive but Unwinnable Arguments

The Hyper-glyIceCreamia

The Log Un-Jam (Sponsored by Polyethylene Glycol)

The Kiddy ADHD Playworld (A Ritalin-Free Zone)

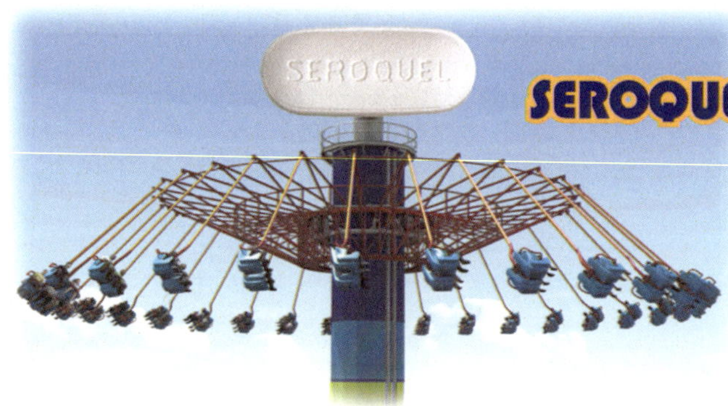


**SEROQUEL SWING**

**Located in Knockemstiff, Ohio. Take the first left off Black Run Rd. and ask for Lefty. He'll tell ya where to go from there.**

You have a habit.

You spend a lot of time on your back.

You don't need no more stinkin' kids.

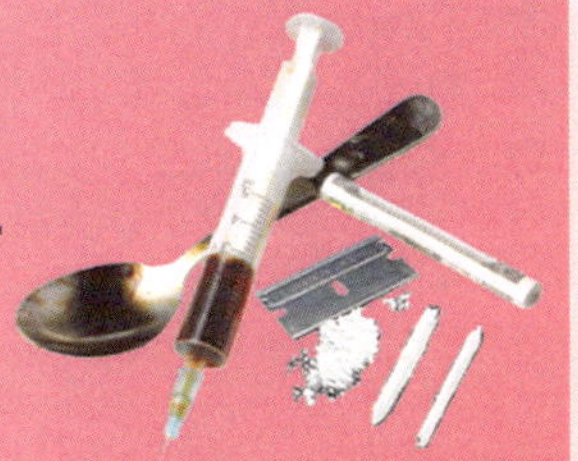

*What's a girl to do?*

**Don't** worry, girlfriend, we've got you covered!

# MethaDon't

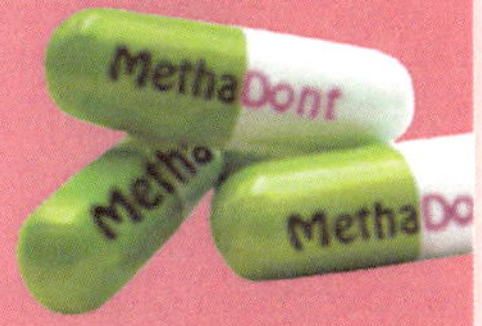


***methadone maintenance plus oral contraception in one convenient dose***

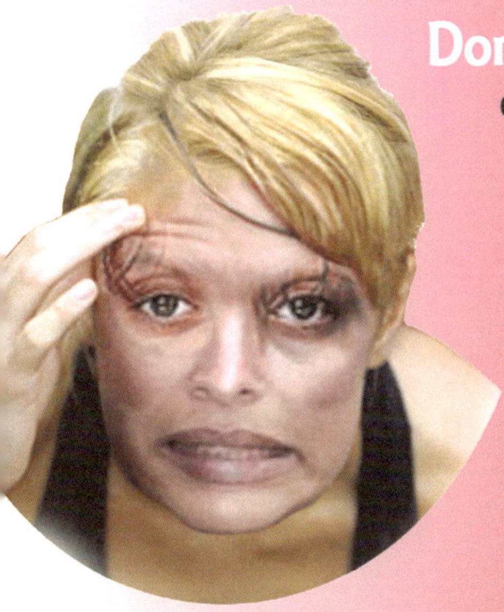

**Don't** miss another pill and end up pregnant. Again.

**Don't** go messin' up your pretty arms with needle tracks.

**Don't** wait. Ask your doctor about **MethaDon't.**

*For the love of all things holy, DO NOT give MethaDon't to your babies to help them sleep.*

**PJ PHARMACEUTICALS**
*The Realistic Drug Company.*
*We're looking out for the taxpayers.*

# MEDICAL MYTHBUSTERS

**Two men mix scientific method with plain old-fashioned ingenuity to figure out ways how to get through their lives as physicians.**

**Watch them as they uncover the truth behind the popular myths and legends of the medical field.**

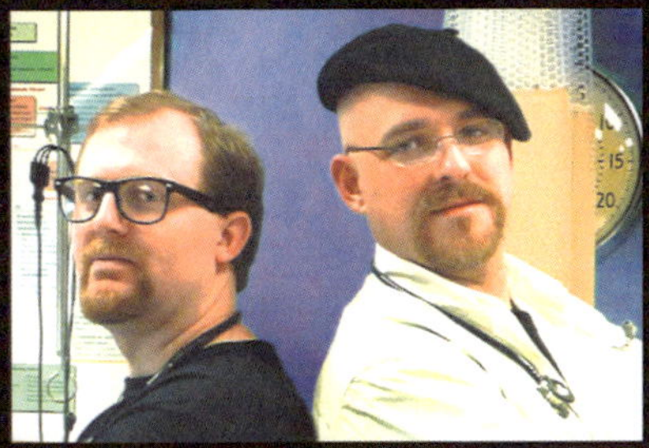

***Who are the mythbusters?***
**VANCE LASSEY & CLINT COLBERG**

**Two physicians, with 13 years combined practice experience.**

**Each week, they take common medical myths and urban legends, and put them to the test!**

**In this week's episode, VANCE & CLINT take on Common Emergency Room Myths!**

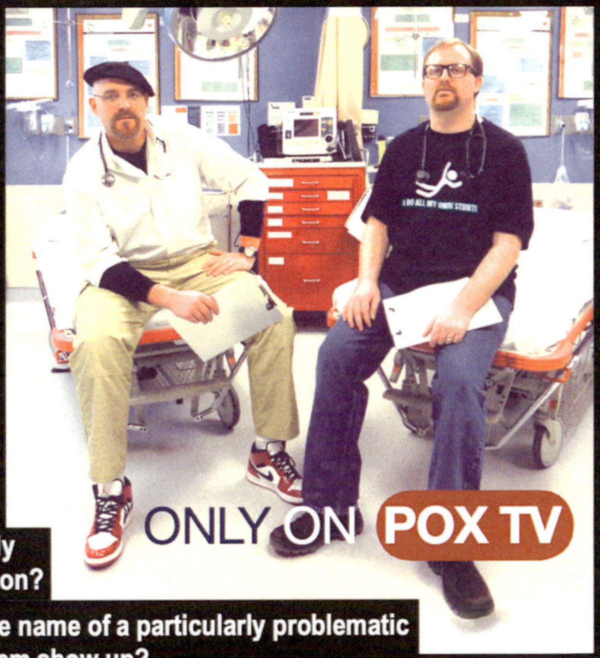


**Does saying the "Q word" (quiet) make it busier in the ER?**

**Do medical diagnoses or problems really tend to present in threes?**

**Does the ER really get busier on a full moon?**

**Does invoking the name of a particularly problematic frequent-flyer make them show up?**

***Join us in future episodes as we go in the search of evidence for mythical diagnoses***

ANOTHER TRUE STORY OF MEDICINE

# VETERANS HEALTH CARE:

I recently underwent an angiogram at the Veterans Hospital in Palo Alto, California. I will not lie to you, the experience was uncomfortable and I had some complications, but the results showed no coronary artery disease. The humor provided by two female student nurses was worth it – *haven't laughed so hard in a while!*

To prepare for the procedure the head nurse instructed the two student nurses to shave the area and apply a 'condom' catheter. The two students nodded they had done this before so the nurse handed an electric razor to one of them and closed the privacy curtain. For a brief moment, the students argued who should shave me. The taller of the two finally relented and brought the shaver toward my crotch. The area normally shaved is in the pelvic area where the thigh pivots at the hip, but for some reason she figured I needed my testicles shaved. She drug the razor across my testicles with a puzzled look, and the other student whispered, *"You need to turn it on, it's electric."* I just laid back, bit my lip and watched in amazement. . . until the now running razor started making diving passes at my nuts, removing tufts of hair and breaking the skin! I envisioned going to the operating room with toilet paper squares all over my privates.

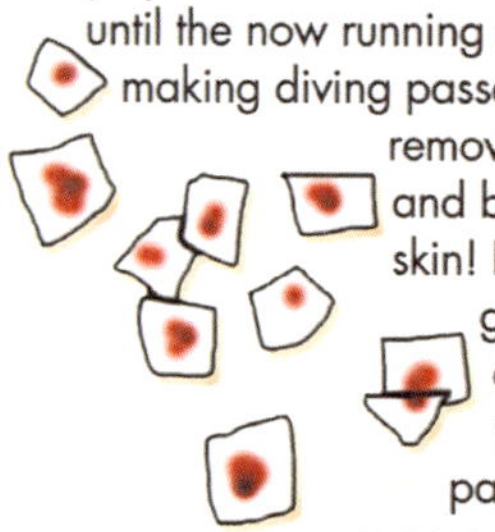

*"Hey, take it easy, those things are tender!"*

She eased up and in a few minutes, there was a pile of pubic hair on the bed. I looked down at what now looked like two squirrels with mange and road-rash. I was really trying hard to hold back the laughter. That's when she followed the fine shaving job with a thorough disinfecting wipe from an alcohol swab! *Jeezus, holy crap that burned,* but I remained quiet. Watching these two was like watching an episode of *Laverne and Shirley.* I thought I'd seen it all, but just then she opened the package to the condom catheter. The room was cold as hell and the head nurse had remarked they keep it cool to protect the electronic equipment. Unfortunately, the male anatomy likes things warm and will shrink in cold weather as mine had done. The nurse looked at the condom catheter, then at my willy with a puzzled look. Without hesitation she reached underneath my nuts and began pumping on the skin of my crotch like she was trying to inflate a *Nike Air* tennis shoe. I don't know if she had seen this technique on a training video or a porno, at any rate she struggled for a minute or two and finally got the condom thingy on. *Oh thank God.* I was about to pee myself as I was still holding back my laughter as best I could. I thought everything was done, they'd leave and I could laugh my ass off, but it wasn't to be.

# WHEN ONLY THE BEST WILL DO.

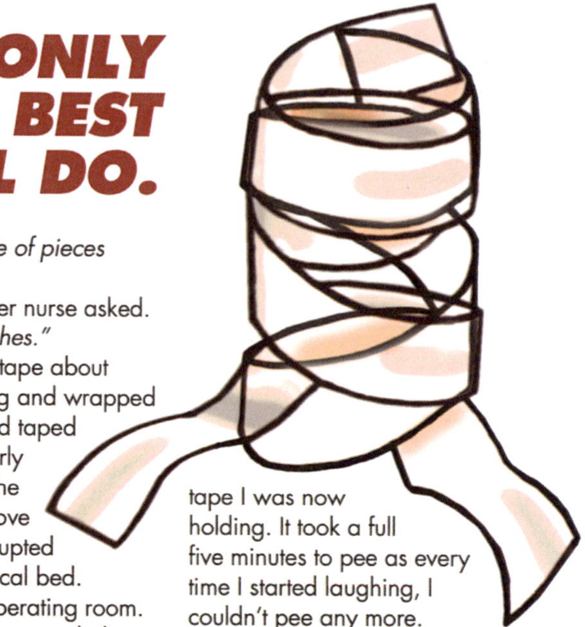

*"Tear me off a couple of pieces of tape."*

*"How long?"* the other nurse asked.

*"Oh, about three inches."*

She tore 2 pieces of tape about seven or eight inches long and wrapped them around my willy and taped the loose ends to my nearly bald nuts. Fear set in at the thought of having to remove the tape, but it was interrupted by the arrival of the surgical bed. I was wheeled into the operating room. The doctor lifted the sheet to scrub the procedure area.

*"What the hell?"* he asked.

*"They didn't shave you?"*

*"Well, they did but it's a long story."*

The doctor grabbed a razor and shaved my leg and performed the angiogram. By the time I got back to the room I really had to pee, but I couldn't go with the condom on and the tape on my nuts. After two hours, the nurse allowed me to go to the bathroom. I must have been in there 10 or 15 minutes when I heard my girlfriend knocking on the door.

*"You okay honey?"*

*"Yes,"* I said feebly as the last of the tape was ripped from my inflamed nuts. I glanced down at my self-performed Brazilian wax and that's when I lost it! I started peeing, laughing uncontrollably and looking at the last remaining pubic hairs stuck to the tape I was now holding. It took a full five minutes to pee as every time I started laughing, I couldn't pee any more.

The next day I had to return to the hospital as there had been some bruising to the procedure area. While I was there, my girlfriend suggested I tell my experience to the head nurse. I started into the story and the nurse began laughing uncontrollably, finally laying her head down on the desk. She was unable to look up for a minute or so. Finally, she stopped laughing.

*"Oh honey, I'm so sorry. You were such a good sport after so much pain."* She began laughing again.

*"What's so funny?"* I asked.

*"Well, they said they knew what they were doing. They performed the same thing on two men the day before you!"* We all had a good laugh." ✚

# X-Ray Files

**If we show you ours, will you show us yours?**

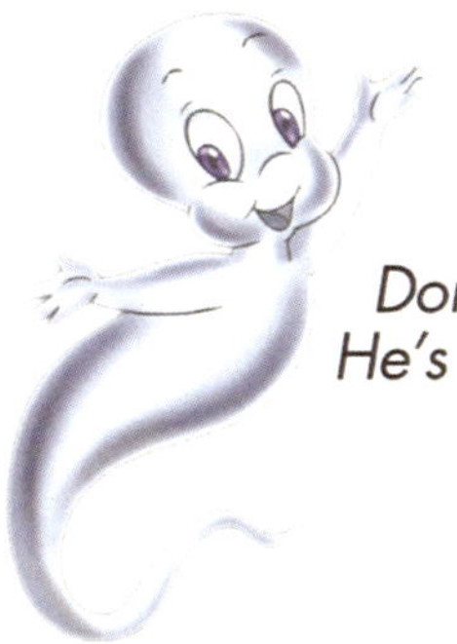

**BOO!**

*Don't be afraid He's friendly . . .*

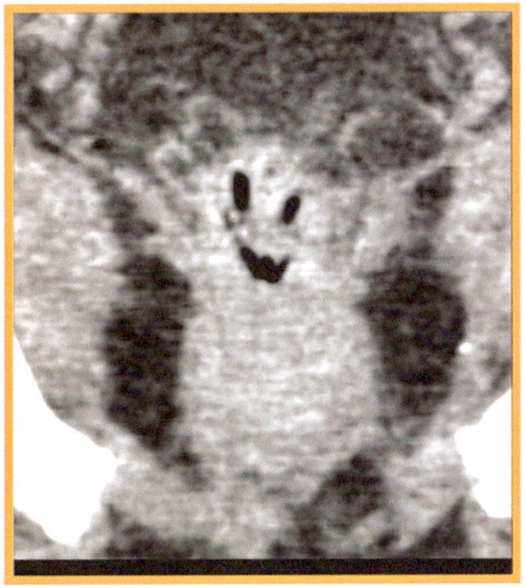

*Here's a patient with a* **GUN SHOT WOUND . . .**

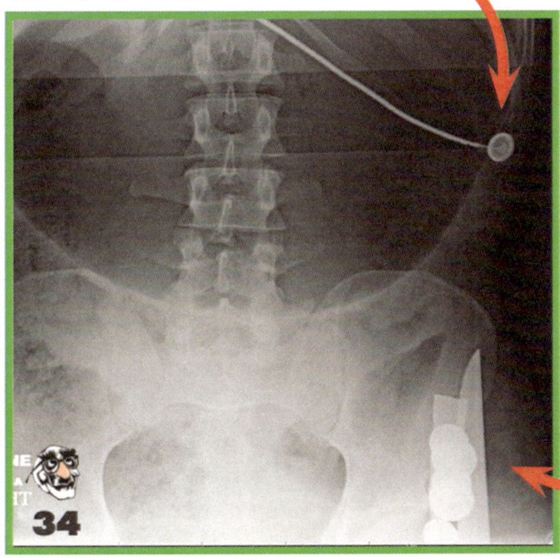

*. . . and possibly a* **STAB WOUND** *in his future based on the objects in his left pants pocket . . .*

*We were told this was a* **PIG FACE.** *It's something, but we can't decide what it is? Any ideas?* Send us an e-mail!

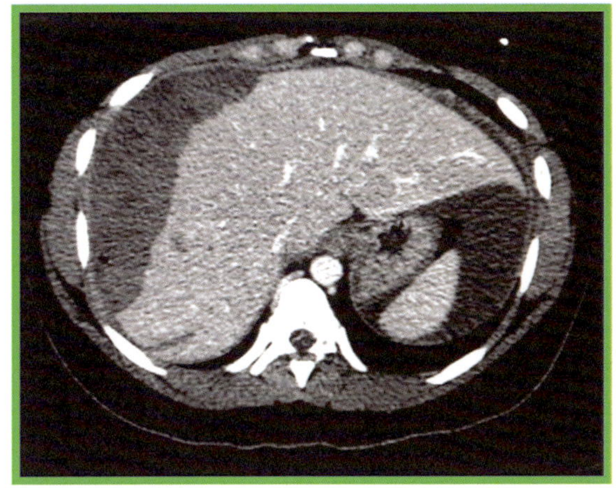

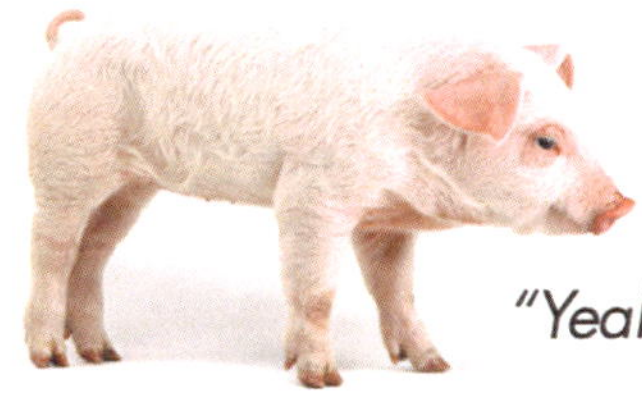

*"Yeah, I don't see it either . . ."*

*Here's a* **CLASSIC** *from our February 2005 issue . . .*

## A HEART IN THE RECTUM for A HAPPY VALENTINE'S DAY!

*Yes, it wrecked 'um. Damn near killed 'um!*

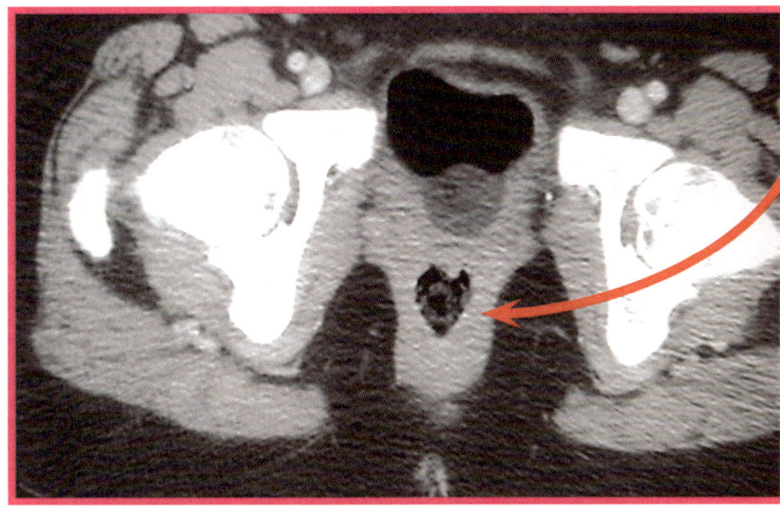

If you're a radiologist, show us your files.
If we use them, you'll get
**A FREE ONE-YEAR SUBSCRIPTION!**

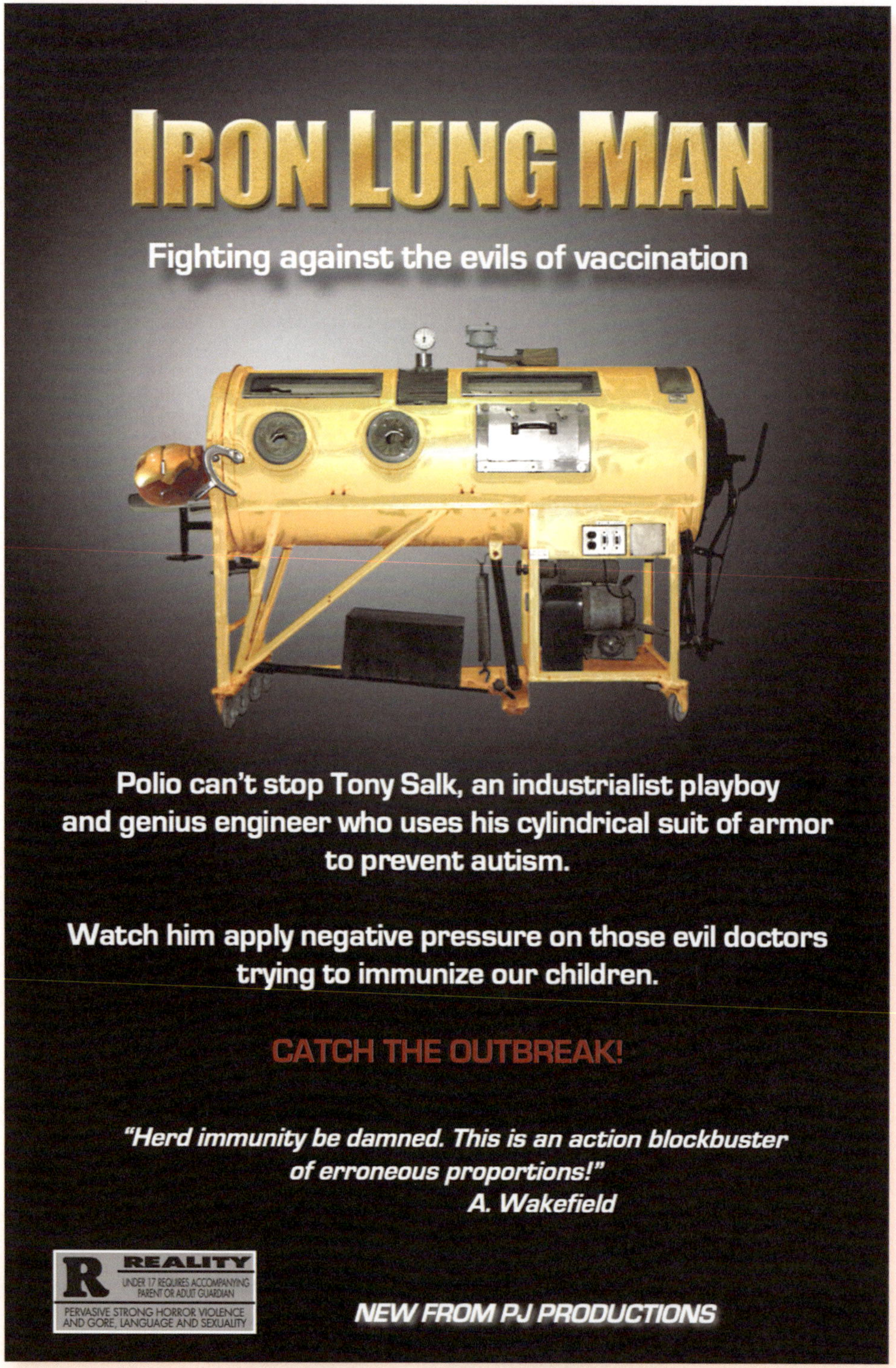


Most doctors are not blessed with tremendous social skills. If you didn't know this, and you are a doctor, then you are one of them, and you're probably a specialist. So just for *you*, the *Placebo Journal* presents . . .

## SOCIAL SKILLS FOR DOCTORS

*This issue's topic:*

# How To Talk To A Referring Primary Care Physician

| What he/she said | What you heard | What he/she meant |
|---|---|---|
| *"I'd like to refer a patient to you."* | *"I'd like to dump a patient on you."* | *"I've tried hard and I can't figure this case out. You've probably seen this before. HELP!" -OR- "This is somatization, but she made me refer her to you."* |
| *"This is a tough case."* | *"I'm too stupid and lazy to figure this case out."* | *"This is a tough case, and this problem is your specialty."* |
| *"Please keep in contact with me so I know what treatements you are trying and so I can continue to manage this patient's care."* | *"Don't steal this patient from me."* | *"After my patients see you, they always come back to me asking what in the hell you told them, because you spent four minutes throwing jargon at them and left the room. I'll need correspondence so I can translate and help you do your job correctly. Believe it or not, our patients don't all have medical degrees."* |
| *"This is a really nice lady."* | *"The patient doesn't have insurance or this is a work comp case."* | *"This is a really nice lady."* |
| *"Sorry about this one . . ."* | *"PUNT. Your turn, jerk! This is what you get for making ten times more money than me!"* | *"Remember when you swore at me on call last week or treated that last patient I sent you so rudely? This patient is impossible to figure out, impossible to deal with, or impossible to spend more than 30 seconds in the room with due to exessive body odor. I think I will send them to "definitive care." Hey, you chose to be at the top of the food chain, so you gotta eat the fare. By the way, this patient has a history of suing doctors, hasn't paid a bill in three years, smokes, and will arrive driving a Lexus."* |

## MORE TRUE STORIES OF MEDICINE

# KNEE JERK REACTION

A couple of years ago I was seeing an established patient back to follow-up on the arthritis medication I had prescribed for her on the prior visit, as well as to follow-up on her other chronic health complaints.

She said, *"I feel just great except I don't really think that* Cialis *you gave me is doing anything."*

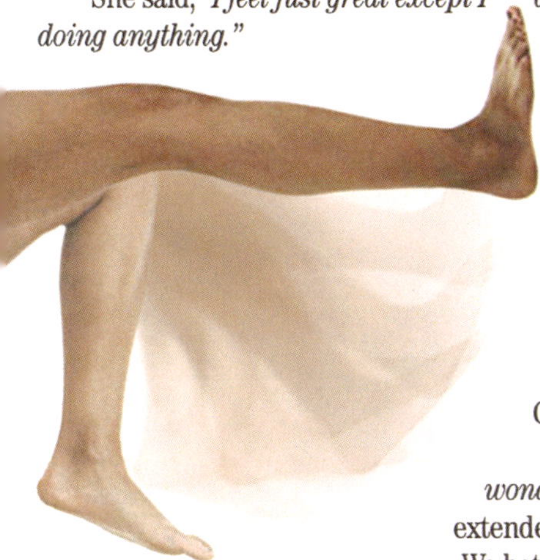

I looked up from her chart with confusion as my mind raced . . . *"Did I give her* Cialis*? Why would I give her* Cialis*? Oh dear, did I make a mistake and write the wrong prescription?"*

I looked back at her chart and confirmed I had dictated at least (and I prayed had actually written) for her to try *Celebrex*.

I tentatively said, *"Do you mean the* Celebrex *for your knee?"*

She blushed and began to giggle. *"Well, no wonder my leg kept doing this,"* she said as she extended her knee with said leg up in the air.

We both laughed until we cried. Understandably, she remains one of my favorite patients as her visits always bring laughter to us both. In fact, she purchased my subscription to *Placebo Journal*. And for the record, I HAD given her *Celebrex* NOT *Cialis*.

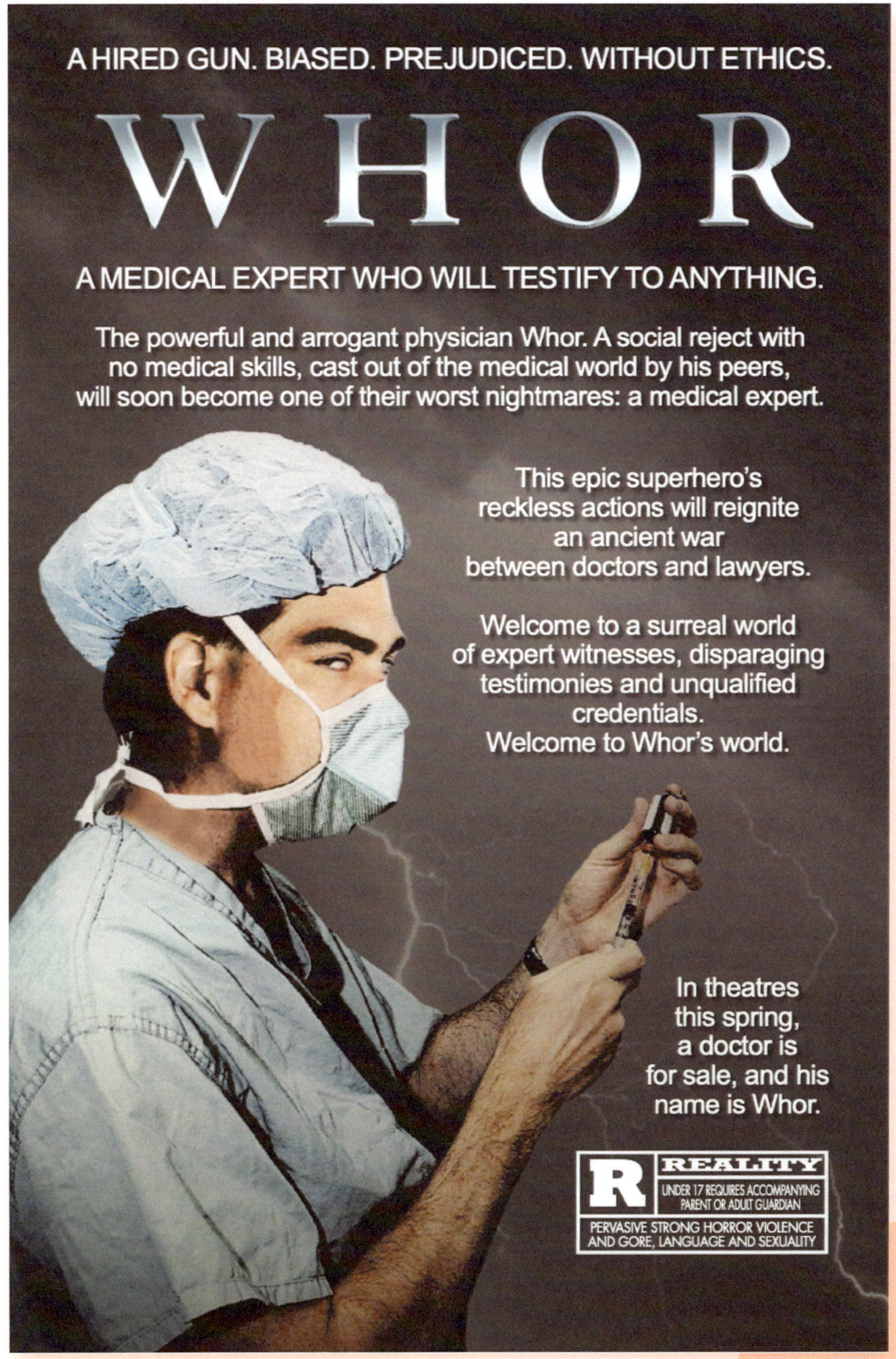

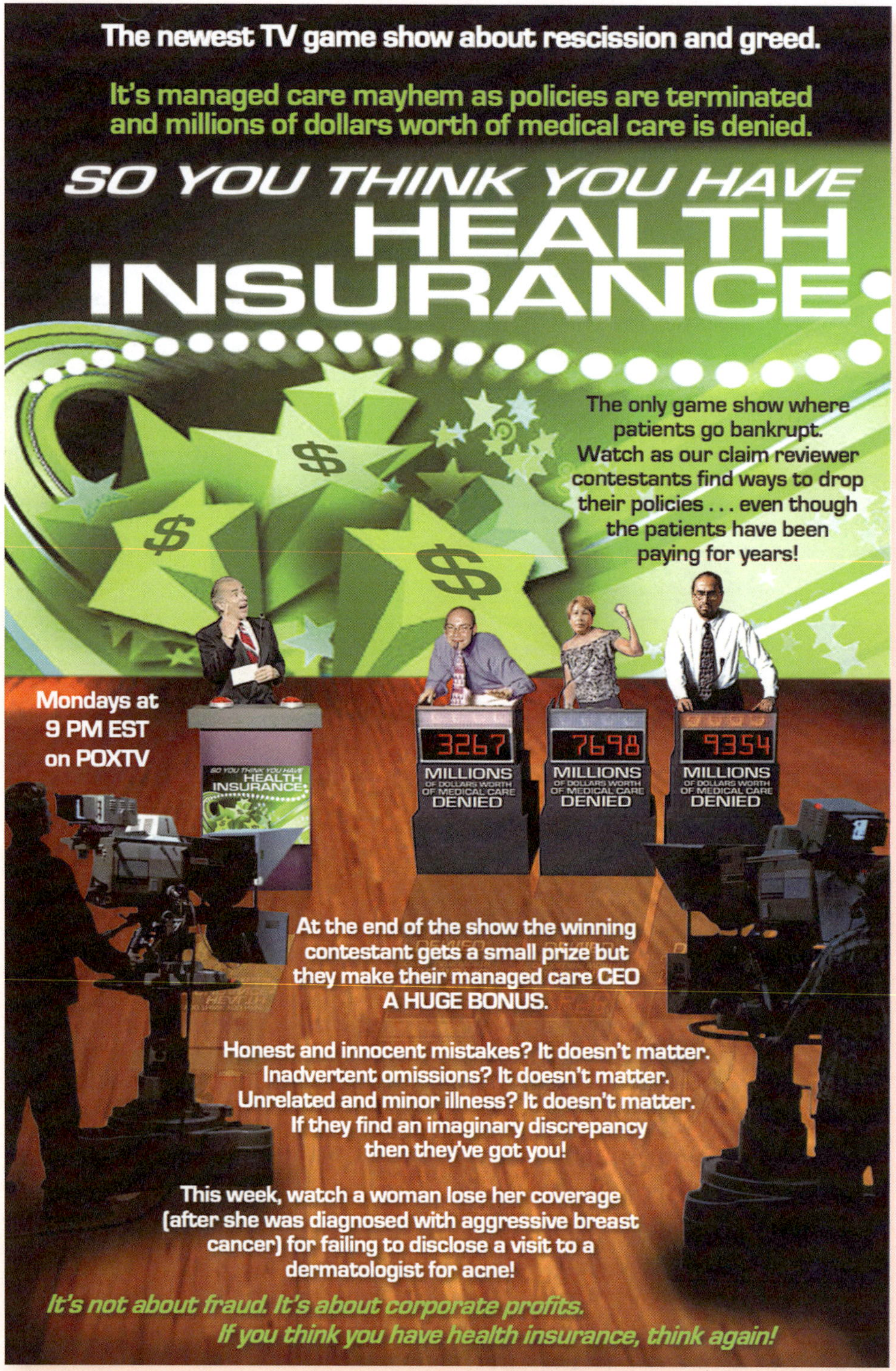
The newest TV game show about rescission and greed.
It's managed care mayhem as policies are terminated and millions of dollars worth of medical care is denied.
SO YOU THINK YOU HAVE HEALTH INSURANCE
The only game show where patients go bankrupt. Watch as our claim reviewer contestants find ways to drop their policies . . . even though the patients have been paying for years!
Mondays at 9 PM EST on POXTV
3267
7698
9354
MILLIONS OF DOLLARS WORTH OF MEDICAL CARE DENIED
MILLIONS OF DOLLARS WORTH OF MEDICAL CARE DENIED
MILLIONS OF DOLLARS WORTH OF MEDICAL CARE DENIED
At the end of the show the winning contestant gets a small prize but they make their managed care CEO A HUGE BONUS.
Honest and innocent mistakes? It doesn't matter.
Inadvertent omissions? It doesn't matter.
Unrelated and minor illness? It doesn't matter.
If they find an imaginary discrepancy then they've got you!
This week, watch a woman lose her coverage (after she was diagnosed with aggressive breast cancer) for failing to disclose a visit to a dermatologist for acne!
It's not about fraud. It's about corporate profits.
If you think you have health insurance, think again!

# DEATH GRIP

Many years ago when I was a third year medical student I did an OB/GYN rotation and I was on the maternity ward. In those days we were only allowed to time contractions (by feeling the patient's abdomen) and take blood pressures. In that age long ago the patients were given demerol and scopolamine (to numb the pain and to supposedly make them forget the pain when it was all over). I was in my scrubs when with my hand on her very pregnant belly. I was attempting to time her contraction.

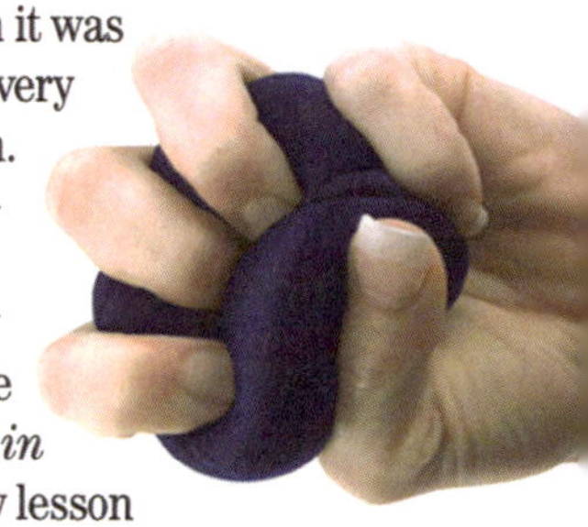

As I was leaning over the side rails trying to accomplish my assigned task, unbeknownst to me (and her) she reached through the side rails and grabbed onto my family jewels with a death grip and didn't let go until the contraction was over. *That was the longest contraction in recorded history (or so I thought).* I quickly learned my lesson *(after I pushed my eye balls back into their sockets)* and never faced the patient again while timing her contractions. I looked silly backing up to the bed but it was safer.

Maybe that's why I went into dermatology and not OB/GYN. ✚

# MARRIED MUCH?

This woman came to the ED after having a fight with her boyfriend. She had been living with him for several years, and he'd never acted this way before. Her wounds were superficial, but she was very upset.

*"So tell me more about what happened,"* I said in my best *Marcus Welby* voice.

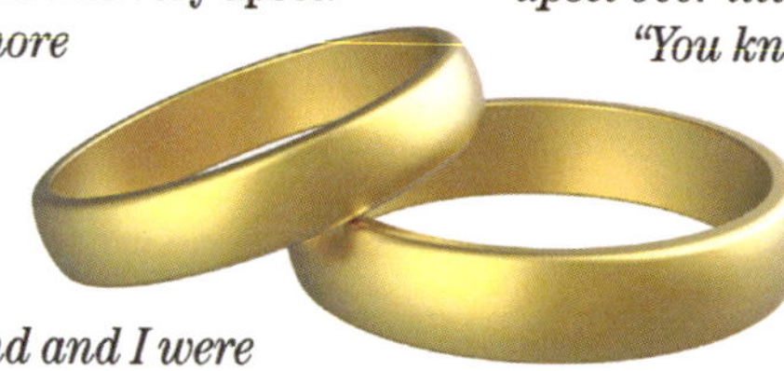

*"My boyfriend and I were fighting and he hit me,"* she sobbed.

*"That's terrible. A man should never hit a woman,"* I said. *"How did the fight start?"*

*"Well, I just got married about three weeks ago,"* she began.

*"Marriage can be tough, especially at the beginning,"* I wisely added, *"Go on."*

*"Well, my boyfriend just gets so upset over little things,"* she said.

*"You know,"* I interjected, *"he's not just your boyfriend anymore. He's your husband now."*

She looked at me quizzically.

*"No,"* she said, *"My husband and I are fine. It's just that when I told my* ***boyfriend*** *that I just got married, he got upset and he hit me."* ✚

## MORE TRUE STORIES OF MEDICINE

# PERRLA

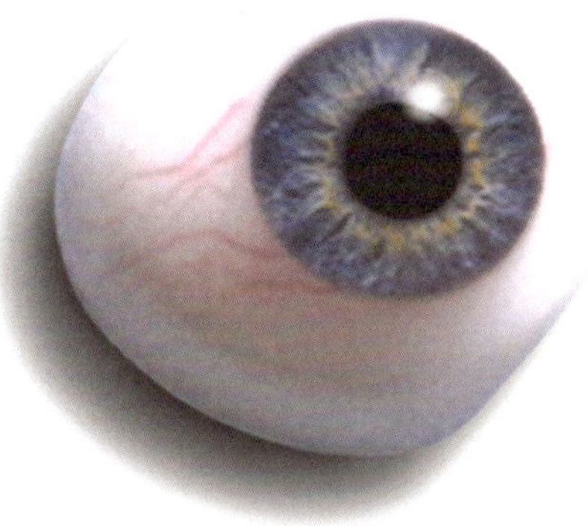

I was working as a locum tenens in an ER and just started my shift at noon. One of the nurses approached me with a report of a patient who needed to be seen soon. She was an elderly woman who fell and had a constricted non-reacting pupil. The local nursing home stated that she "possibly fell" two days before they brought her in. The story goes on to say that she was found on the floor of another resident's room. There were no witnesses, no complaints by the patient, and no injuries were noted. They decided not to send her to the ER at that time but instead decided just do "neuro" checks. When the patient complained of not being able to see, a nurse noticed some blood coming from her right eye. She then noted that the patient had a "small and sluggishly reactive" right pupil and had her sent to my ER.

Upon seeing the transfer sheet, I noticed that one of her ten diagnoses was "dementia." When I began to question her however, she seemed pretty alert and oriented. She did complain of some nausea as well as not being able to see out of the right eye. Otherwise, she was fine.

Upon examination, I found some fresh blood on the eyelid and at the lateral margin of the orbit. The pupil was indeed constricted, not reactive and not reflecting light. The source of the bleeding turned out to be small pinpoint area under the upper conjunctiva. Inspecting the area closer on the upper part of the eye, I found numbers and letters. ***It was a prosthetic eye!!!!!***

When I asked the patient how long she had had a fake eye, she stated, *"I have a fake eye?"* I guess that dementia label was accurate. Doing some review of the chart I found no record of blindness in the patient's nursing home history. The kicker was that on the supposed "neuro" check sheets they were filling out, the box for "pupils equal and reactive to light" had been checked off. Someone may want to get a refresher medical course! ✚

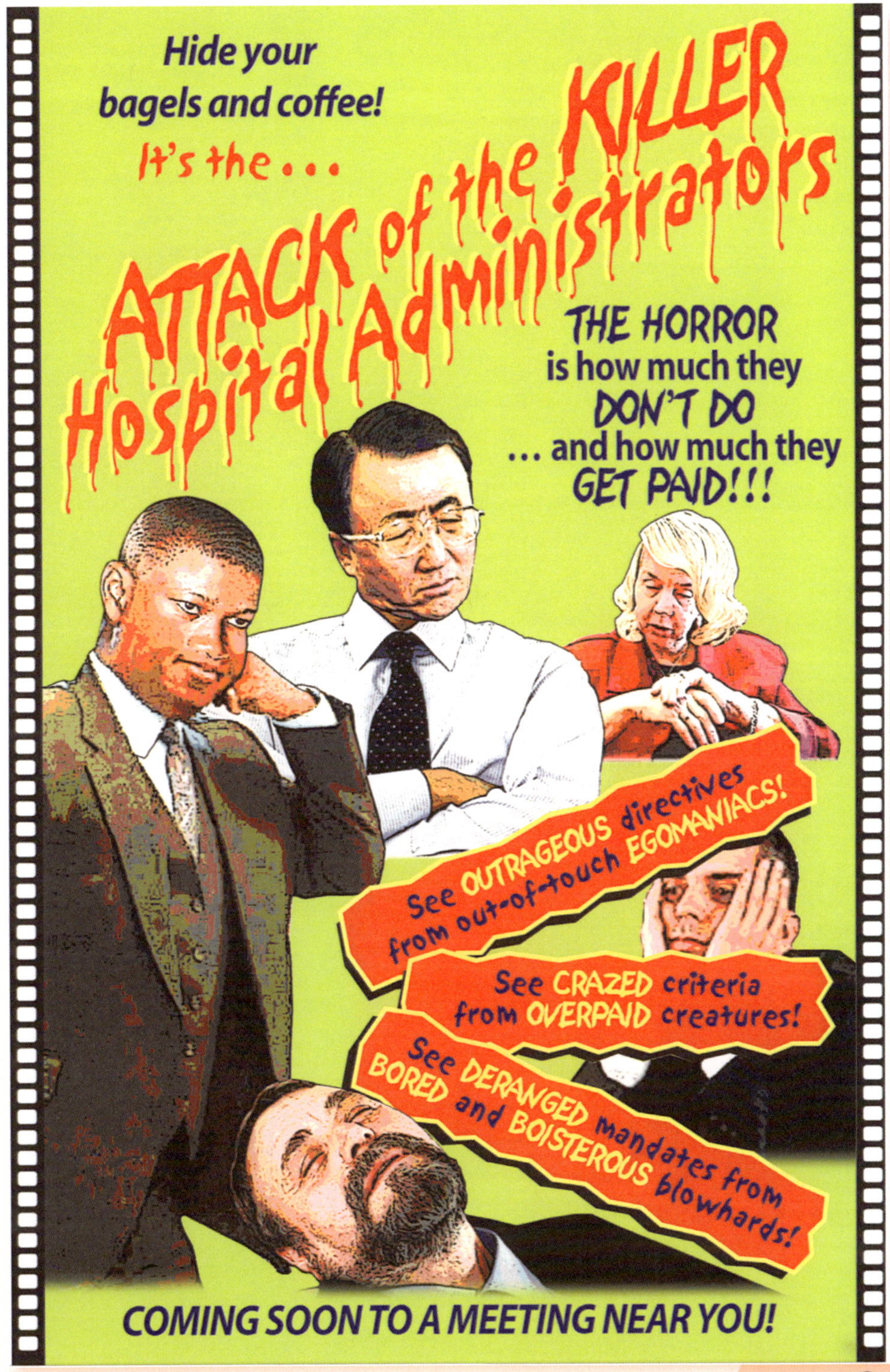
Hide your bagels and coffee!
It's the...
ATTACK of the KILLER Hospital Administrators
THE HORROR is how much they DON'T DO ... and how much they GET PAID!!!
See OUTRAGEOUS directives from out-of-touch EGOMANIACS!
See CRAZED criteria from OVERPAID creatures!
See DERANGED mandates from BORED and BOISTEROUS blowhards!
COMING SOON TO A MEETING NEAR YOU!

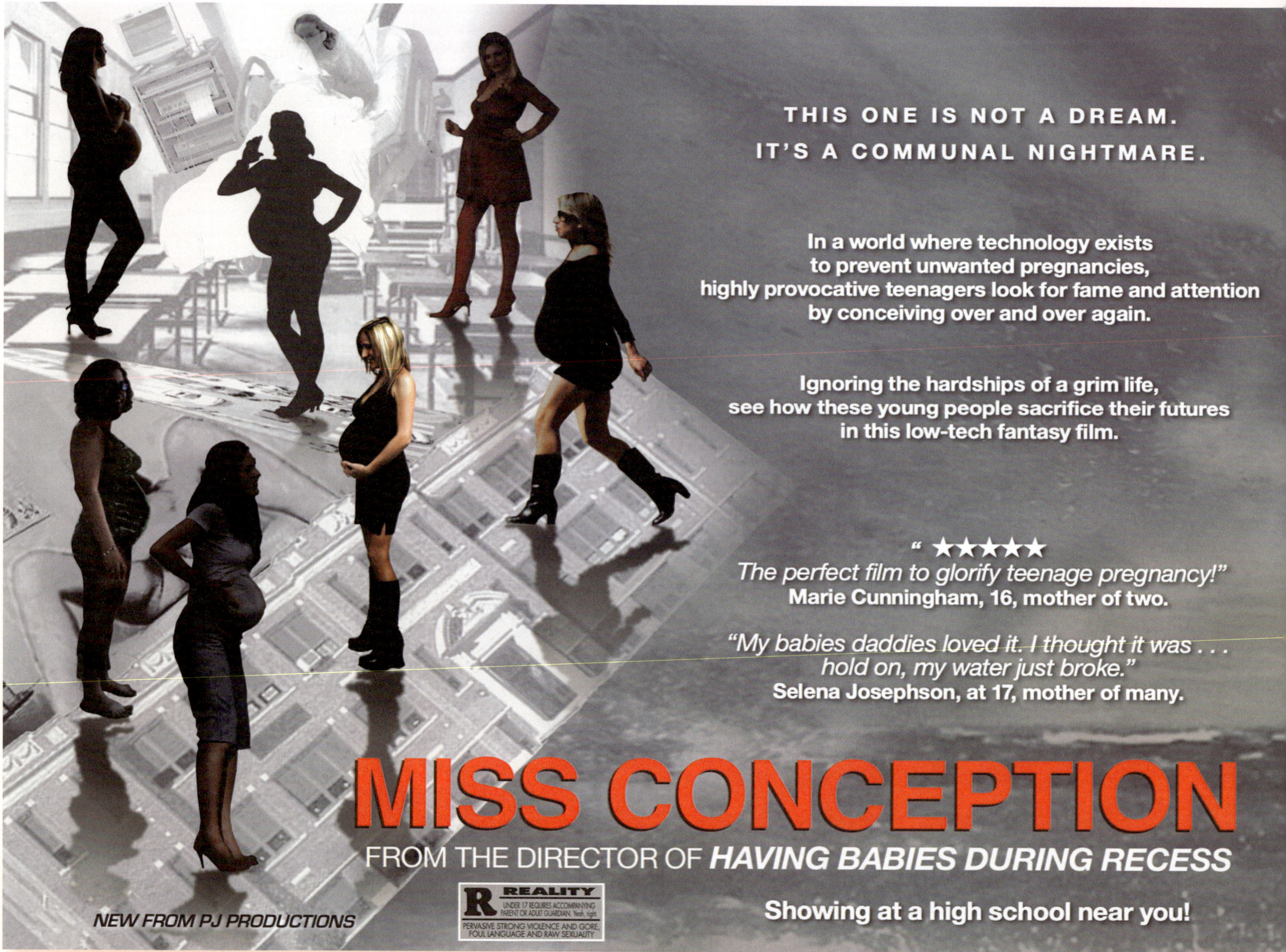
THIS ONE IS NOT A DREAM.
IT'S A COMMUNAL NIGHTMARE.
In a world where technology exists to prevent unwanted pregnancies, highly provocative teenagers look for fame and attention by conceiving over and over again.
Ignoring the hardships of a grim life, see how these young people sacrifice their futures in this low-tech fantasy film.
" ★★★★★
The perfect film to glorify teenage pregnancy!"
Marie Cunningham, 16, mother of two.
"My babies daddies loved it. I thought it was . . . hold on, my water just broke."
Selena Josephson, at 17, mother of many.
MISS CONCEPTION
FROM THE DIRECTOR OF HAVING BABIES DURING RECESS
NEW FROM PJ PRODUCTIONS
R REALITY
UNDER 17 REQUIRES ACCOMPANYING PARENT OR ADULT GUARDIAN. Yeah, right.
PERVASIVE STRONG VIOLENCE AND GORE, FOUL LANGUAGE AND RAW SEXUALITY
Showing at a high school near you!

## PEDIATRIC MEDICAL ALGORITHM OF REALITY

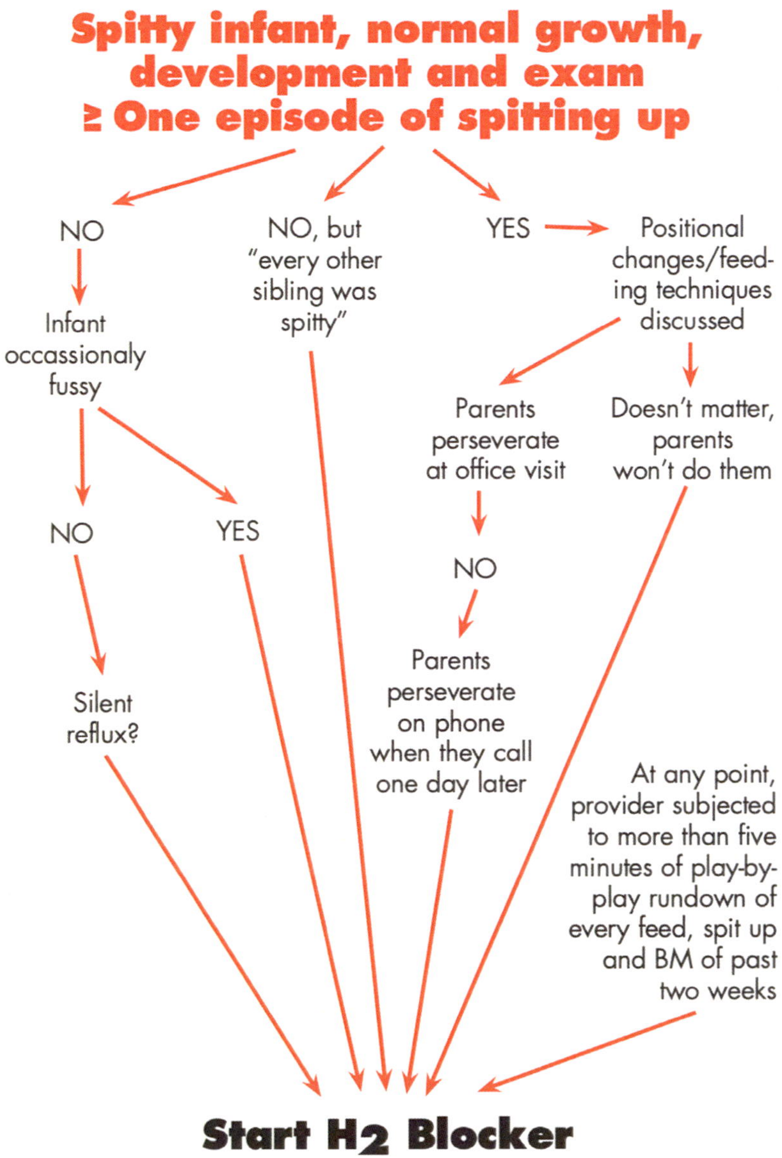


MORE TRUE STORIES OF MEDICINE

# IT PAYS TO BE HONEST

Back in the days when anesthesiologists did interviews in the hospital, I was trying my best to get some history from the next morning's patient. Every time he tried to answer, his wife interrupted with a correction or embellishment. After I had gleaned all of the information that was forthcoming, I asked the patient if he had any questions.

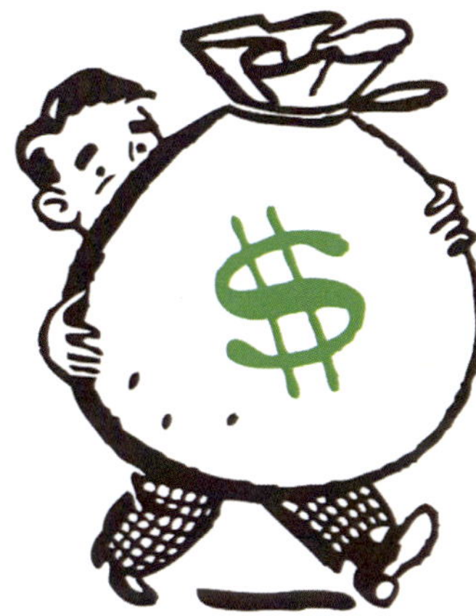

He asked, *"About what time will we start tomorrow?"*

I replied that the staff would come to get him about 5:30 a.m. (This was at 10:15 p.m.).

At this, his wife clasped her hands over her chest and said, *"Oh doctor, what drives you doctors to work such long hours?"*

Glancing up from my note, and in a matter-of-fact tone, I replied, *"Greed, ma'am, insatiable greed."*

The patient in the other bed, apparently taking this all in with his eyes closed, sat up and exclaimed, *"That's the first honest thing I ever heard a doctor say."*

Apparently, the patient appreciated my candor because he requested my anesthesia for his next surgery. ✚

*From an actual OB resume we received . . .*

**"Developed marketing strategy to double obstetric births in county over three years."**

*What kind of strategy would that be?*

Public service announcements promoting the virtues of teen sex.

Sponsoring free hotel rooms for after prom activities.

Pornos in the high schools.

Importing generic contraceptives from China.

*I haven't heard if the strategy succeeded.* ✚

# MY FAVORITE MUNCHAUSEN

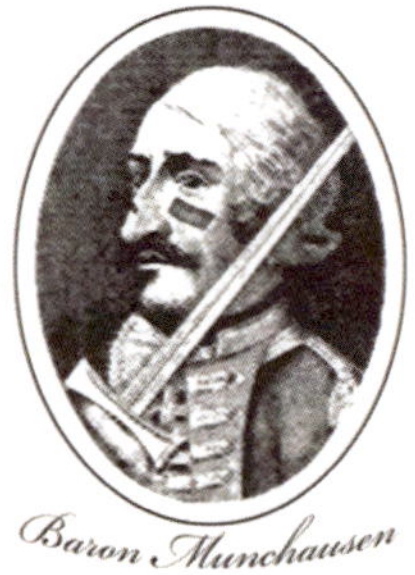

*Baron Munchausen*

*EDITOR'S NOTE: The editors find the* ***Munchausen Syndrome*** *intriguing in an odd way. Publishing these stories may aid some physicians to diagnose these patients with a factitious disorder. We in no way want to make fun of people with psychiatric disorders. Munchausen By Proxy is child abuse and thus we will not publish any of those stories for that reason.*

## A Whole Latte Arrhythmias

Antigua was a 34-year-old female who was very active in the medical world. Heck, she even taught the Advanced Cardiac Life Support (ACLS) class at the hospital. That is not to say that she didn't have her own medical problems. She did suffer with hypertension, asthma and depression. Her biggest problem, though, was the constant palpitations she was getting. Sometimes she felt her heart almost beating out of her chest and it drove her crazy. The EKGs never found a thing so her doctors decided to use a cardiac event monitor. Luckily they did find some tachycardia on the tracings but still felt an electrophysiological study was needed. Wouldn't you know it, there were periods of atrial fibrillation and atrial flutter found and she was placed on some special medication and sent on her merry way. *But it was not to be.*

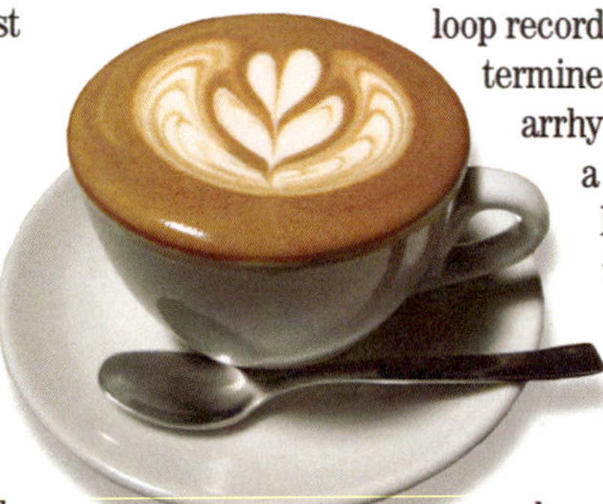

Antigua came back to her doctor's office soon thereafter with more complaints of palpitations. She even self-recorded some EKG tracings from her ACLS class which again showed the atrial fibrillation and atrial flutter. *What the heck was going on here?*

Her doctors decided to implant a loop recorder to truly determine the cause of her arrhythmia. This is not a simple procedure. It is costly and intrusive but Antigua was worth it. The day they were to put that in she was found to be agitated and sweaty. *Was she just nervous?* A quick EKG in the clinic prior to the implantation did show a ventricular tachycardia. *Things were getting worse!* Labs showed some abnormalities including a severely low potassium. The doctors investigated further and found an excessive amount of methylxanthime in her blood and urine. *Hmmmm, that's weird?*

Following up on this they found caffeine levels that were six times normal and actually in the toxic range. *What the hell was going on here?*

The doctors approached Antigua about this caffeine overdose but she would have none of their accusations. With some more prodding, a psychiatric consultation, and a little luck the doctors discovered that Antigua more than just loved her caffeine and this was not just a simple coffee addiction. No, Antigua had a nasty habit of ingesting a toxic dose of caffeine pills prior to seeing the cardiologist in order to cause the heart rhythm problems. *Another case of Munchausen solved by our heroes!*

Though Antigua would not agree to be admitted to the hospital to fix her psychiatric ails, she did promise to go to an intense outpatient treatment center. No one believes she ever went. Miraculously enough, Antigua's palpitations did go away prior to discharge right around the time they discovered her caffeine problem. Who knows if they will come back but next time you have your ACLS taught at your local hospital by a jittery instructor you may want to be ready with those paddles. It could be Antigua and she may go into V Tach right in front of your eyes!

Liberally embellished from the Journal of Electrocardiology, 2011 Mar - Apr; 44 (2): 229-31. ✚

### ANOTHER TRUE STORY OF MEDICINE

## NEW TERM LEARNED

After a long shift in our urgent care dealing with several truly bizarre lab results on top of all the usual craziness, I was more than ready to take off my thinking cap. As I headed down the hall from my office, the next shift's nurse (Donna) stepped out of a room directly into my path, causing me to pause for a second. That was just long enough for my nurse (Joanna) to look up and come running, *"Oh, Dr. D., I have one more lab for you!"*

I jokingly said to Donna, *"Thanks for blocking me,"* to which Joanna added to her, ***"Yeah, thanks for doc blocking'!"***

✚

(Note that the names have been changed to protect the innocent - and the guilty!)

DIAGNOSTIC AND STATISTICAL MANUAL OF MENTAL DISORDERS

# A DSM ENTRY WE'D LIKE TO SEE

## *DSM-IV-TR* DIAGNOSTIC CRITERIA FOR 666.0 PERI-CALL DYSPHORIC DISORDER

### *Diagnostic Features*

The essential feature of ***Peri-Call Dysphoric Disorder (PCDD)*** is an intermittent loathing for ones job that is ordinarily liked, and a loathing of the knowledge that the disorder itself alters ones personality, even if only temporarily. This must occur in a rhythmic fashion for a period of not less than six months starting six months from the beginning of one's job (Criterion A). While suffering from the effects of PCDD, Individuals generally describe their mood as, *"Shut the hell up, can't you see that I'm busy and haven't slept in two days?"* When asked about that statement later when not under the effects of the disorder, the patient (usually a physician) will not remember having said it, but admit to having felt *"horrible at the time."* During periods of symptomatology from PCDD, the individual must display at least two of the following additional symptoms: Suicidal ideation, homicidal ideation, narcissism, binge eating disorder, or feelings of hopelessness (Criterion B).

During the six month period after the onset of symptoms, any symptom-free intervals can last no longer than the longest interval between multiple-day on-call periods at the individual's place of work (Criterion C).

The diagnosis of PCDD is not made if the individual does not have to go on call for his or her job, or if they never have to leave their home or even get out of bed while on call. Further exclusion is made if the individual makes more than $250,000 a year for a job that includes call, because average psychiatrists at that point simply don't feel sorry for you and won't make the diagnosis no matter how miserable you are.

### *Specifiers*

#### *Pre-Call Dysphoric Disorder Subtype*

This specifier should be used if the onset of the symptoms occurs within seven days of starting a long call shift. Despite the fact that the individual is not on call, the knowledge of the unpleasantness that is forthcoming creates a general atmosphere of anhedonia similar to the way a good kid feels walking down the hall to the principal's office after being sent there for the first time. Such individuals will typically have further issues as the call period begins.

#### *On-Call Dysphoric Disorder Subtype.*

This specifier should be used when the symptoms are particularly severe during the period of call. Frequently the individual suffers from sleep deprivation, binge eating, and saying a host of things he or she will regret later.

#### *Post-Call Dysphoric Disorder Subtype*

This specifer is typically used when the individual suffers from extreme sleep deprivation after a period of call, and is not given time to rest before going back to the routine work schedule. It includes a period of guilt over the binge eating while on-call which is typically answered by further binge eating and guilt.

#### *Combined-Type Peri-Call Dysphoric Disorder Subtype*

This specifier should be used pretty much always, and is for when the three above subtypes all apply around a single call period. The physician who qualifies for this diagnosis should be kept away from weapons of any kind.

TABLE 1

**INDIVIDUAL MUST MEET ALL OF THE FOLLOWING:**

a. Have intermittent hatred for his or her job even when they usually like it, which causes a change in personality that causes unease.

b. Have a job with intermittent long sleepless call periods for at least six months, and the symptoms in Section A must occur with a week of them.

c. Make less than $250,000 per year.

**INDIVIDUAL MUST EXHIBIT TWO OF THE FOLLOWING SYMPTOMS, DURING OR WITHIN ONE WEEK OF A CALL PERIOD:**

1. Suicidal ideation
2. Homicidal ideation
3. Narcissism
4. Binge eating disorder
5. Feelings of hopelessness

Individual must have no symptom-free intervals which last longer than the longest interval between multiple-day on-call periods.

**INDIVIDUAL MUST EXHIBIT 10 OF THE FOLLOWING 16 CRITERIA WITHIN ONE WEEK OF A CALL PERIOD:**

1. Sudden urge to read recruiting junk mail, even from correctional facilities
2. Ataxia (walking like one is drunk)
3. Excessive irritability
4. Anorgasmia (or other sexual dysfunction when scared the phone will ring during sex)
5. Dysarthria (slurred speech)
6. Sense of impending doom
7. Unexplained and unwanted urge to treat co-workers (nurses/administrators) rudely
8. Auditory hallucinations (usually anti-hospital administration voices)
9. Poor memory
10. Delusion that living in a cardboard box under a bridge with no responsibilities looks pretty damn good
11. Caffeine abuse
12. Difficulty concentrating
13. Overwhelming feeling that every patient is lazy, a hypochondriac/somaticizer, a drug seeker, or simply inexplicably intentionally coming in specifically to ruin your day
14. Longing for isolation
15. Mood swings
16. Excessive fatigue (falling asleep at stop lights or while dictating or writing.) ✚

## PJ MEDICAL ALGORITHM OF REALITY

# MEANINGFUL USE

Does your medical office meet the criteria for Meaningful Use? Not sure? Let's find out.

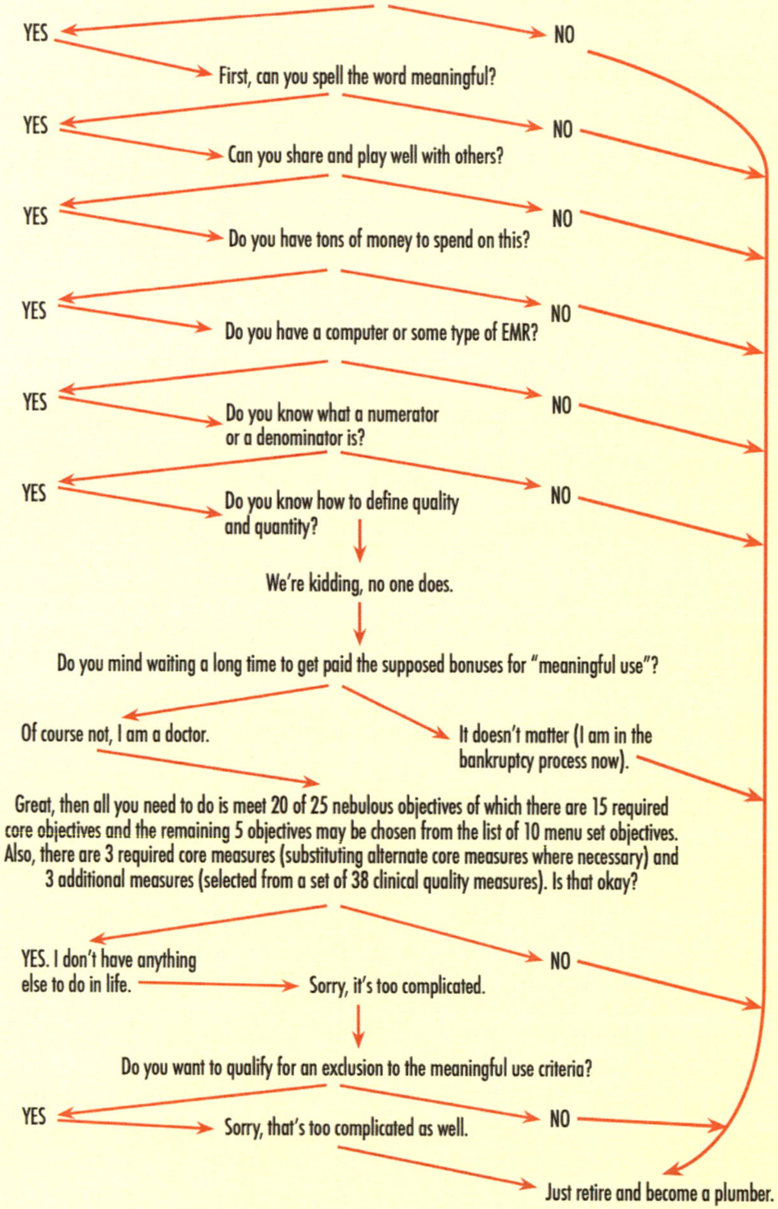


# PROGRESS (?) NOTE

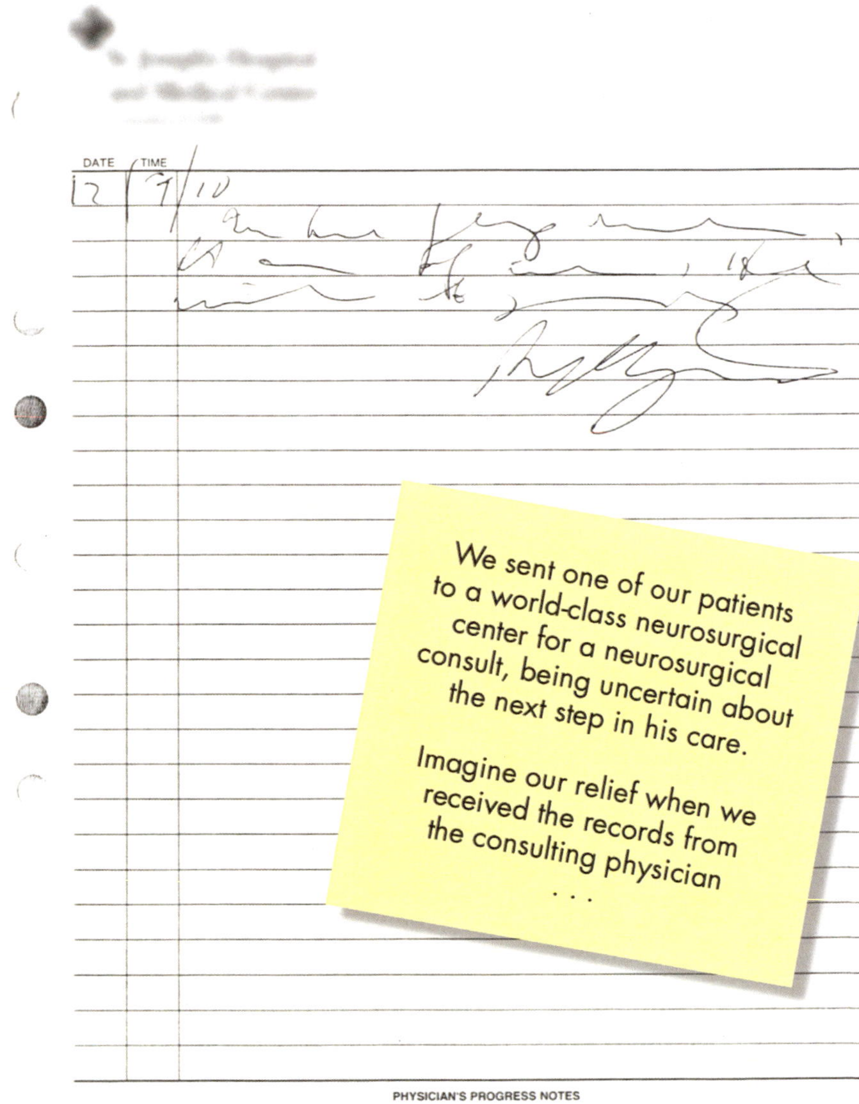


*Editor's Note:* For some people, typing or dictating may actually be worth it.

### ANOTHER TRUE STORY OF MEDICINE

# THE ROUNDABOUT

I had been a unit medical director at the VAMC in 1980. I broke my middle metatarsal one night and awoke in the morning with a swollen foot. I could not put on a shoe. I dressed and hobbled to my car. I pulled up into the VAMC parking lot and hobbled, not to my office, but to the PT gym. I asked to borrow a set of crutches and possibly a cast shoe. The therapists got the items, but the department supervisor showed up. She needed an authorization. She sent me to Employee Health. It was about a quarter of a mile away in this building. I prepared for a round of hopscotch and made it over there.

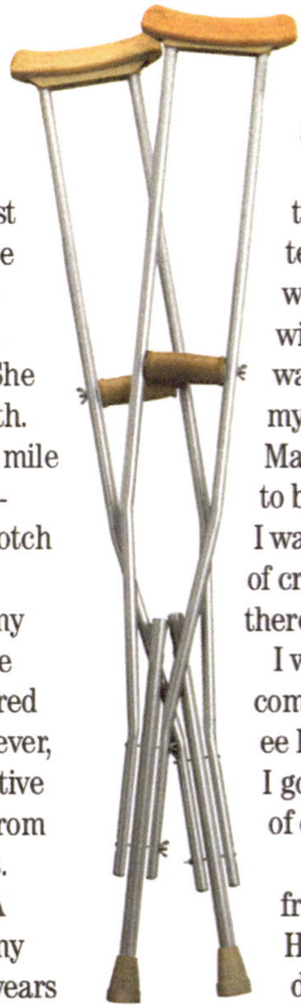

The intake nurse got my history and then denied me care. The injury had occurred at home. Fortunately, however, I spent my two years on active duty preventing Missouri from being invaded by Arkansas. I slowly retreated to the VA intake clinic. I explained my injury. I showed my three years of orthopedic training and diagnosed a third metatarsal fracture of my left foot. I prescribed rest, elevation and non-weight bearing with a set of crutches. The intake clerk agreed, but since I was an employee of the VA, I had health insurance. I, as a former member of the Army of the United States, was to go to my personal physician for care. However, I was not allowed to return to work without a work release from my physician and clearance from Employee Health. As a good former soldier, I followed orders and left. I went to my car and drove home.

Once home, I contacted a doctor I knew in an urgent care center. Before I could leave, my pager went off (cell phones were not yet widespread). The clinic manager was angry. I had left without seeing my patients in the amputee clinic. Many had traveled a hundred miles to be seen. I explained the scenario. I was told that he would get me a set of crutches and to get my ass back there. I did so.

I was met by the clinic manager accompanied by a member of Employee Health that told me to leave until I got a doctor's note and my own set of crutches.

I left again and went to my friend at the urgent care center. He got the x-rays confirming my diagnosis. I got the crutches and the cast shoe.

I returned to the VA just as the workday was ending. My clinic was rescheduled. My friend called that night and laughed. He said that this is what will happen if the government ran health care. He was a soothsayer. ✚

# Malapropisms

Submitted by Readers of the *Placebo Journal Blog*

● *"The patient was bean bagged while in the ambulance,"* instead of being bagged.

● *"The sheets were stiched in place in preparation for transport,"* instead of the sheaths were . . .

● *"Medical degree from Two Lane."* Must be a driving school near Skidmore.

● *"Assessment: Erectile dysfunction.
Plan: See Alice."*

● Had a woman tell me her husband had been on *"the lemon tree"* (telemetry).

● Also been told *"I have the myalgies"* (fibromyalgia).

● A woman went to the doctor and after examining her, he told her that she had a deficiency in her womb and if she ever had a baby, it would be a miracle. She went home and told her husband that the doctor said she had a fish in her womb and if she ever had a baby, it would be a mackerel.

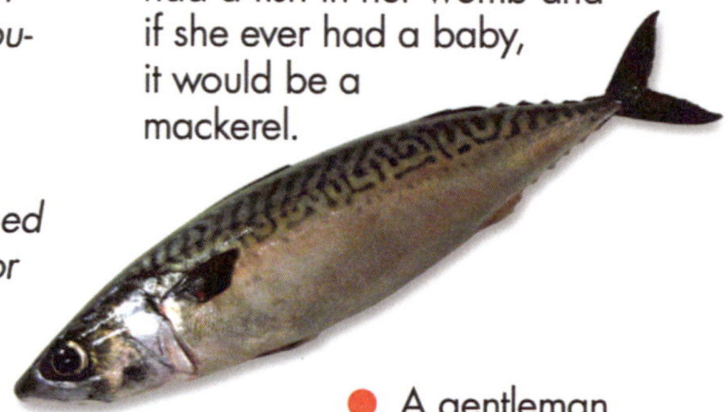

● A gentleman told me he had had Romantic Heart Disease, and pollen in his colon.

● I recently saw a patient with a history of "tickelitis."

● While admitting a man to the hospital, he told me to make sure they know he sleeps with a PAP smear on his face (CPAP).

● *"I have a headache, I need some purple Jesus."* (Percogesic)

● *"It's pussy!"* said the mother of a child whose spinal wound had purulent drainage. And yes, that's exactly how she pronounced it (but with a spanish accent).

● *"I had the chicken pops."*

● *"I had a tuba ligation."*

● Then there's the really common "rotary cup" injury.

● A patient told me that he had had a tube placed to drain VD of the chest (collapse of the lung).

● We had a patient call and ask for a refill on her Premium Vaginal cream (as opposed to the generic kind, I'm sure. The real brand is *Premarin*).

● A patient asked that I renew her Rx for birth control pills. She said she was on Ortho No man. This should be quite effective.

● I had a mother in the ER tell me her son had *"neurotic fibromas"* (neurofibromatosis).

● I had a patient at the VA once tell me that he was told by his doctor that he had *"some roaches"* in his liver . . . Obviously he meant something different, but no less serious . . .

● I had a mother tell me that her daughter was referred to the Endo Clinic because she had Public Hairs. Another mother told me that she was concerned about her infant son's *"meat"* (meatus or part of the penis).

● *"The patient is a 45-year-old sexually frustrated female who presents with left shoulder pain."* (I have no idea what the consulting orthopedic surgeon actually said, but I am pretty sure *Dragon Dictation* got it right).

● As a by-product of speech recognition text that I was editing in my role as medical transcriptionist – *"Highland calves"* instead of hyaline casts. ✚

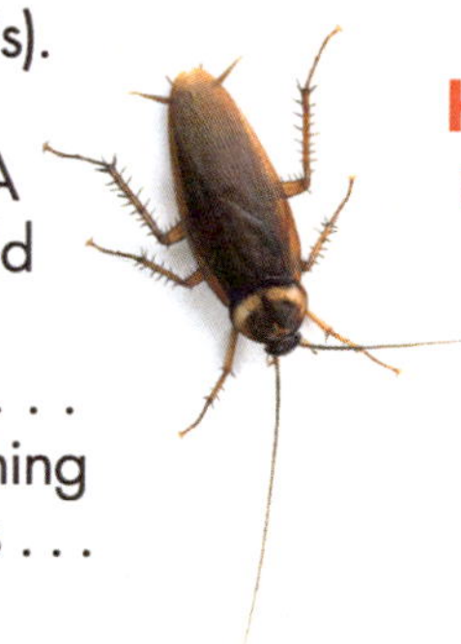

**If you've heard a funny malapropism, submit it to placebojournal.blogspot.com**

***PJ Electronics* Introduces The World's First**

# AEDD

**(Automatic External Doctor Defribrillator)**

You've seen them walking down the hospital corridors.
You've seen them staring aimlessly at electronic medical records.
You've seen them sleeping in the doctor's lounges.
The blank stares. The lack of emotion. The smell of burnout.
Physicians, slowly but surely, all dying inside.
***Now there is a cure.***

***The Automatic External Doctor Defibrillator (AEDD), when used properly, automatically diagnoses job-threatening burnout and shoots 3000 joules of electricity through an ailing doctor's soul.***

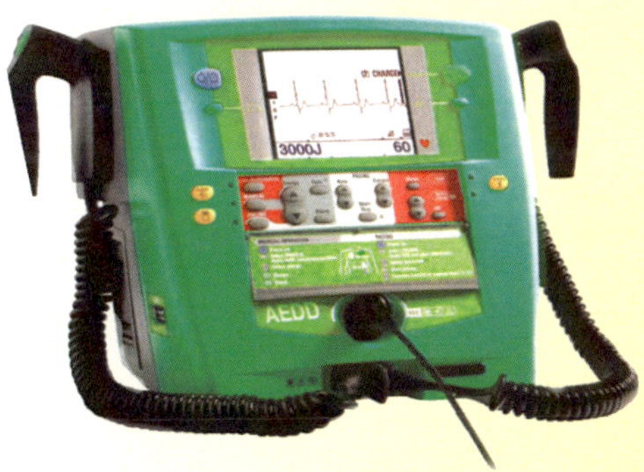

**Perfect for:**

♥ Bitter doctors
♥ Angry doctors
♥ Impaired doctors
♥ Doctors who have become administrators
♥ Doctors whose career has destroyed their marriage and made their kids hate them
♥ ER Doctors (let's be honest, their souls were sucked out before residency was over) ♥ Psychiatrists (no explanation needed)
♥ Doctors in favor of government-run health care (to shock some sense into them) ♥ Older doctors trying to keep trophy wives satisfied
♥ Younger doctors trying to keep trophy wives satisfied

## Only $499

***Order now and get a free EpiDoc Pen that you can use to treat those resistant cases!*** ✚

# TOP EIGHT MOST CREATIVE DRUG/ALCOHOL TEST EXCUSES

## *BY PEOPLE OTHER THAN CHARLIE SHEEN*

**❽ *"I was eating deer meat and the deer were grazing on weed."***

**❼ *"My brother needed a ride. I couldn't kick him out of the car and he rolled up all the windows and started smoking weed."***

**❻ Went to *Earth, Wind and Fire* concert. *"It was just blowing around everywhere."* (was really Earth, Coke and Fire concert).**

**❺ *"This is not right. I want a retest. I never used the heroin! The only way this could be positive is if it went through my skin."* (So you are holding heroin in your hand but you don't have a problem?)**

**❹ *"Isn't it legal here?"* (No, sorry, we're not in Canada – didn't you notice there was sun?)**

**❸ *"I was waitressing and had my water out and someone replaced my water with a Margarita. I hardly ever drink and didn't notice what had happened."* (Wow, how long did it take you to notice the water was citrus flavored?)**

**❷ *"I'm a fermenter. My body makes alcohol. There's only like seven of us in the whole world."* (I actually heard someone say this and I didn't laugh out loud.)**

**❶ *"I never used meth, but my boyfriend did and then we had sex . . ."* (insert innocuous physician question here) *". . . Well it WAS oral sex."* (This one is NOT made up, but gathered from the emergency room.)** ✚

## TRUE STORIES OF MEDICINE

# SATANISM

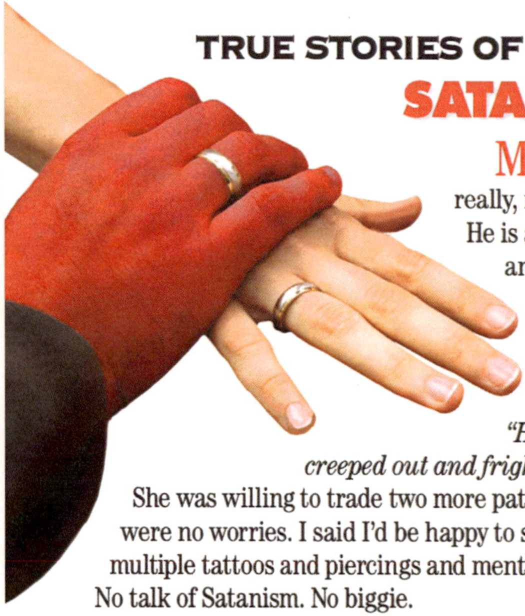

My colleague told me that she really, really didn't want to see Mr. Z. He is a young man with a back injury, and he is a worker's comp patient . . . like pretty much everyone. I asked if he was mean to her or what happened . . . She was kind of embarrassed and said, *"He's a Satanist. I just get too creeped out and frightened when I see him."* She was willing to trade two more patients for him and I said there were no worries. I said I'd be happy to see him. I saw Mr. Z. He had multiple tattoos and piercings and mentioned that he was doing better. No talk of Satanism. No biggie.

So I told my dad the story. I thought it odd my colleague was so frightened of a person of a different faith . . . even if it was Satan. After all, Christian, Jewish, Hindu, Moslem – none of their deities have ever come out of the sky instantly and hurt (or help for that matter) anyone recently. *Why should Satan be any different?*

I was feeling pretty proud of myself when my dad hit the nail on the head.

*"Sonya, of course you're not scared of Satan – you were married to him for 15 years!"* ✚

# "MY CONDOLENCES"

One problem with being a primary care practitioner and caring for geriatric patients is that every few weeks one of your charges passes away. I got into the habit of once a year going up to the local stationery shop and picking up maybe six "so sorry for your loss" and a half dozen "in this time of grief," and a few "if there's anything I can do" cards to send to the grieving families. I put the stack on the counter and a cashier, who I didn't recognize, said, *"Excuse me, why are you buying so many condolence cards?"*

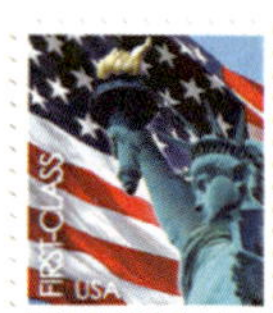


I explained that I was the doctor down the street, and I sent them to patients' families. She retorted, *"You must not be very good."*

My explaining that this stack was not just for that week didn't seem to improve my skill status in her mind. ✚

# FIRST NIGHT ON CALL

A century or two ago when I was a third year medical student, I was assigned my surgical block at an affiliated suburban hospital. On my first night on duty the on-call room phone awakened me - for the first time in my budding career as a physician. What follows is the verbatim dialogue with the very concerned nurse.

*"Mr. Boyd swallowed the contents of his* Foley *(urine catheter) bottle."*

*"So?"*

*"Will it hurt him?"*

*"No, it's sterile,"* I responded.

Prolonged silence.

*"What's the problem?"* I asked.

*"I don't know how to record it. Is it input or output?*

*"Just write both."* ✚

# REALLY NEED TO LISTEN

In 1962, the year of my internship in NYC, I sat for the National Board exam which was required at that time for licensure in many states. Part of the exam consisted of a physician-proctor observing the candidate taking a history and doing a physical exam on a real live patient. Hospitals where the exam was given would trot out patients for this event and frequently, after a few encounters, these patients would become pretty savvy as why they were called in.

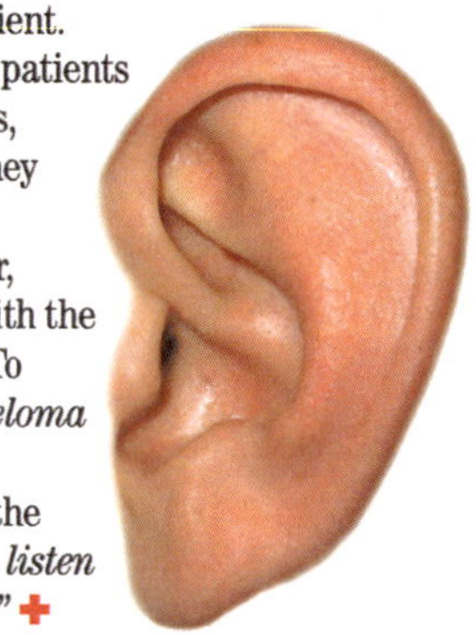

After my patient, accompanied by the examiner, entered the room I introduced myself and led off with the usual, *"What seems to be the problem?"* approach. To which, my patient responded, *"I have multiple myeloma and SBE."*

After the appropriate pause, I turned to the examiner and stated, *"Osler said that if you listen to the patient, he'll give you the diagnosis."* ✚

# FUN MAZE

**Help the managed care CEO find his bonus.**

START HERE

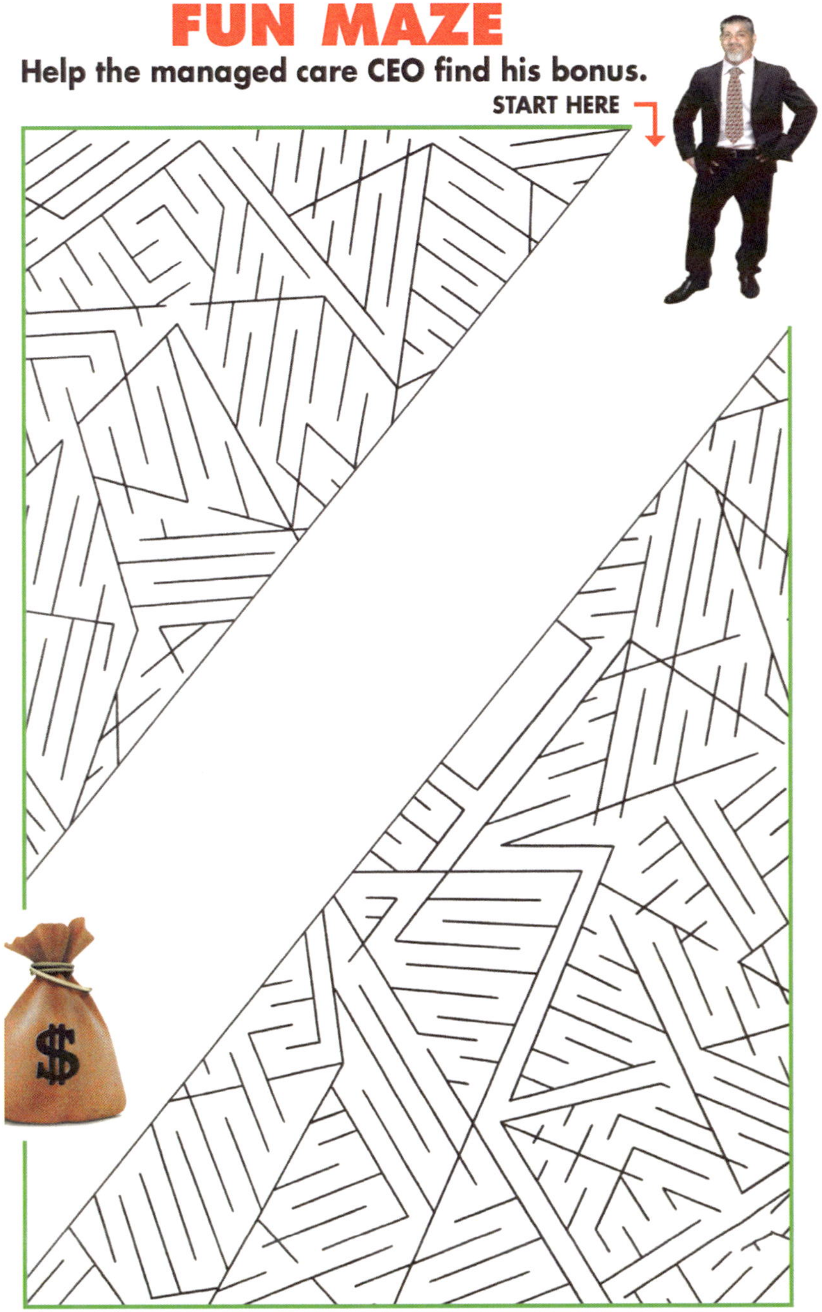

# VOCABULARIA AMERICANA

## HERE ARE SOME REAL PATIENT MALAPROPISMS.

***"Lost my natures"***
(impotence)

***"Fireballs on my eucharist"***
(fibroids on my uterus)

***"Pain in my testamints"***

***"Sick as hell anebia"***
(sickle cell anemia)

***"Smilin' Mighty Jesus"***
(spinal meningitis)

***"Ministrations"***
(every 28 days)

***"Ah feels lots better after my bible movement."***

***"I haven't demonstrated for three months and I think I'm stagnant."***

***"My suppessary is stuck!"***

***"I've had trouble with my prosperous gland."***

***"I'm fixin' to get loose."***
(diarrhea)

***"Electrocuted 1959, haven't been able to feel since."***

***"I have to be castrated."***
(catheterizrd)

***"My eyes roll up every time I think bad thoughts. I quit work in 1946 because my eyes rolled up every Monday."***

***"Very close veins"***

***"Cerebral hemmarhoids"***

***"I had a drawing up of my penis that cut my wind off."***

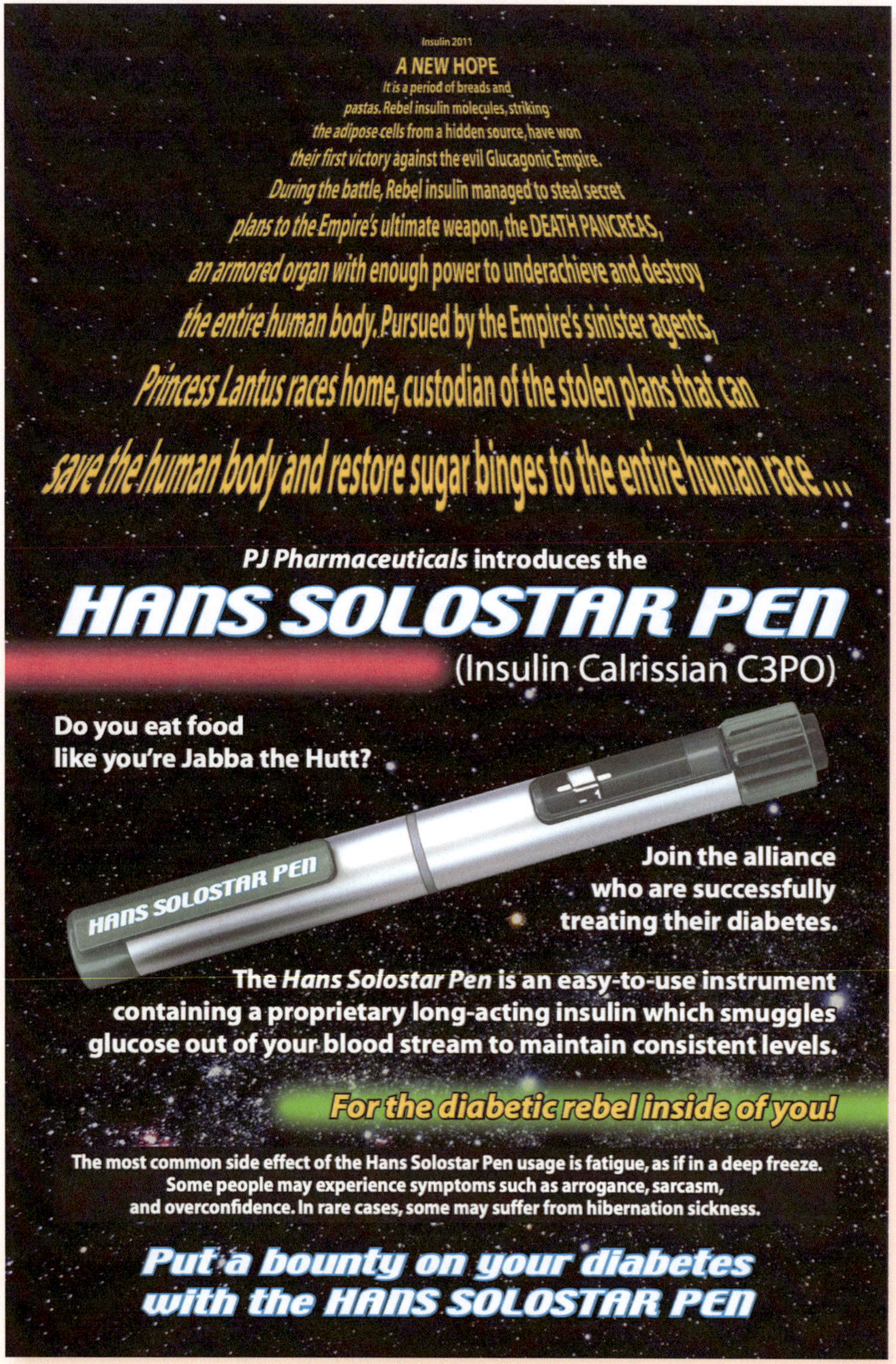


# MORE MANAGED CARE MADNESS

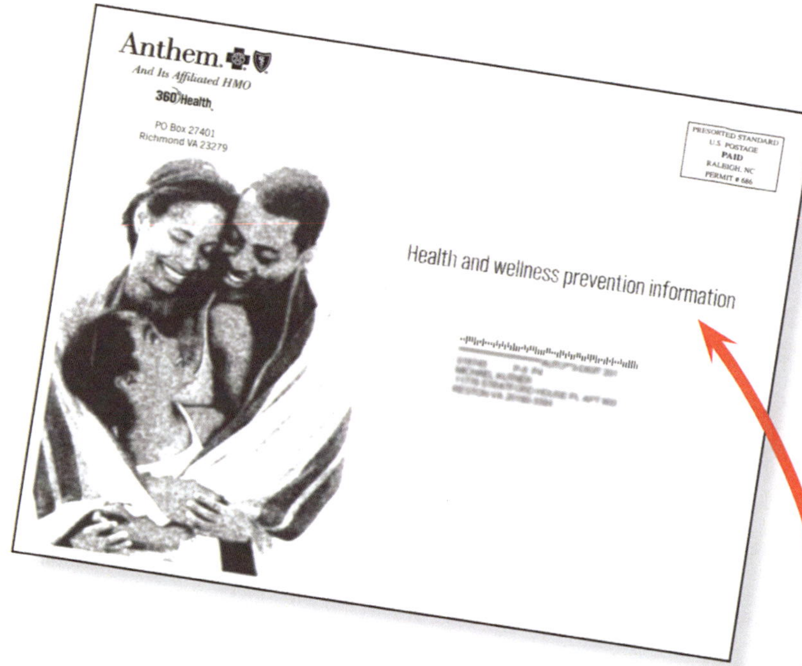


Health and wellness prevention information

*"Looks like* Anthem *has a new goal . . .*
*preventing health and wellness.*
*Sounds about right."*

MORE TRUE STORIES OF MEDICINE

# LOVE STORY

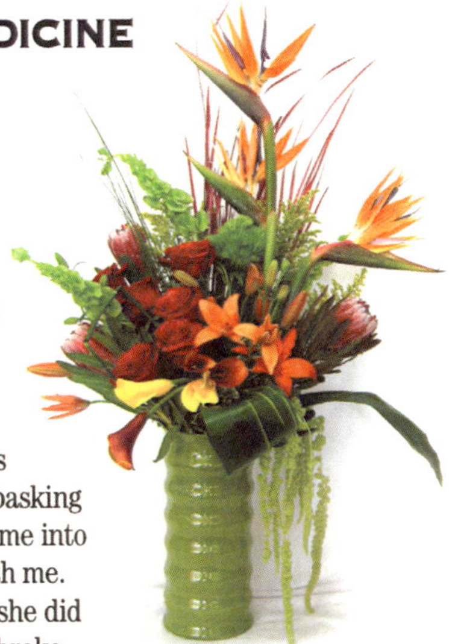

As a student I was lucky enough to get a patient with a good laceration that I got to repair on my own! The guy was a nervous wreck and a bit of a weenie but I got him laughing and relaxed so the procedure went beyond textbook.

A couple days went by and I received a beautiful bouquet of roses and other exotic flowers with a thank you note. A couple hours after I was basking in my glory and exotic scents, one of the nurses came into my office to tell me the police wanted to speak with me. I told them to send them back to the office which she did with a funky grin on her face. Apparently this guy broke into the florist's shop and stole the flowers and the store wanted them back.

End of the story is not only did I lose a beautiful thought but he never came back to get his sutures out. *Where could he be????* ✚

# NOT A SMART CALL

I work in the ER so it seems I've heard and seen everything. Alas, some days I'm shocked anew. A 34-year-old woman came in, accompanied by her mom. She said she'd smoked marijuana *("just two hits!")*, and was feeling very anxious, and she said her heart was *"pounding out of her chest."*

*"Do you think it could have been laced with something?!"*

Oh, and by the way, her boyfriend (not her husband, mind you; he works out of town) is a cocaine dealer, and he's the one who gave her the weed.

*Hmmmm . . .*

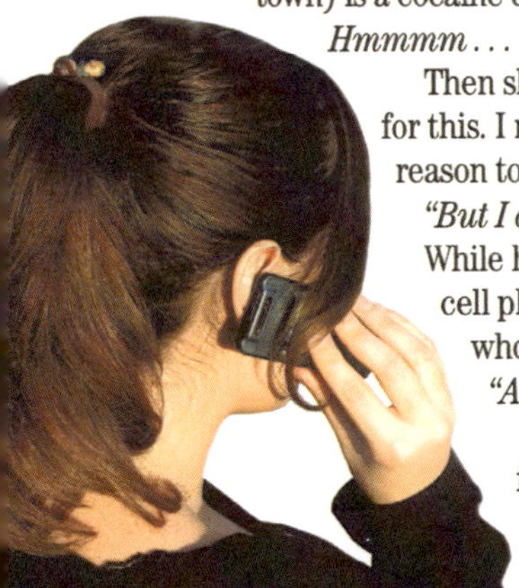

Then she asks if she's going to get in trouble with the cops for this. I reassured her that we're not the cops, and have no reason to call the police about this.

*"But I called them,"* she says. *Whaaa . . .?*

While her mom was driving her in, the patient was on her cell phone with the police department, telling them the whole story! Apparently she said to the dispatcher, *"Are you going to tell the cops about this?"*

The dispatcher replied, with as straight a face as possible, *"Ma'am, we ARE the cops, and YOU called US!"* ✚

**NEW from PJ PRODUCTS**

*TrichoPhiten*™

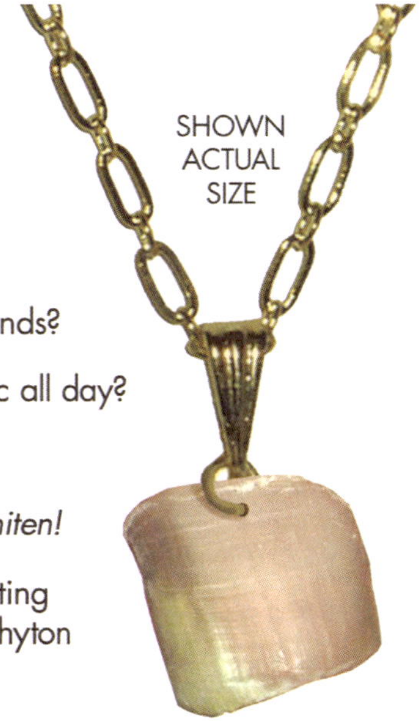


Having trouble making it through rounds?

Getting tired of seeing patients in the clinic all day?

Is surgery making you sleepy?

Then you need the power of *TrichoPhiten!*

We have a secret method of harvesting the right toenails with the right trichophyton fungal species.

*TrichoPhiten* is the only one with natural onychomyGOODNESS built right in.

**Remember, only elite doctors wear *TrichoPhiten.***

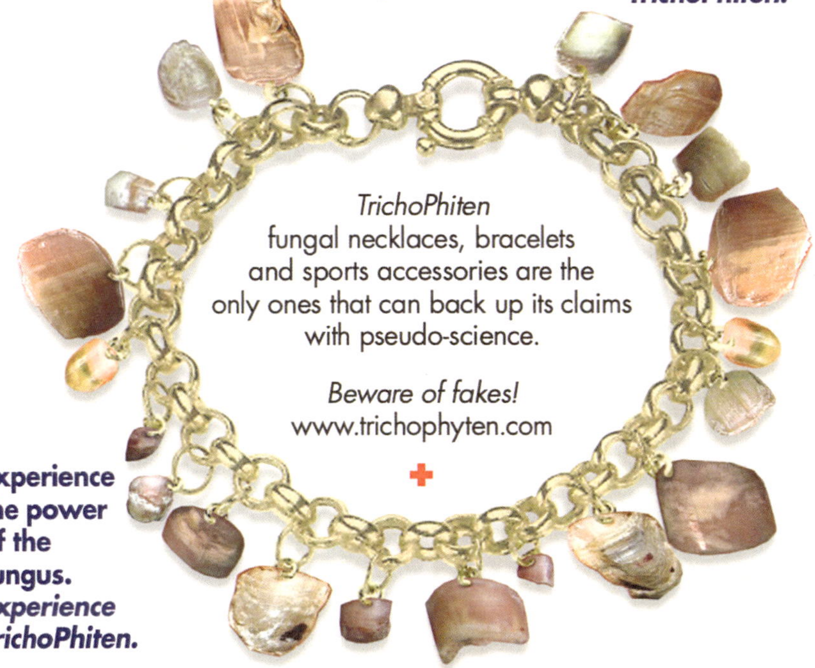

*TrichoPhiten* fungal necklaces, bracelets and sports accessories are the only ones that can back up its claims with pseudo-science.

*Beware of fakes!*
www.trichophyten.com

✚

**Experience the power of the fungus. *Experience TrichoPhiten.***

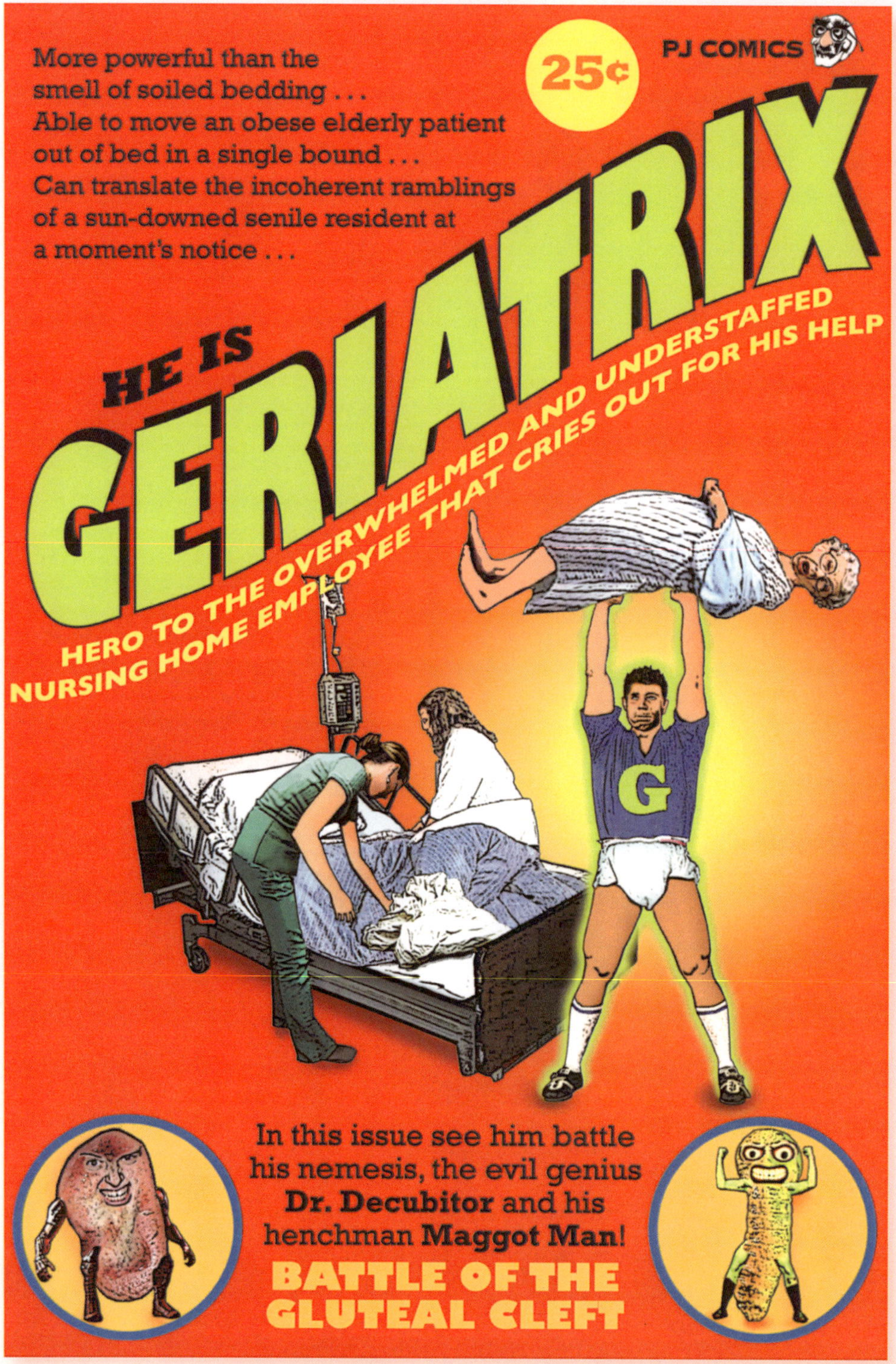


*New from PJ Physician Support Products*

# The Intern/Resident NOT-ON-CALL SLEEP KIT

You've heard it before: *Sleep when you can.* With the ***PJ Not-on-Call Sleep Kit***, you can really maximize those few hours of sleep. Our product comes with a 95% no-interruption guarantee!

***Our amazing kit includes:***

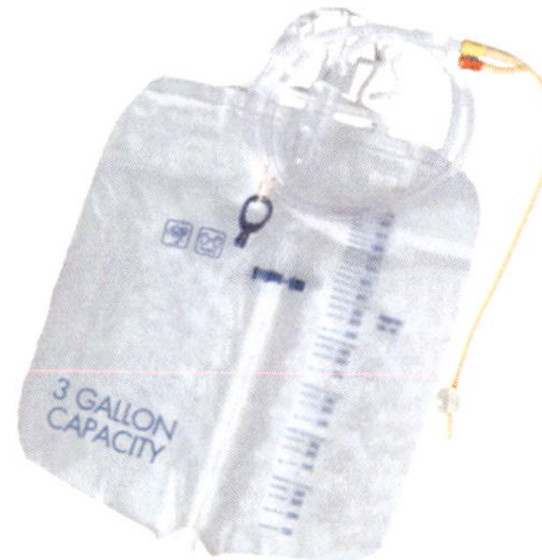

Urinary catheter with 3-gallon collection bag

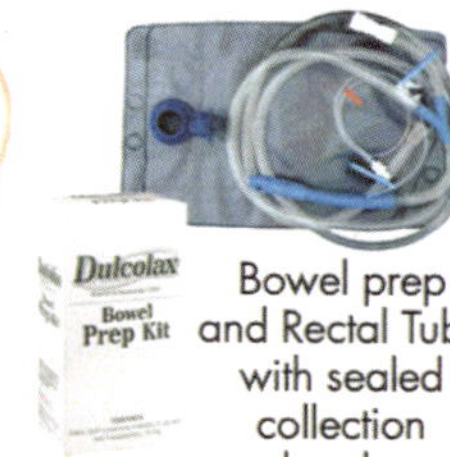

Bowel prep and Rectal Tube with sealed collection chamber

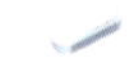
Sleeping Pill (just in case you need it)

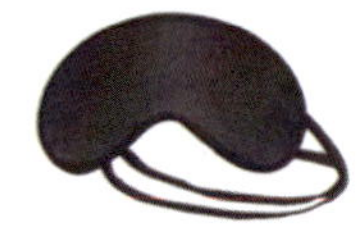
Eye mask

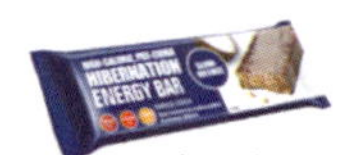
High-calorie, pre-coma, slow-release "hibernation" energy bar

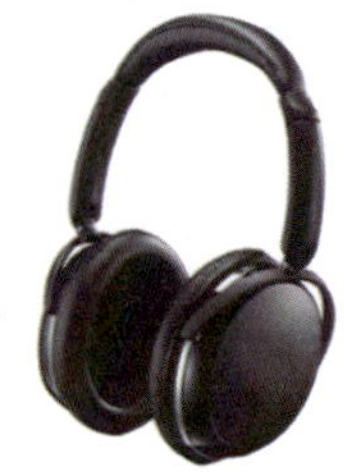
Noise-cancelling headphones

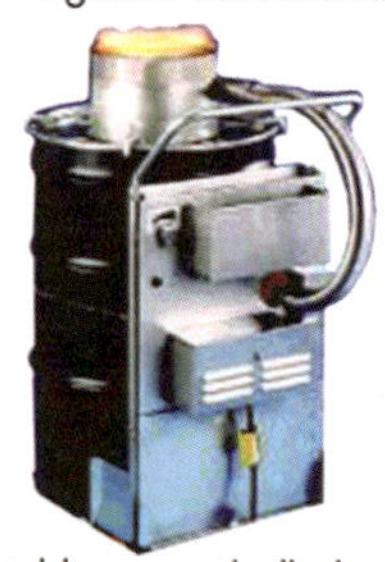
Portable pager/cell phone battery incinerator

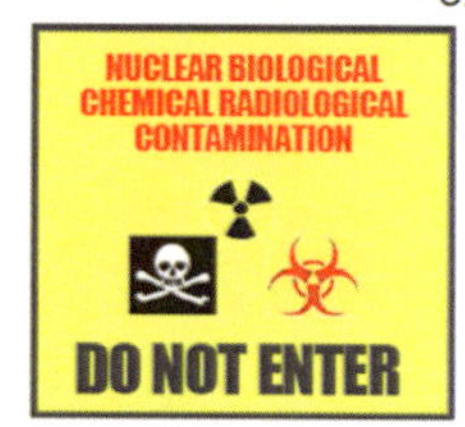

Door sign

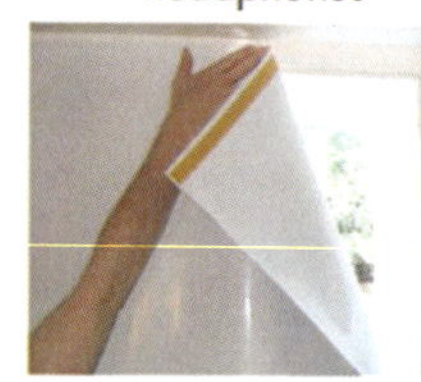
Black-out stick-on window shade

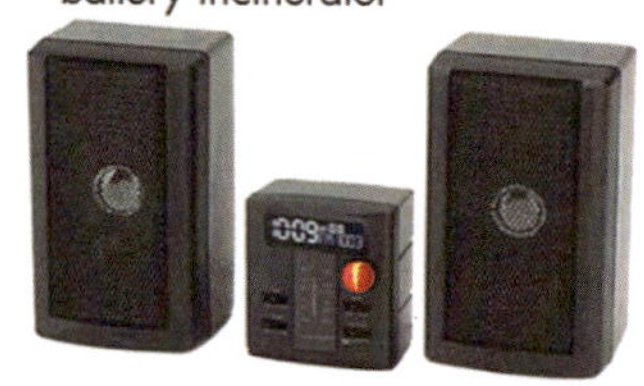
Alarm clock with power amplifier and dual 18" subwoofers, with optional electric shock setting

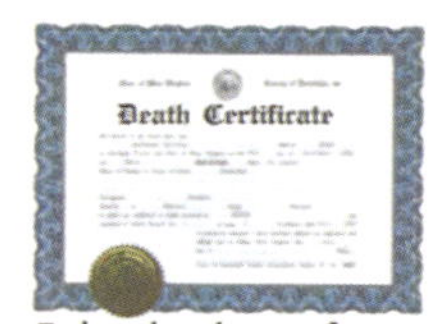

Fake death certificate

***Look for our post-call extracranial anesthesia hammer coming out next month!*** +

## CATCH ME IF YOU CAN

I was working in the psychiatric emergency room and was called to do a consult to the medical ER. The patient was intoxicated and needed psychiatric clearance prior to going to inpatient detox. I interviewed him and he said he had been taking tranquillizers. I asked him the name of his psychiatrist and he said, *"Dr. Frank Abagnale."*

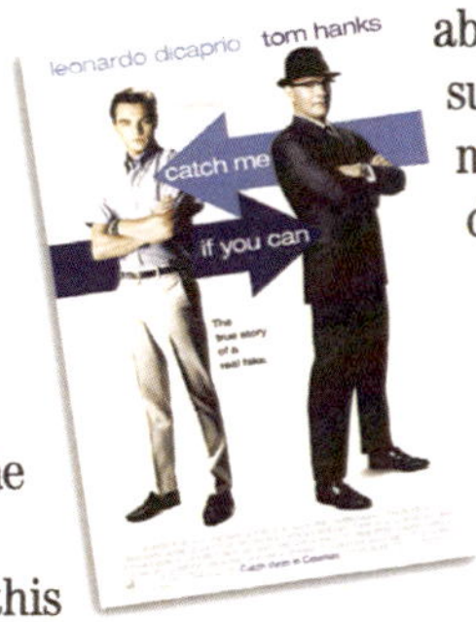


I probed further and the patient became very vague – he couldn't recall where this doctor practiced or what his phone number was. As I walked back to write up the consult, a light bulb went on. *"Frank Abagnale"* – wasn't that the name of the character in the film *Catch Me If You Can,* an excellent Spielberg movie starring Tom Hanks and Leonardo DiCaprio, about a young con artist who successfully fakes having many careers, including a doctor and a pilot?

I returned to the patient and asked him about the coincidence. He burst out laughing. *"Ya caught me, doc. You're good. Nah, I didn't see no shrink. I buy my pills on the street . . . but wasn't that a great movie???!!!"* ✚

### TRUE STORIES OF MEDICINE

## COUPON

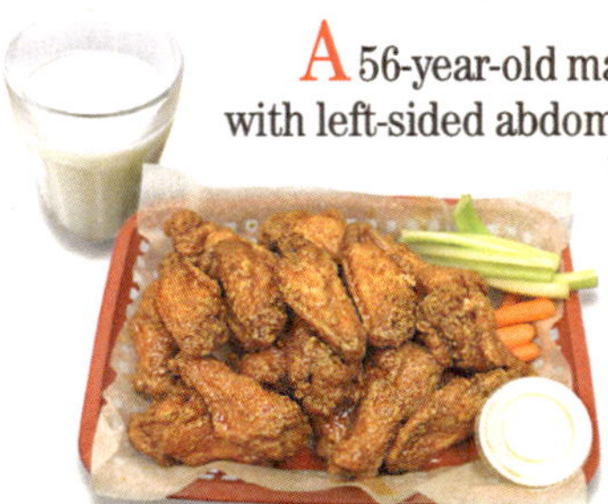

A 56-year-old male with a history of diverticulitis came in with left-sided abdominal pain he was having for about four days. It wasn't too bad, but was annoying and hurt with deep breathing. He did not have any diarrhea and the abdominal exam was positive only for some left-sided pain on palpation.

He thought he might feel better if he could clean himself out and he suggested he might eat some greasy chicken wings and milk, since he had a lactose intolerance. In the meantime, I was writing out a prescription for *Levaquin* to treat his obvious diverticulitis and commented, *"I think I have a coupon* (given out by the drug company) *for this."*

He queried, ***"For the wings?"*** ✚

# GonStar™

**The world's most comprehensive in-vehicle sexual safety service.**

**An Actual Conversation:**

"GonStar, how can I help you?"

*"Yes, GonStar, I am in the back seat and we are about to get busy. Does this person I am with have gonorrhea?"*

"Can I have some more information?"

*"Sure."*

"What is his name?"

*"(Whisper – What is your name?") His name is Barry."*

"What is his full name?"

*"(More whispers) Barry Fenderblick."*

"Hold on one second . . . (delay). Ma'am, are you still there?"

*"Yes, GonStar."*

"We are recommending you pass on this one."

*"Thank you, GonStar."*

"You're welcome. Is there anything else we can do for you?"

*"No, thanks."*

***We can keep you disease-free in ways you never thought possible.***

**Whether you have just met someone or suspect your spouse may be harboring something bad "down under," GonStar is there for you when you need us most.**

**GonStar's ability to track your partner's STD status (gonorrhea, Chlamydia, herpes and more) is 94% accurate.**

***Our methods are proprietary but our diagnostics and results are legendary.***

*GonStar services require vehicle electrical system (including battery), wireless service and GPS satellite signals to be available and operating for features to function properly. Subscription Service Agreement required.
Visit www.GonStar.com for more information.

# sickly bandz®

The perfect fashion accessory
for your favorite medical disease.

## patients everywhere are going WILD over sickly bandz!!

These colorful rubber bands are made of bisphenol A* and are die-molded into many different fun shapes. Some will even return to their original shape when you take them off your wrist.

Our Organ Failure Collection

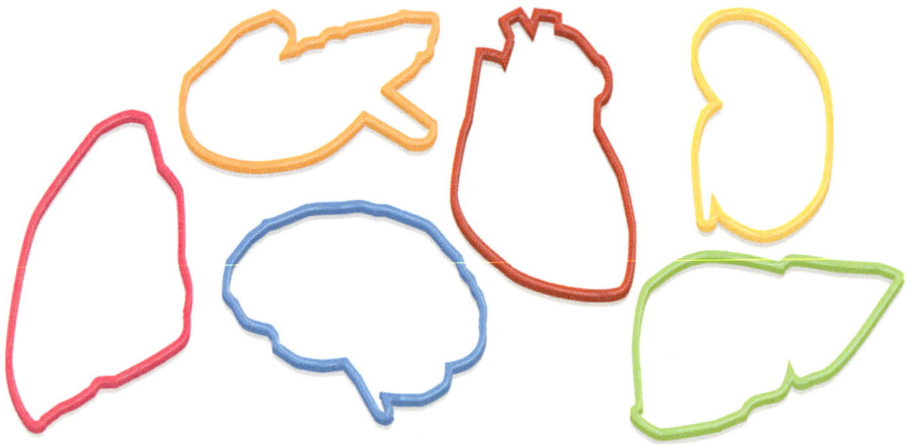

**This chemical could cause behavioral and neurological problems in the developing fetus and young children.*

## COMING SOON

Sickly Bandz that represent behavioral and neurological problems in the developing fetus and young children!

collect 'em

trade 'em

show 'em you're sick!

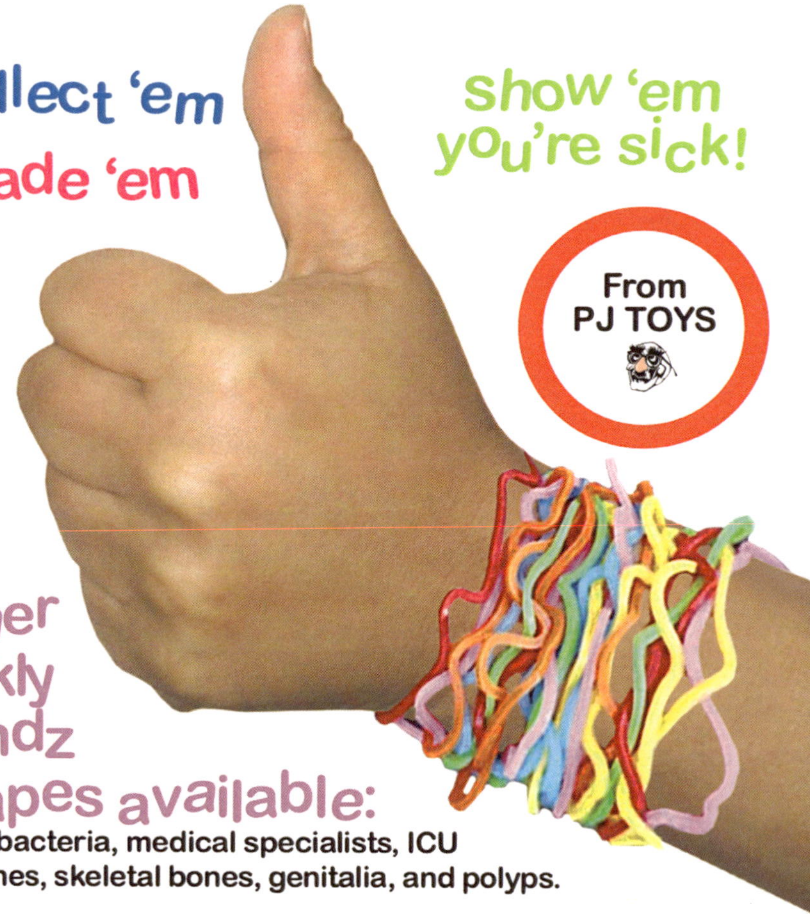

From PJ TOYS

## other sickly bandz shapes available:

STDs, bacteria, medical specialists, ICU machines, skeletal bones, genitalia, and polyps.

*"Everyone at my AA meeting had their Sickly Bands on. Most had the liver failure one but I had the liver and the heart failure bands!"*

Remo Milkin

*"I got mine when I was in detox. Now I use it to tie off my arm when I shoot up black tar heroin. Thank you Sickly Bands!"*

Shania Johnson

## available at hospital gift shops everywhere!

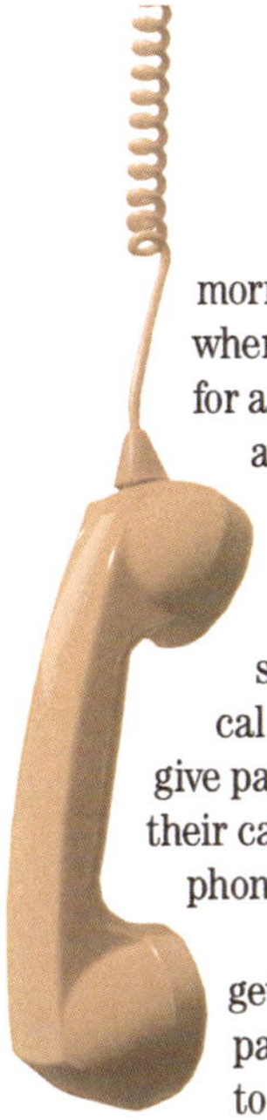

## AMS . . . ANOTHER TRUE STORY

I was trying to get through rounds in a timely manner and had my morning planned out in my head. My nice plans were quickly demolished when I got a page from a nurse on a unit that I hadn't scheduled to visit for another couple of hours. One of my patients was behaving strangely and the nurse wanted me to come and evaluate the patient's **a**ltered **m**ental **s**tatus. Irritated that my calm orderly morning was being threatened, I headed to the unit.

The patient was alone in her room when I arrived, and even more strange was that she was having a conversation on the phone. In typical patient fashion these days, my presence was ignored. I usually try to give patients the benefit of the doubt and give them a moment to complete their call and hang up. Only this patient continued to chatter away on the phone about her flower beds and such.

By this time I was thoroughly annoyed – at the patient for not getting off the phone – and at the nurse for calling me to evaluate this patient for an "**a**ltered **m**ental **s**tatus." So I cleared my throat and moved to the end of the bed. I still received no acknowledgement from the patient. I moved to the side of the bed and was prepared to pry the phone from her knobby little hands if necessary. It was when I reached the head of the bed that I realized she had the phone upside down and was talking into the earpiece.

I offered up a silent apology to the nurse I had been cussing out in my head and went to work. ✚

## COMMON

I was a third-year medical student and was in the operating room "assisting" the resident with a lower extremity amputation. The resident isolated the neurovascular bundle and pointed to the posterior tibial artery and asked me to identify it. I was a bit tired and wasn't able to quickly separate artery anatomy from nerve anatomy and couldn't remember if it was just the "tibial artery," or the "posterior tibial artery," or the "common tibial artery." So I decided to be vague and go for the lowest common denominator and answered "tibial artery."

Trying to coax me into being more specific, he asked if the patient had more than one tibial artery. Without even giving a second's thought to my answer, I blurted out, *"Of course, she has one in her other leg."*

How in the world I survived surgery without a slap or two upside the head I'll never know. ✚

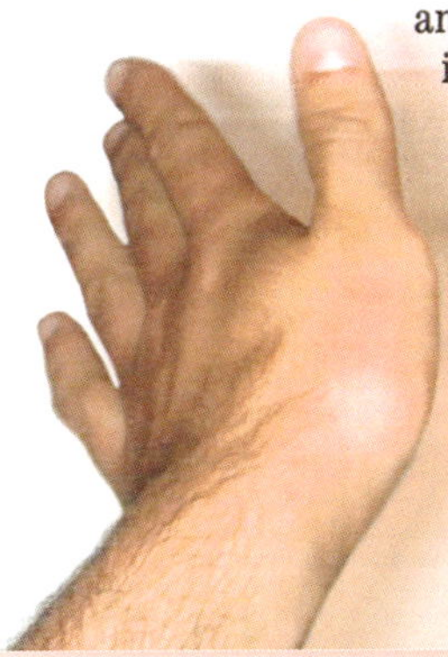

## The world's first approved Rotund Rump Inhibitor

# Assiphex™
## Urphatazole

Losing weight is hard.
Gastrointestinal distress is painful.
ASSIPHEX combines the two
to allow you to lose the weight
you always wanted –
by destroying your stomach lining.

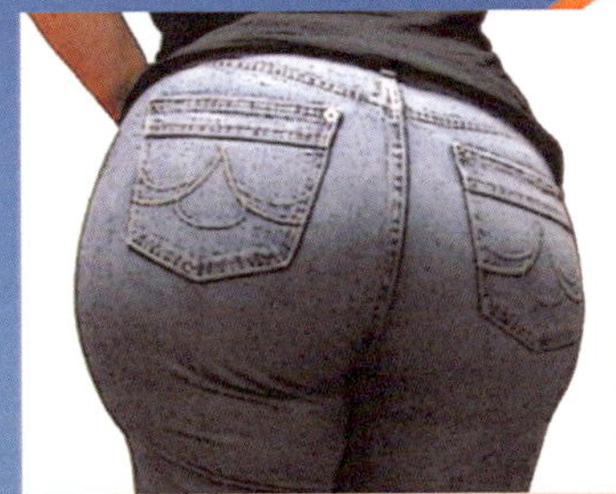

Before ASSIPHEX

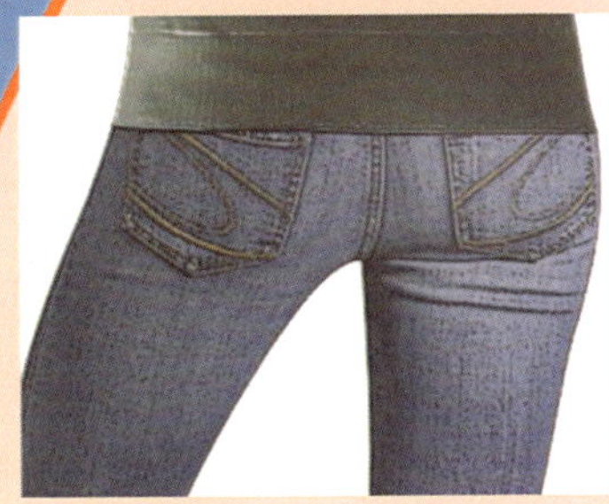

After ASSIPHEX

Did you ever notice how much weight people lose when they go through a case of cholera or some other gastroenteritis? We did. There are many chemicals and foodstuffs in this world that do a lot of damage to your stomach and intestines.
PJ Pharmaceuticals has harnessed this magic and put it in a pill. Sure, we have failed before (CYANARA) but we never stop trying. Neither should you.

Ask your doctor about ASSIPHEX.
Our two varieties, spicy jalapeno or Thai pepper, put the Grrrr in GERD.

Who needs this medication?
- Americans
- Lazy people
- You

*When normal dieting doesn't work then maybe you just need a good kick in the ASSIPHEX!*

Spread the word and get a free colostomy bag (which you will eventually need) on us. If your baby's got too much back then tell her about ASSIPHEX and we will send her a complete starter set of adult diapers.

PJ PHARMACEUTICALS
The Realistic Drug Company

Remember, when everything else fails you can still lose your mass effects with ASSIPHEX.

*IMPORTANT SAFETY INFORMATION: ASSIPHEX has a very poorly established safety profile. ASSIPHEX has been known to cause heartburn, a bad taste in your throat, and belching but that's not all! Most people get diarrhea, nausea, abdominal cramping and so much more!! In fact, if you don't get seriously injured or die taking ASSIPHEX then we will be pleasantly surprised.*

# X-Ray Files

**If we show you ours, will you show us yours?**

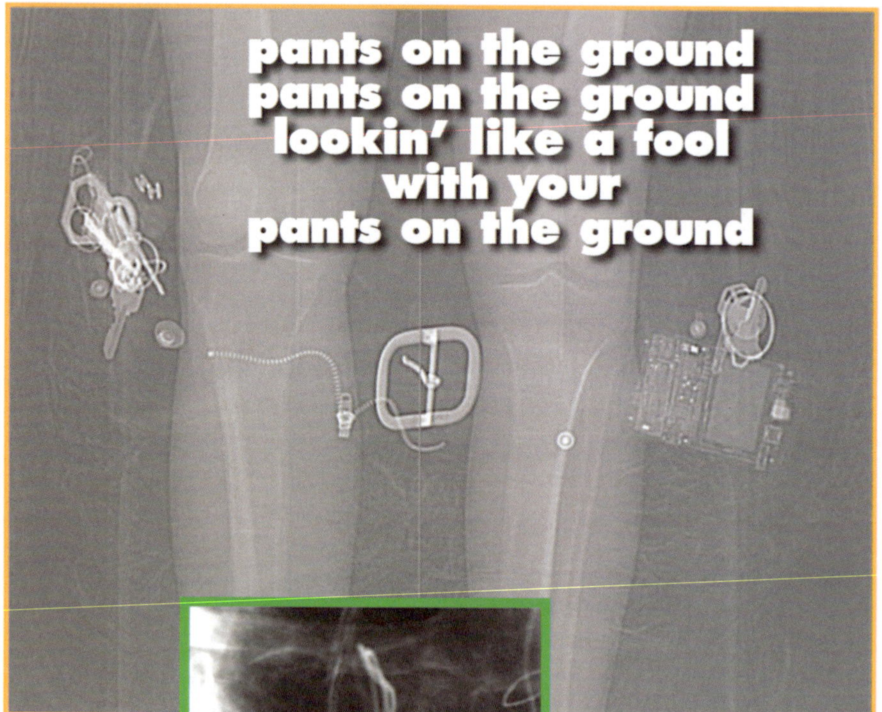


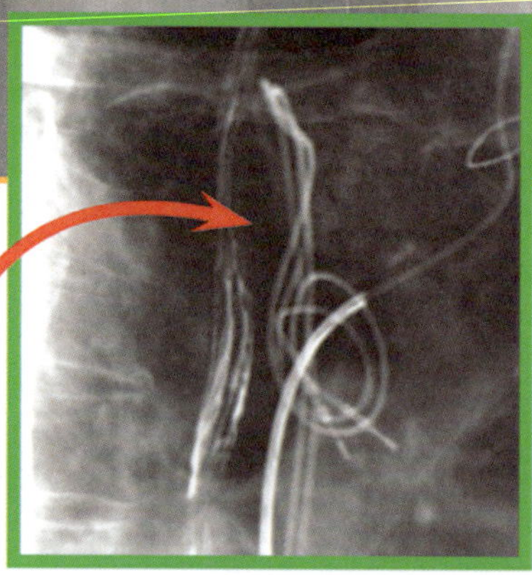

*We don't know if this patient is* **MUSICAL** *but the pacemaker wires apparently sing in the treble clef.*

## NOW AT THE ZOO

*We have* **ANGEL FISH**

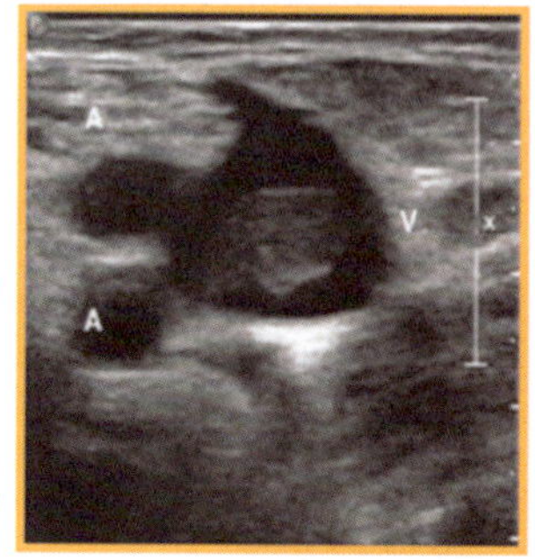

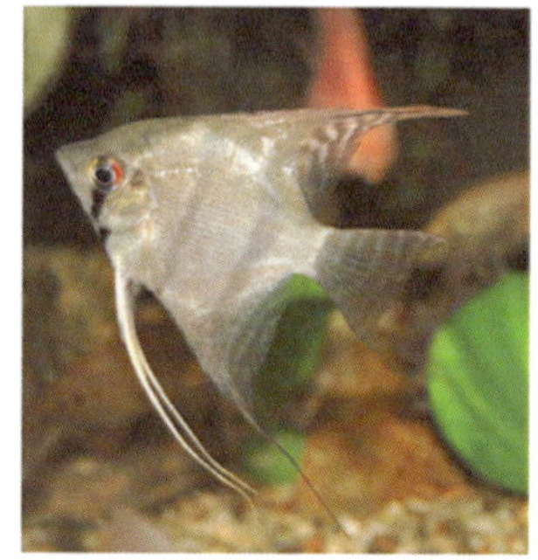

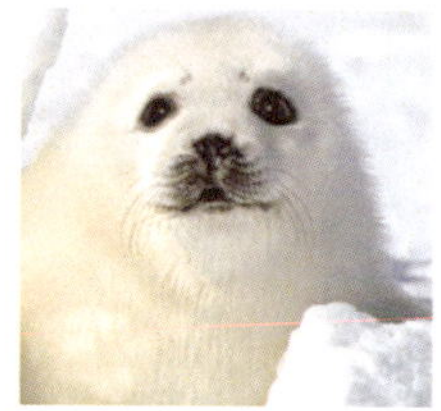

*And a* **BABY SEAL** *on an ultrasound.*

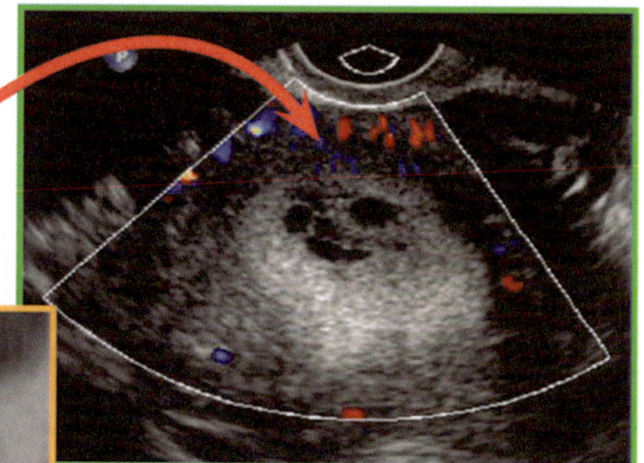

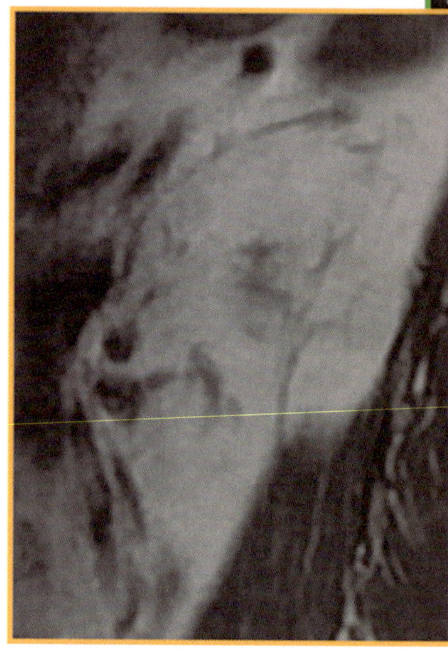

*We also have an* **OLD ENGLISH SHEEPDOG** *on an MRI of the spine.*

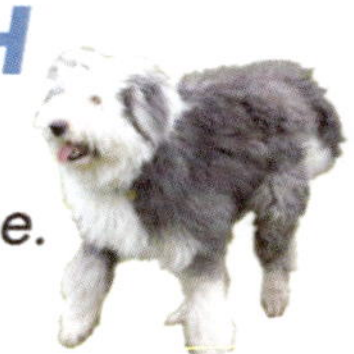

*And we even have a* **PTERODACTYL.**

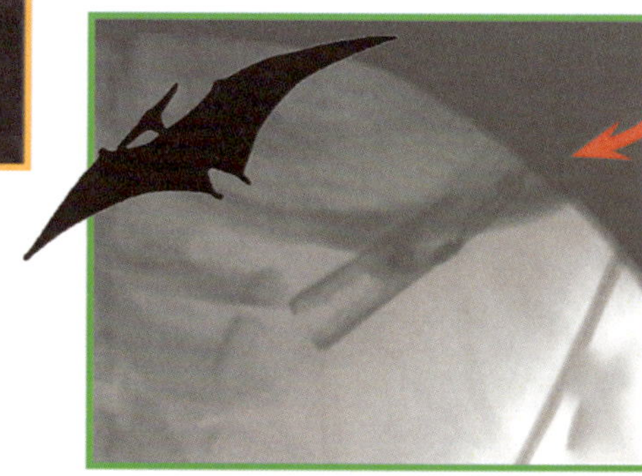

If you're a radiologist, show us your files. If we use them, you'll get **A FREE ONE-YEAR SUBSCRIPTION!**

NEW

# onguysa

(sexagliptin)

You have taste. You have style. Unfortunately, you now have diabetes. *PJ Pharmaceuticals* dares to be different with its first "orientation-targeted" medication. For the diva who has diabetes, we have your drug.

*The discriminating diabetic medication made just for gay men.*

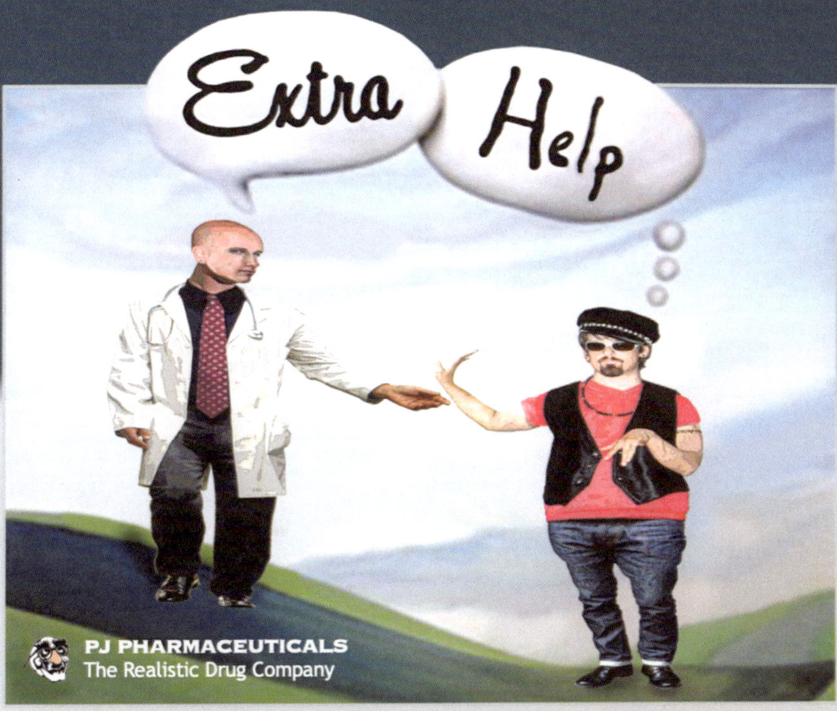


*Onguysa* is a prescription medicine that belongs to a class of medicines called DP-4 inhibitors. *Onguysa* lowers blood sugar by helping the body increase the level of insulin after a fabulous meal.* So invite some friends over, mix a few cocktails, order in delivery, and tell them you're taking *Onguysa*!

Come out to your doctor and tell him you want to be *Onguysa*! Who knows, maybe your cute doctor takes *Onguysa* as well?

*Onguysa* comes in its own pill purse. *It's neat. It's fashionable.* And it dares you to be a real boy. You can even choose from a wheel of gay colors even *Crayola* can't mix up!

* Use *Onguysa* as directed. Take *Onguysa* by mouth one time each day exactly as directed by your doctor. Do not change your dose and swallow more *Onguysa* without talking to your doctor.

Society for Universal Quality And Statistical Standards

# SUQASS

***Say goodbye to the art of medicine and say hello to quality.****

We believe in quality medicine and the key to quality medicine is using the word quality over and over again. Quality standards. Quality doctors. Quality staff. Quality hospitals. No one knows quality like a quality organization which is known not only for judging and grading quality but reinforcing and remunerating quality as well.

**SUQASS** is a biased, for-profit organization that accredits and certifies the quality of thousands of health care organizations and programs in the United States. **SUQASS** is easily influenced to accredit and certify any medical business that will:

1. Pay.
2. Say the word "quality" ten times fast without making a mistake.
3. Pay.

## MISSION STATEMENT

**SUQASS** is recognized nationwide as a symbol of quality that reflects an organization's commitment to meeting certain quality standards as long as those standards stand for quality. Like you, we have no idea what that means.

## VISION STATEMENT

Treating people as numbers and not people.

So if you want your organization to look good to patients, to the media, to insurers, and even the government then you want to **SUQASS**.

**Call 1-555-ISUQASS now** and let our team of quality information specialists evaluate your organizations quality indicators to see if you qualify to be graded as:

- High quality
- Higher quality
- Highest quality

***We are SUQASS! Do you SUQASS?***

* Studies have shown over and over again that quality indicators have never been proven to improve the healthcare system. Though pay-per-performance programs claim to use evidence-based medicine to justify its existence, there are no studies showing any evidence that the concept of pay-for-performance works. ✚

## PROOF OF DIAGNOSIS

A young mom brought her 6-year-old to see my partner for kindergarten immunizations. The child went bonkers and had to be restrained by three nurses to get her shots. This is not unusual, but even after the shots were given, the kid continued to get progressively more riled up, until she was throwing a full-scale tantrum, which looked funny coming from a 6-year-old, not a 2-year-old.

This continued to escalate, with the child throwing every piece of medical equipment she could grab, slamming doors, and punching walls. Swinging at and often landing solid punches in her mother's face, Mom did little to prevent the violent outburst or stop her from breaking stuff or throwing tongue depressors and gauze pads all over the room.

My colleagues often engage in the classic nature/nurture debate when we see kids behave in such a manner. Today the debate was unnecessary, because the mother answered it for us as they left the clinic, screaming child in her arm: *"Yeah, we usually* **have** *to give her* Mountain Dew *when she gets like this. That's how we proved she has ADHD."* ✚

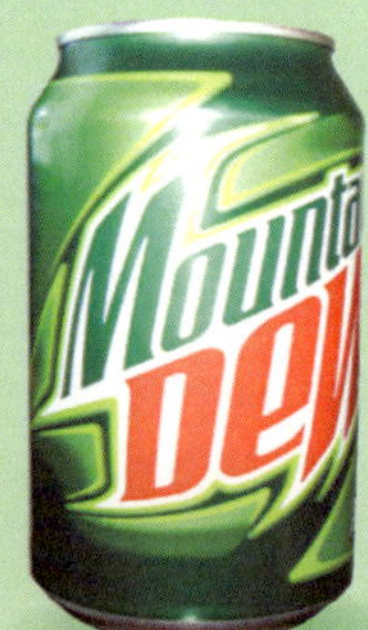


## HAVE A COKE ON ME!

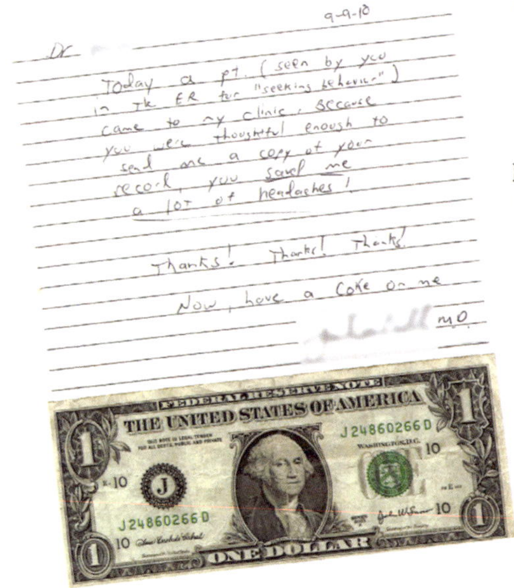
9-9-10

Dr. [illegible]

Today a pt. (seen by you in the ER for "seeking behavior") came to my clinic. Because you were thoughtful enough to send me a copy of your record, you saved me a lot of headaches!

Thanks! Thanks! Thanks!

Now, have a Coke on me

[illegible] MD

I recently saw a chronic pain patient in my ER. **First red flag.** I noticed she'd driven past two hospitals to get to mine. **Second red flag.** Before I even saw her, I pulled her drug profile from our Board of Pharmacy, and spoke to her physician. She'd received multiple narcotics from several providers. Her doctor told me she was a relatively new patient. He shared with me that she was frustrated with this doc because he had the audacity to ask her to provide old records from previous providers.

When I went to see the patient, she assured me she had no new injuries, and this was her chronic pain. She also lamented that her current doctor wouldn't write her for any pain medicine, so she was switching to Doctor #2.

I confronted her in the lie. Her husband said, *"Well, at least she's not lying about the pain she's having."* Needless to say, I sent her on her way. I sent a copy of my dictation to both Doctor #1 and #2.

A few days later I received the note above from Doctor #2.

*What a cool guy!* ✚

*Do you have any male patients who are drama queens?*

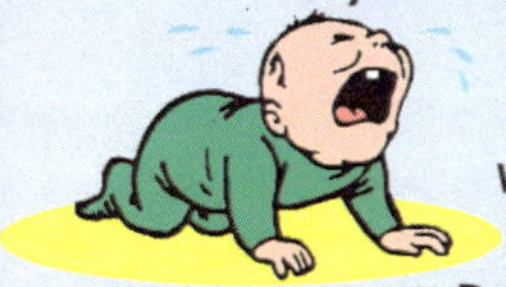

*Are you amazed how some men whine over the tiniest of symptoms?*

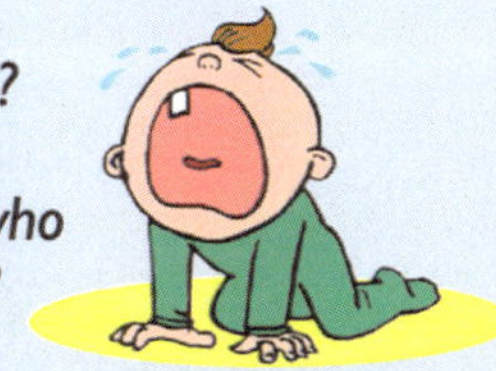

*Do you see some men in the office who chronically complain over nothing?*

*Do you sometimes want to pretend you are Don Corleone and slap the patient across the face while yelling,* "You can act like a man!"

PJ Pharmaceuticals *introduces its newest medication to treat all of the above and it is called:*

# SBAP-18U

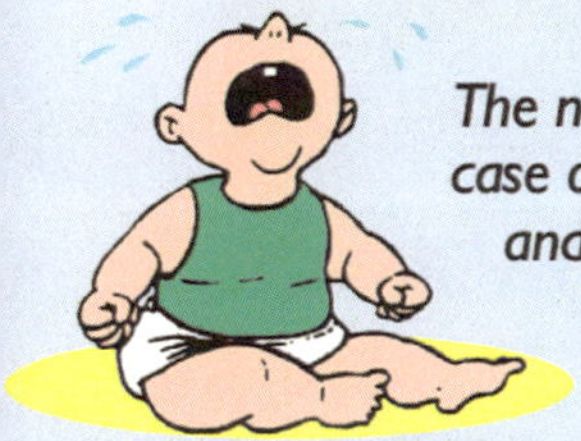

*The next time one of your male patients comes in for a case of a missing backbone, offer him the SBAP-18U pill and send him on his way. Tell him it will cure all his ailments and make him come to his senses.*

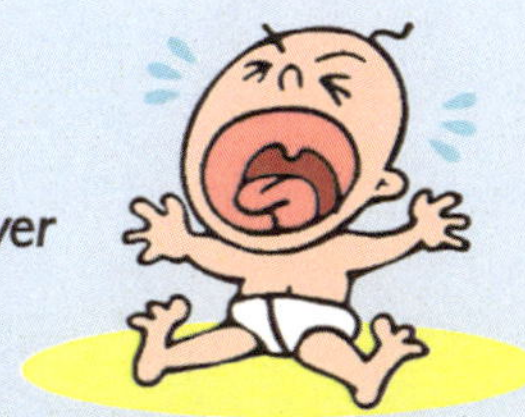

*SBAP-18U stands for "Stop Being A Pussy," and he will be alerted to this when he retrieves the placebo drug at the pharmacy. Sure, he may never return but maybe he will get the message and, well, stop being such a pussy. And if he transfers his care, who gives a crap?*

**You can only win with SBAP-18U!***

"When I read the box and saw what ***SBAP-18U*** stood for I was really mad. I even yelled out loud. Now my throat hurts and I think my back is acting up. Do you think I have something serious?"

**Kyle Werner**, age 31

* **PJ PHARMACEUTICALS** *The Realistic Drug Company* is not responsible for patient complaints to the Board of Medicine, patients firing their doctors, or patients doing physical harm to their doctors. Since these male patients, by definition are pussies, there really is a minimal chance any of this will happen.

# What is one thing you should NEVER ask your doctor?

*All True Answers from Readers of the* Placebo Journal *Blog*

- ***"Are you married?"*** and a follow-up question, ***"Would you like to go out sometime?"*** *(Totally gross when you have just heard about some very personal medical issue and likely inserted your finger into one of that person's orifices.*
- ***"Did I wake you?"*** (From a patient calling you in the middle of the night.)
- ***"Don't you have any samples of those Oxycontin pills?"***
- ***"What is a normal blood alcohol level?"*** *(*Umm . . .zero.)
- During a physical exam, never ask, ***"So what are you thinking about?"***
- ***"Hey, what do you use for your erectile dysfunction?"***
- ***"Doctor, is it okay if I pay you with a goat and two chickens?"***
- ***"Can you fill out these (enter any number) papers for my workplace?"*** (Usually at the end of the visit.)
- ***"Does this gown make my butt look fat?"***
- ***"Can you loan me a couple of dollars until payday?"***
- ***"I just moved into a new apartment, can I get a note that says air conditioning is medically necessary?"***
- ***"Can I get a note stating I need to keep my dog for mental health reasons?"***
- ***"Will you spread my cheeks so I can pass gas?"*** (This actually happened to my husband – a physician.)
- ***"I saw this drug advertised on TV and I want a prescription for it."***
- ***"Can you fill out my FMLA form and by the way I need to take it with me and oh, I left it in the car and there's also the refill for my husband and the school form for my child and my other child needs . . ."***
- ***"When is your baby due?"***
- ***"Will you sleep with me and give me an honest opinion of how good I am in bed?"***

# X-Ray Files

***If we show you ours, will you show us yours?***

**MR. MAGOO** thinks he's looking into **A MIRROR . . .**

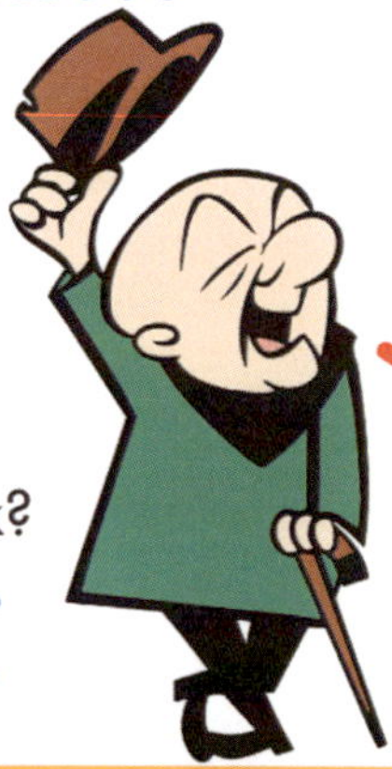

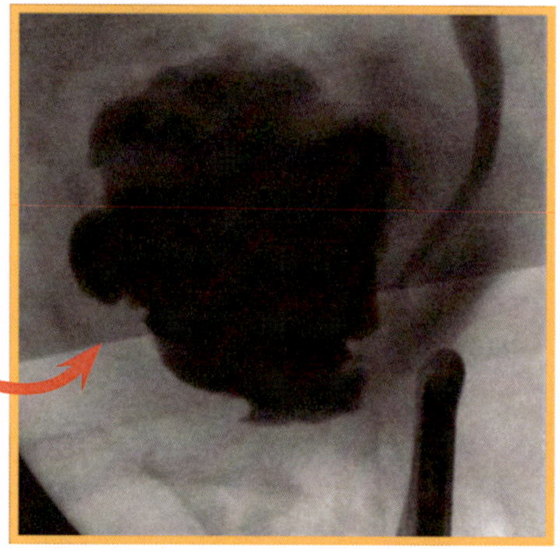

In the mood for a snack? **ASK MR. PEANUT.**

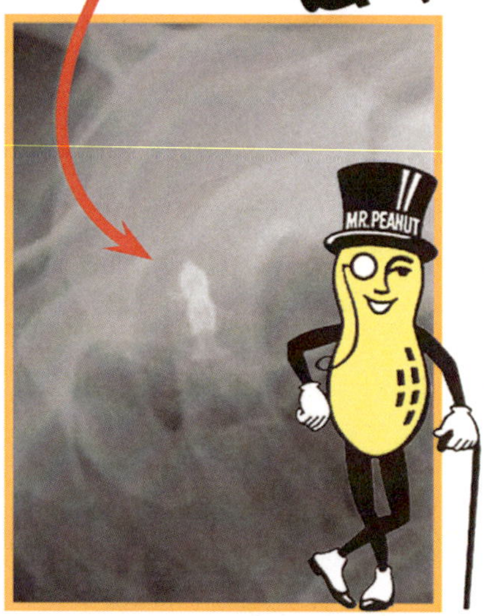


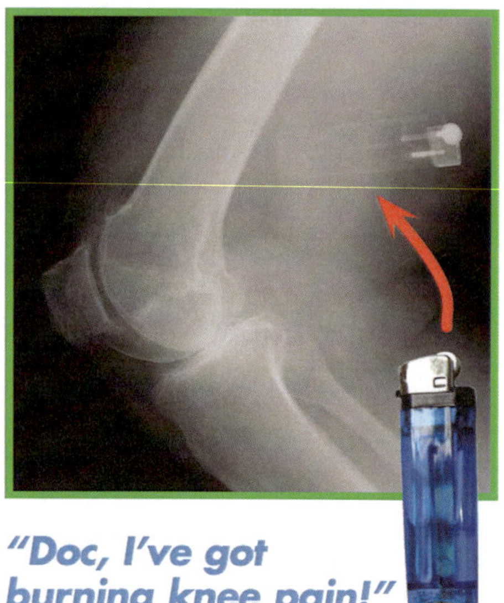

***"Doc, I've got burning knee pain!"***

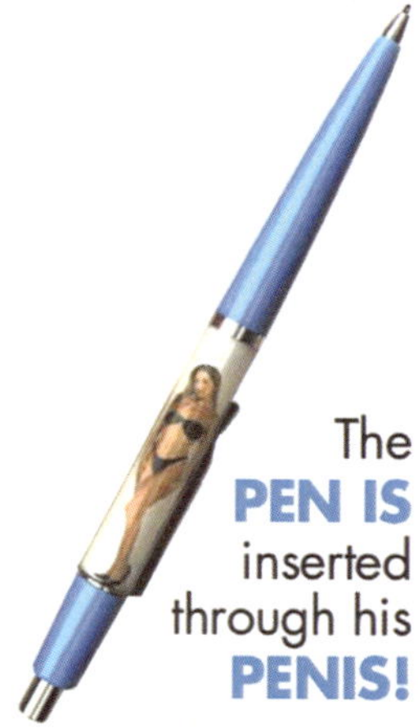

The **PEN IS** inserted through his **PENIS!**

***Yikes!!!***

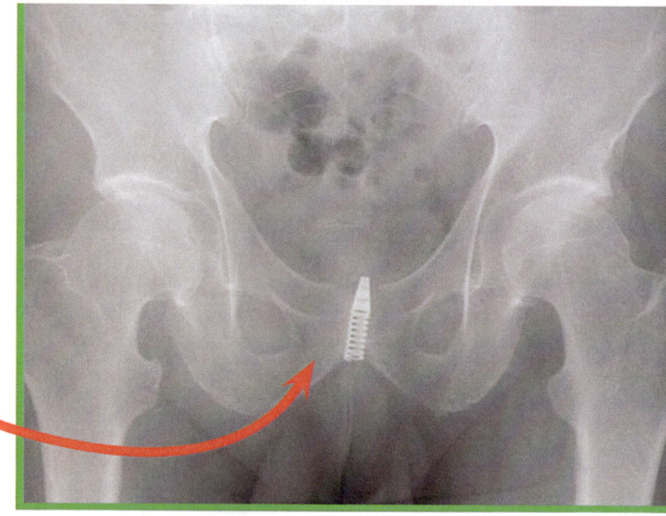

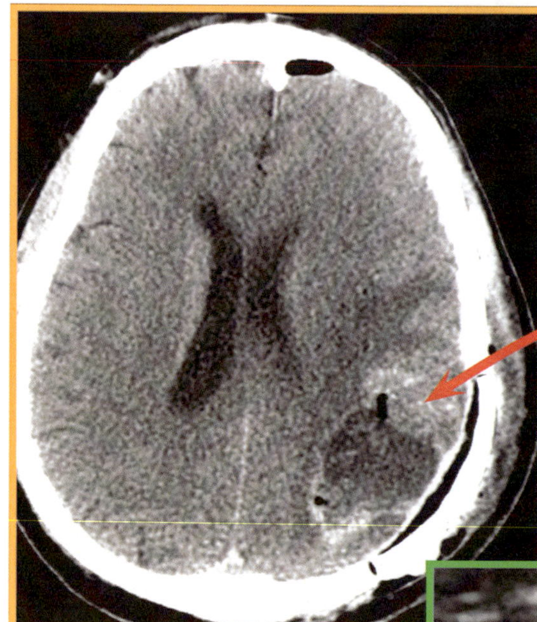

Here's a ***LIONESS HEAD*** on a brain scan . . .

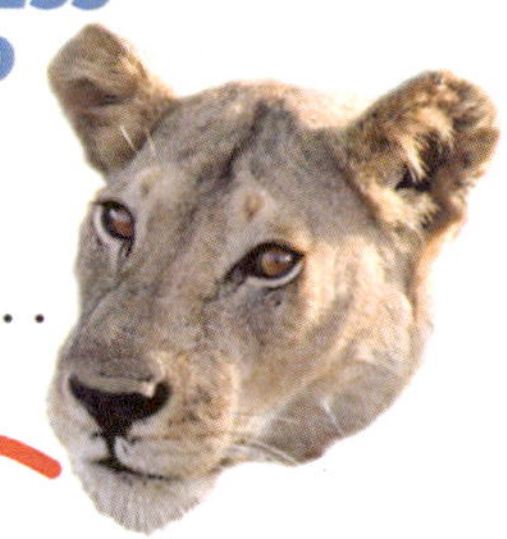

. . . and a ***POODLE*** on an ultrasound!

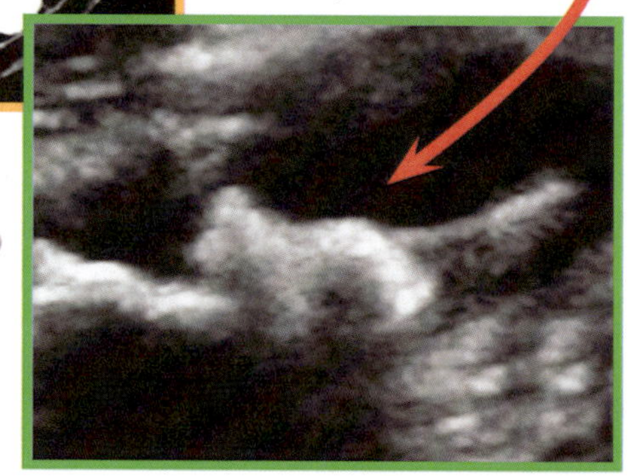

If you're a radiologist, show us your files. If we use them, you'll get a **FREE ONE-YEAR SUB-SCRIPTION!**

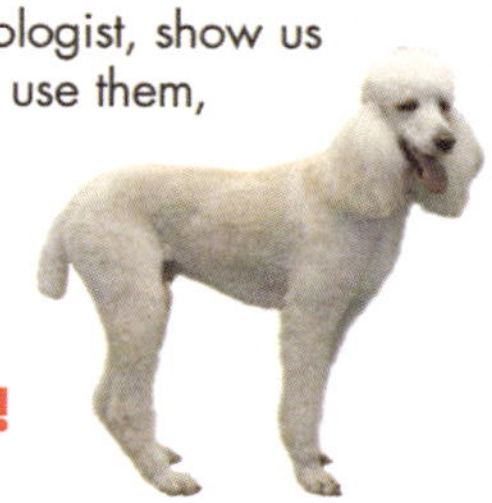

## ANOTHER TRUE STORY OF MEDICINE

# BELLY LANDING

Jack Murphy, all 300 pounds of him, shook like a bowl of *Jell-O* when he laughed. *"You gotta help me here!"* he pleaded. *"C'mon Doc! You can do it!"* he said, *"If you give me a sterile needle, I'll do it myself!"*

*"You know I can't do that, Mr. Murphy. We're not set up for surgery in this office,"* I said, gesturing with my palms up at the tiny office – an office the residents had rumored to be a converted janitor's closet. An exam chair, a small desk, and a gurney completely filled the limited space. In the fall of 1973 this one very small room was the Department of Ophthalmology at our VA hospital.

*"You can't send me home like this!"* he said, pointing to his right upper eyelid. *"It's ripe, Doc!"*

His right eye was swollen completely shut, and there was a yellow mass pointing anteriorly on the eyelid. He was right; it was ripe and ready for incision and drainage.

*"It's a chalazion,"* I said.

*"A shillelagh?"* he questioned.

*"Keh-lazy-en,"* I said phonetically, *"I think it comes from a Greek word for lump."*

*"It sounds Irish,"* he said as he was laughing.

*"Besides,"* I added, *"I don't even have an assistant to help me. I am alone here."*

*"Maybe you can find a good looking nurse on the ward to help you?"* he suggested.

The eye clinic was staffed by a single second-year resident from the university. There were no receptionists, no secretaries, no assistants and no nurses. Its primary function was to provide cataract surgery to the veterans and intraocular surgical experience for the ophthalmology residents. This chalazion was too trivial for the operating room – which required an admission to the hospital – yet it loomed as a major procedure for this tiny room; nevertheless, he needed it lanced.

*"I'll be back,"* I said, and leaving Jack in the room, I wandered down the hallway of the neurology ward. I had received help from the ward nurses on occasion and I was hoping to enlist a volunteer assistant. This day, unfortunately, they were all too busy with admissions to help me. But then I spotted Mary.

Doe-eyed Mary, the new clerk at the nursing station on the neurology ward, had only been working at the VA hospital for a few weeks. She had told me that she was interested in going to nursing school, but secretly she wondered if it would be an appropriate choice for her. Extremely shy and reticent, in her early 20s, she had confided to me that she was worried about her reaction to blood.

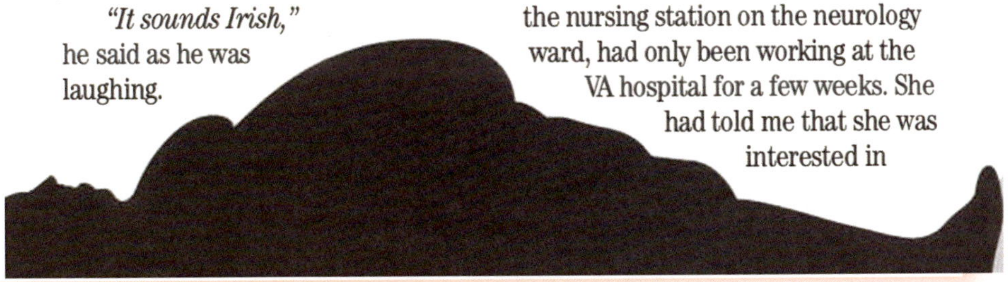

*"No worries,"* I reassured her, *"all of us had that doubt."* I told her that as a Special Forces physician I had helped to train Green Beret medics – and even these battle-hardened veterans initially had their doubts. She just needed some experience, and we were going to provide that for her.

*"I'm not so sure,"* she said.

*"Oh, you'll do just fine,"* I said, *"You don't even have to look unless you want to."*

*"O.K,"* she replied hesitantly, still worried.

We walked back to the eye clinic at the end of the hallway and I introduced my patient to my new assistant. *"Mary, thanks for helping Doc,"* Jack said, *"he really needs an extra hand to do this,"* pointing at the festering mass on his eyelid. I could not see in the dimly lighted room that she had already begun to pale.

By re-arranging the room we were able to create a surgical suite of sorts, albeit a tiny one. The gurney was moved away from the wall to the center of the room, allowing just enough space for Mary to squeeze between it and the wall. Jack was lying supine on the gurney, a goose-neck lamp arched over his chest, a sterile field draped over his massive abdomen – in lieu of a Mayo stand. I sat on a stool at his head, my back against the closed door of the room. I hoped no one was claustrophobic.

Carefully I arranged the instruments on the sterile field which was balanced at the apex of Jack's girth: a syringe of lidocaine, a large chalazion clamp, forceps, a curette, scissors and a scalpel. Mary opened a sterile pack of gauze and cotton-tip applicators and I placed them on the field. After a *Betadine* prep we were scrubbed, gloved, and ready to go.

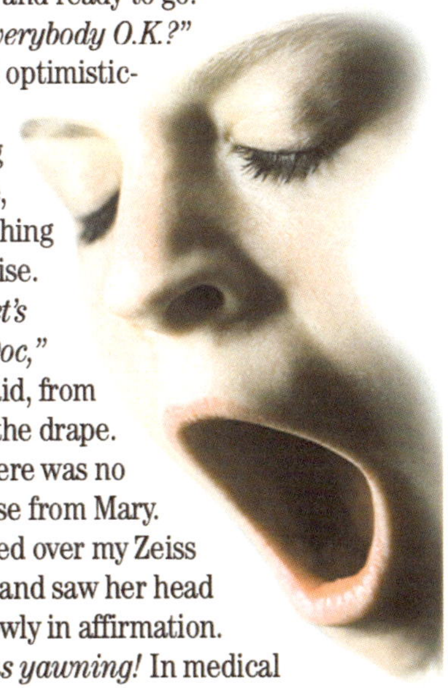

*"Everybody O.K.?"* I asked optimistically, sensing trouble, but wishing otherwise.

*"Let's do it, Doc,"* Jack said, from under the drape.

There was no response from Mary. I glanced over my Zeiss loupes and saw her head nod slowly in affirmation. *She was yawning!* In medical school I had been a phlebotomist in the blood bank; I remembered that yawning was not a sign of boredom in the blood bank. *"Uh oh,"* I thought.

We almost made it. The chalazion, under pressure from the clamp,

*continued on next page*

A hard-nosed dermatologist tries to find out if there is anything more to his job than just treating acne.

# TRUE ZIT

## A COMEDONE BROS. MOVIE

See how Dr. "Zoster" Cogburn searches for that one

**TRUE ZIT**

that will make his career worthwhile.

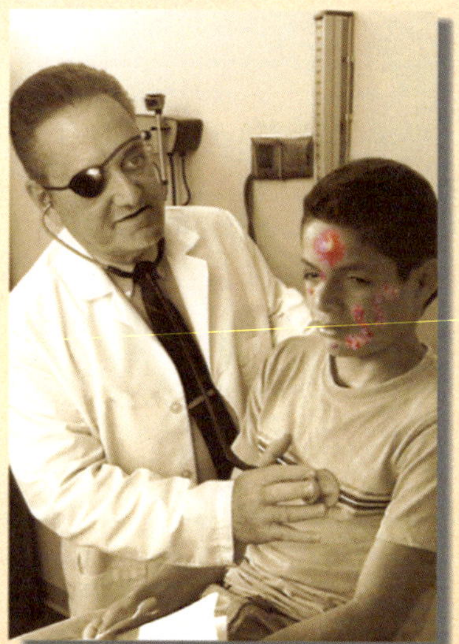

## REFLECTION

Maybe getting paid a ridiculous amount of money isn't really worth it?

R — REALITY — UNDER 17 REQUIRES ACCOMPANYING PARENT OR ADULT GUARDIAN — PERVASIVE STRONG HORROR VIOLENCE AND GORE, LANGUAGE AND SEXUALITY

*COMING SOON TO A THEATRE NEAR YOU.*

# PJ MEDICAL GRAPHS OF REALITY

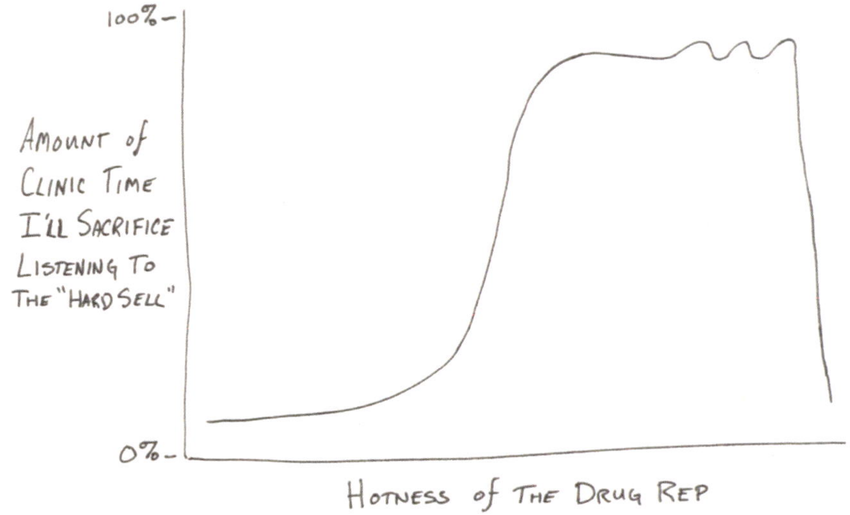


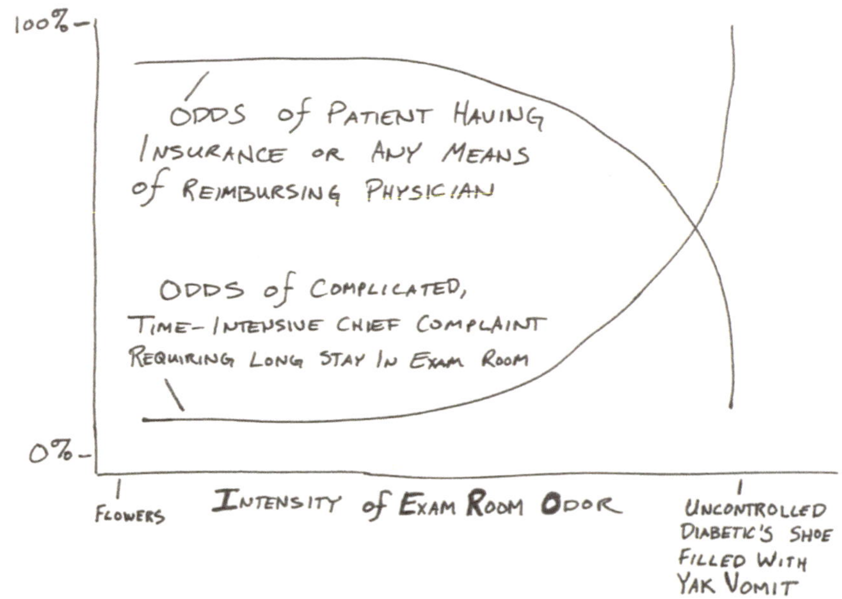

## TOP TEN THINGS THEY DIDN'T TEACH US IN MEDICAL SCHOOL

**10** Practicing medicine is the easy part. It's all the other crap that grinds you down.

**9** You might have gone into medicine because you like people, but medicine will beat that out of you.

**8** Not all little old ladies are nice.

**7** It is your responsibility to remind otherwise fully functional adult patients of their appointments.

**6** There is medical decision-making and then there is insurance decision-making.

**5** Don't argue with any patient about anything if you can help it.

**4** Every antibiotic and pain medication argument takes 10 minutes off a physicians life.

**3** When a patient says, *"Doctor, you are the only one who has helped me . . . you are the only one who understands . . ."* Run Like Helll!

**2** You will never have as much credibility as the patients' aunts' neighbors' friend.

**1** The Triple Auscultation Point, i.e. where the heart, abdomen and lungs can all be heard in 10 seconds with one stethoscope application, is going to eventually be too detailed an exam for what managed care wants us all to do.

# AndroMousse™

(testosterone hairstyling product)

**The first androgen-containing hairstyling product that not only gives you the extra volume and shine you crave but it also increases your testosterone level!**

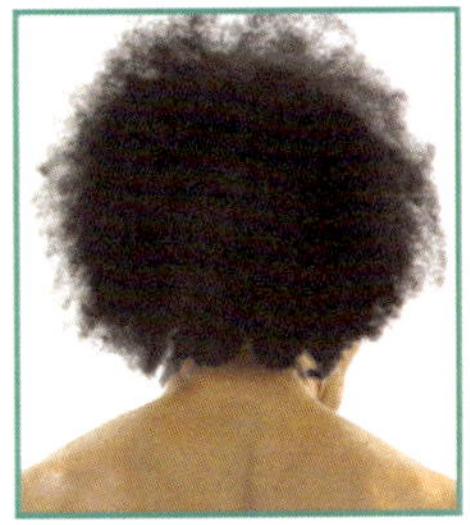

BEFORE

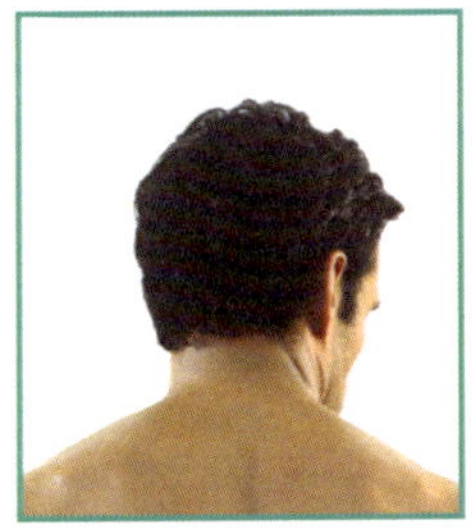

AFTER

Low testosterone, medically known as hypogonadism, occurs when a man doesn't produce enough of the hormone testosterone. Up to 13 million men in the United States may have low testosterone. Even more disturbing, almost 20 million men have simply atrocious hairstyles.

**AndroMousse will:**

- Increase your energy
- Improve your mood
- Increase your muscle mass
- Improve your erections
- Give your hair that luscious shine and softer look that you won't find in a gel.

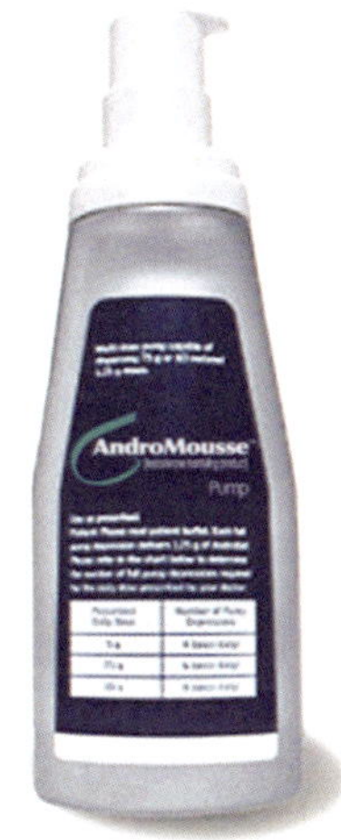

**Isn't it time you fix your low T and your low G (glamour)?**

Also available:
**AndroMousse Gray** and **AndroMousse Curls & Waves**!

Our new pump dispenses a whipped-cream like dollop of **AndroMousse*** equal to 25 mg of testosterone as well as: Water, Alcohol Denat., PVP/VA Copolymer, Hydrolised Wheat Protein,PG-Propyl Silanetriol, Cocamidopropyl Hydroxysultaine, Methylparaben, Fragrance, PEG-60 Hydrogenated Castor Oil, Sodium Chloride, Phenoxyethanol, Sodiun Hydroxide, Butylparaben, Ethylparaben, Isobutylparaben, Propylparaben, and Denatonium Benzoate.

* This product is not for bald people. The most common side effects of **AndroMousse** include: increased red blood cell count, headaches, increased blood pressure, and bed head.

**PJ PHARMACEUTICALS**
The Realistic Drug Company

# American Family Practitioner

## INFORMATION FROM YOUR FAMILY DOCTOR

### Physical Activity: What You Should Know

**Please note:** The information presented is the best we could make up. Depending on our mood, this could always change. Some of this material is not suited for anyone.

**Do I really need physical activity?**

Yes. It is good for your heart and lungs. You will live longer and feel better.

**Who should exercise?**

Everyone benefits from exercise. There should be no reason to stop you from trying but you should consult your doctor if you have heart trouble, high blood pressure, arthritis, or if you feel dizzy often or have chest pains.

**Aren't you just covering your ass by writing that?**

Yes.

**How much physical activity do I need?**

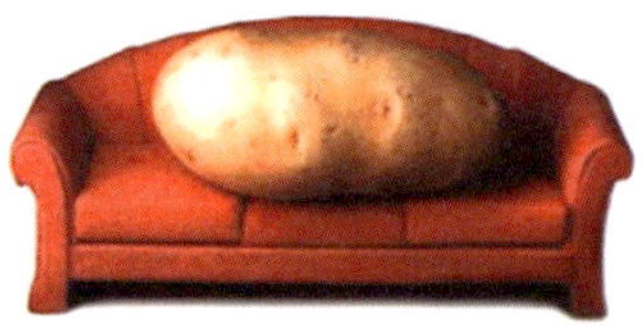

Probably a lot more than you are getting now. Most people need at least 30 minutes of cardio at least five days a week. If you are like most Americans you are getting, on average, none.

**What types of physical activity should I do?**

There are many activities that you can do. These include:
• Joining a gym • Walking • Dancing • Biking • Hiking • Rollerblading

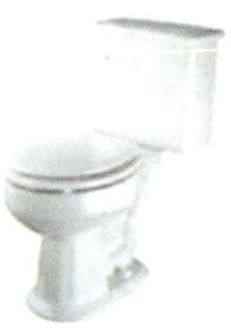

**Does having a bowel movement or looking for food in the fridge count as exercise?**

No.

**Do I have to work hard?**

It probably will be more effective if you give it some effort. There is a reason that the word "work" is included in the term "workout."

**But I don't want to work hard.**

Then why are you even reading this?



**Can't I get some machines to do the work for me?**

Unfortunately, you have to actually participate in the exercise. There was what was called "toning" machines that were promoted as exercise and all you had to do was lay there and let the machine move you around. They were found to be a rip-off and did not accomplish a thing.

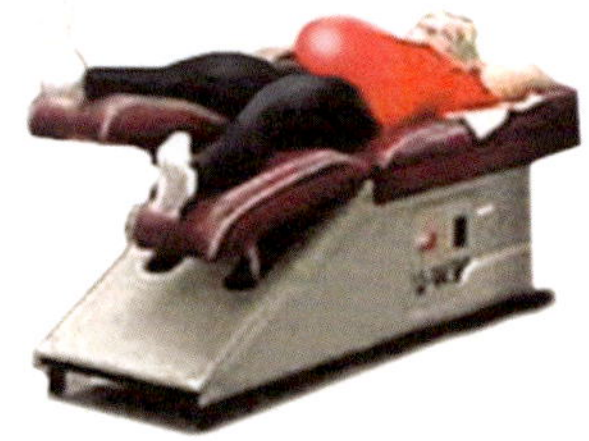

**Where can I buy one of those machines?**

Did you not just read what I just wrote? They don't do anything except cost you money!

**Can you buy them on *eBay*?**

*Oh, my God. You're not going to exercise, are you?*

**No.**

Great. Do you have any more questions?

**Are there any pills that can make me look better, give me the effects of exercise and solve all my problems?**

You'd be better off buying those ridiculous toning machines.

**Really?**

Yeah, you can find them on *eBay.*

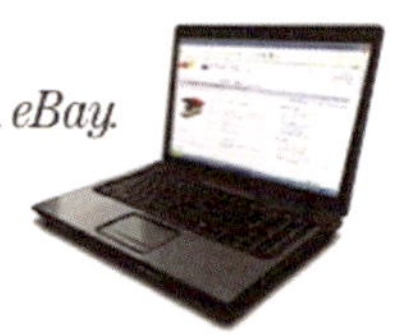

**Thanks.**

*This handout provides a general idea of this topic. Not everyone will like what they read. For those people, we recommend talking to your own family doctor.*

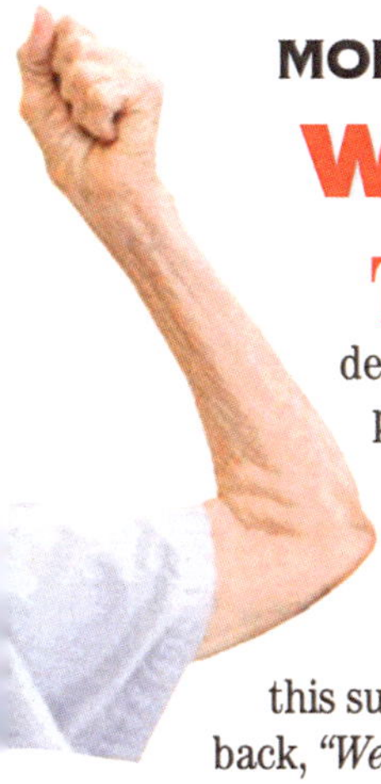

### MORE TRUE STORIES OF MEDICINE

## WHIPPER SNAPPER

This story comes off best if you understand I work in a deep Appalachian rural town. As my nurse escorted my oldest patient into the office, I complimented her youthful stride – *"No cane, no walker! Look at you!"*

Her daughter bragged, *"She just celebrated her 96th birthday last week!"*

I replied that my grandmother would be turning 98 this summer. The patient (I think suspecting a challenge) whipped back, *"We oughtta get together and WRASTLE."* ✚

## TIGHT

A gynecologist with a medical group that saved money by using minimally trained transcriptionists once dictated a report on a lady with atrophic vaginitis that had narrowed the cervical os so much that he couldn't get a sample brush in to test for cancerous changes.

What he said was, *"I was unable to perform a Pap smear due to the patient's having a very tight os."*

The transcriptionist, being unfamiliar with "os," typed the word in her vocabulary that sounded closest to it.

It makes sense . . . we all know how difficult those tight-assed patients can be. ✚

## BPMs

We had a patient come in because his new defibrillator had fired several times during sex. The interrogation showed no arrthythmia, just sinus tachycardia in the 170's. One of my colleagues said, *"175 BPM during sex? I must have been doing it wrong all these years!"* The defibrillator was reprogrammed to tolerate a higher rate, and he was discharged home to continue *"doing it right."* ✚

## AMAZING THINGS PATIENTS SAY

*"Did you check your temperature?"*
**"Not with a thermometer."**

*"How are your blood sugars after meals?"*
**"You mean when I check them?"**

A patient was given *Rozerem* for insomnia. She read the PDI and was upset when she learned it could cause erratic behavior, like "sleep sex."
She said, **"It's been 10 years since I've had sex. If I'm going to have it, I want to be awake!"**

**"I don't never, not not have pain!"**

*"How many brothers do you have?"*
**"I never counted."**

A female patient asked, **"Did that stool test check for my prostate?"**

**"My dog has a thyroid problem, is it contagious?"**

**"I only eat one breakfast in the morning."**

**"Is that pill an accelerator to slow things down?"**

**"I didn't know I was blind in my left eye!"**

**"In the past, tampons gave me headaches. I switched to pads. They gave me a rash. I switched back to tampons. Can Toxic Shock Syndrome do this?"**

**"I'm walking the same distance but it's farther now."**

*"How is your pain?"*
**"It's more constant."**

**"He needs to know EVERYTHING, the ins and outs of a duck's ass!"**

**"I didn't take anything for the back pain because I didn't want it to go away."**

**"When I pinch my nose closed after I spray the medicine in it, do I breathe in through it?"**

**"I've been trying to get pregnant to have a baby."**

**"The cough is less deep, depth-ness wise."**

*"Your blood sugars are higher lately. Are you eating more?"*
**"What do you mean?"**

**"The pain goes all the way up my back to where my breasts are!"**

**"I was rear-ended from behind."**

*"How is your pain on a scale of 1to10?"*
**"In the middle of a 7."**

**"I seem to have a hitch in my giddy-up!**

**"I'm outside a lot, off and on."**

**"I need some Monstacillin for this cold."** ✚

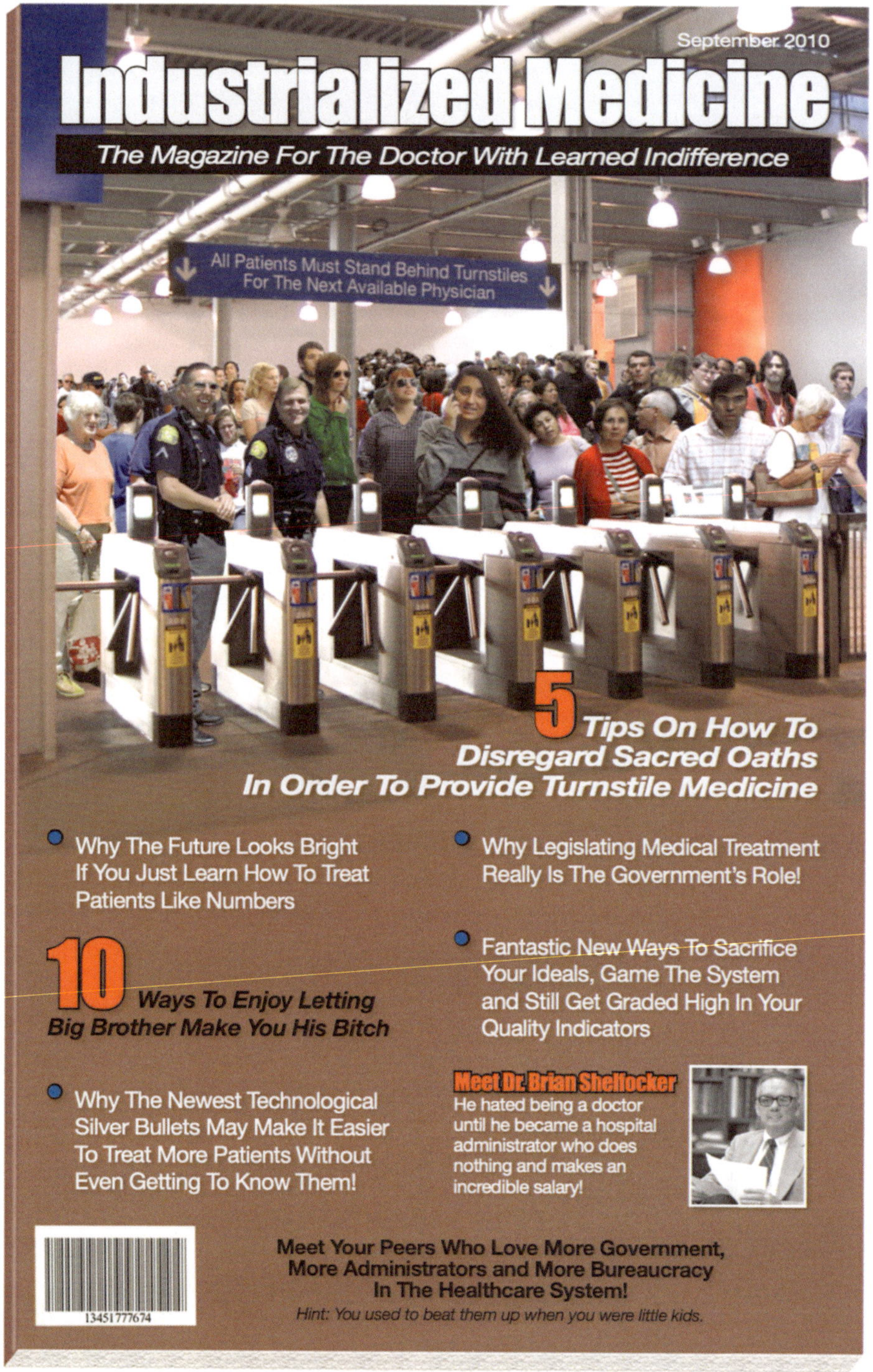


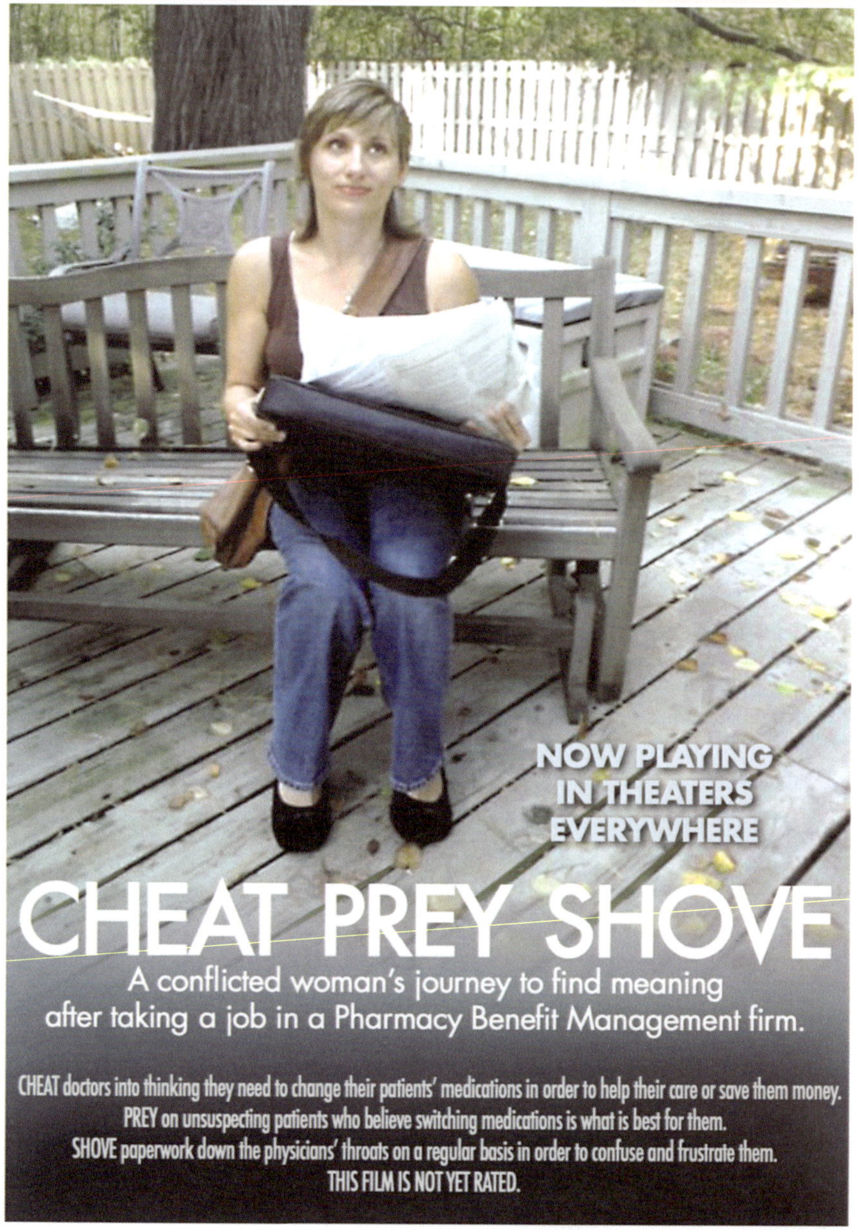


*"Three little words soon to be on every doctor's lips.*
*That and "Go f#ck yourselves!"*

Ann Grayson, MD

*"I hated the book and the movie made me even more nauseous.*
*Why do these companies exist, anyway?"*

K. Sebelius

# 25 GUARANTEED WAYS PATIENTS CAN TICK OFF THEIR DOCTORS

Submitted by readers of the *Placebo Journal* Blog

**1.** Ask him to wait just a second while you finish reading the last paragraph of your romance novel or finish your cell phone call.

**2.** Eat garlic and onions for lunch. Keeps the doc on her toes.

**3.** Change the baby's diaper and leave it open in the wastebasket.

**4.** Need babysitting, no problem. The nurses have time to keep your kids amused while you have your pelvic exam. Yell a lot through the door. Helps set the mood.

**5.** Bring in articles from magazines, off the web, or neighborly advice to diagnose your own symptoms.

**6.** Talk or text something very funny while the doctor makes his exam. Keeps you busy while he does his thing. Also allow the doctor in on the conversation. He'll love you for it.

**7.** Need to vomit? Why worry about even trying to make it to the trashcan or bathroom? Just let it fly . . . then the doctor can really see that you are indeed sick. No, really sick. Don't worry about the clean up. Isn't that what nurses are supposed to do?

**8.** As your doctor leaves the exam room after your visit, ask him if he has a second to fill out your FMLA papers.

**9.** Try to convince your doctor that the three months worth of prescription medication that he wrote for you eight months ago just ran out.

**10.** Leave your cell phone on the counter where the doctor sits and ask a friend to call during your visit and have your phone ring loudly playing any John Phillip Sousa march.

**11.** Tell the medical team treating your cancer that you want only "natural" methods instead of the surgery and chemo they recommend. But as your condition worsens, tell them that you're "not a quitter" and want every possible life-sustaining treatment, CPR and all.

**12.** Take forever to remember how many siblings you have. Take even longer to know their ages or health status.

**13.** Don't answer a yes/no question with a yes or no. Tell a long story instead.

**14.** Try to cram as many complaints as possible into one office visit. Demand to be referred to a different specialist for each of them on the grounds that primary care docs are just HMO gatekeepers and can't be trusted to do anything right.

**15.** Whatever course of treatment is recommended, grumble that *"Dr. Oldstyle never did it that way."* (This works better if Dr. Oldstyle has been dead for a while).

**16.** Communicate location of pain by waves of one or both hands; report that your problem has been present for *"a while"* and that *"they did some kind of tests at that other hospital."* Forget name of hospital, along with test results and procedures done.

**17.** Bring an unrequested fecal sample to your appointment, in a plastic baggie.

**18.** Tell the doctor your spouse is a nurse or respiratory therapist and that she has already diagnosed you with whatever and you just need him to get the prescription.

**19.** Tell the doc how much you hate the health care profession and how malpractice premiums aren't really that expensive.

**20.** Debate with the doctor about how to treat a problem because you *Googled* it or saw a video on *You Tube.*

**21.** Brag about the lawsuit you are currently suing another doctor for (especially when it's the same thing you are asking the doctor to do and he would do it the same way as the first doctor).

**22.** Every time you go to see your doctor, complain about new and unusual symptoms that are totally different than the symptoms on your last visit which have now gone away.

**23.** Avoid all forms of personal hygiene for a minimum of two days before your appointment.

**24.** Tell your doctor that everything's fine today, but two weeks ago you had severe abdominal pain, diarrhea, a pounding headache, fever of 103.7, you were vomiting your guts out, shortness of breath, whirling dizziness, with some blood in your stool. You took some *Tylenol* and in two days felt like normal. Then ask, *"So, doc, what do you think I had?"*

**25.** Tell your doctor that the sharp stabbing pains in the middle of your abdomen have been going on for *"a while."* Let him figure out if it's a short while or a long while, and how short or how long. ✚

*"I was so "in" to it, I just couldn't put it down – my tractor rusted and the weeds grew up around me! I, however, am relaxed from laughing and enjoying my* **PLACEBO JOURNAL."**

*As seen on* Facebook/Placebo Journal Fans

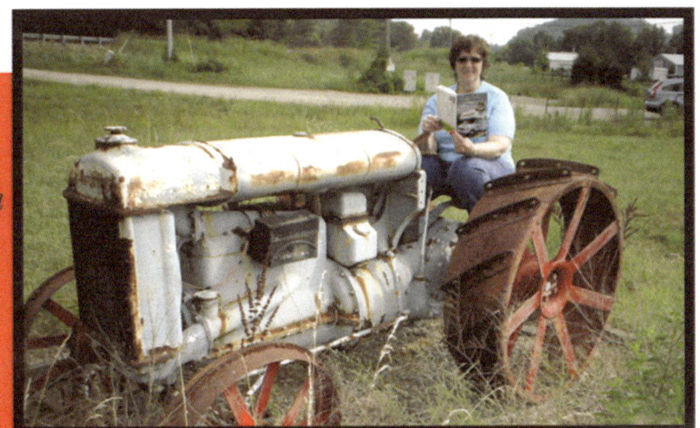

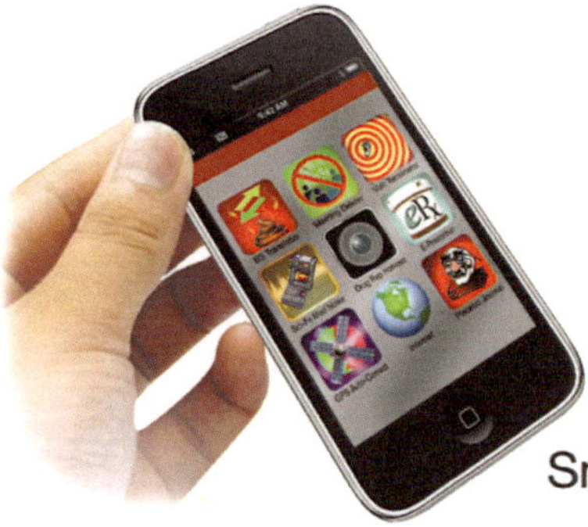

*Placebo Mobile Media Products* Is Proud To Present Our 2010 Fall Lineup Of

# APPS for DOCS

Smartphone Apps for Medical Professionals, Compatible with All Smartphones and Operating Systems!

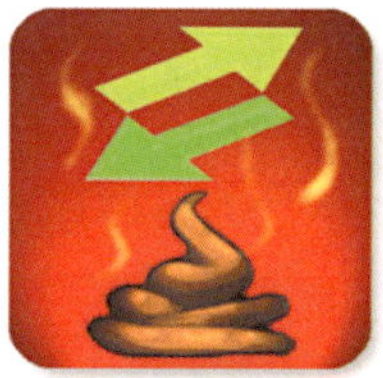

**PATIENT BS TRANSLATOR APP** Automatically decodes a patient's words into their actual wants. • *"I have trouble getting to sleep,"* becomes, *"My other doctor cut off my* Xanax *supply."* • *"I'm allergic to* Toradol *and ibuprofen,"* becomes, *"I want some oxycodone."* • and *"I am here for personal reasons,"* becomes, *"I slept with a hooker a few nights ago and now it burns when I pee."*

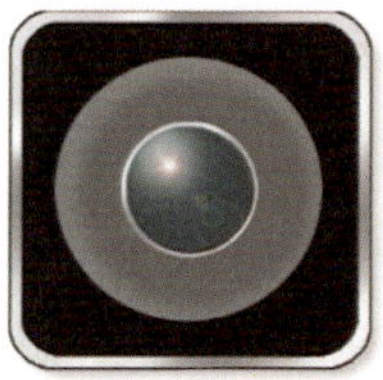

**DRUG REP HOTNESS SMARTPHONE CAMERA PLUGIN** Your smartphone camera automatically photographs your drug reps *(if you have any left these days)* and gives them a score from 1-10. It e-mails the score to the drug rep, so he or she knows how likely you are to listen to them at all or prescribe their drug.

*X-ray vision camera phone sold separately.*

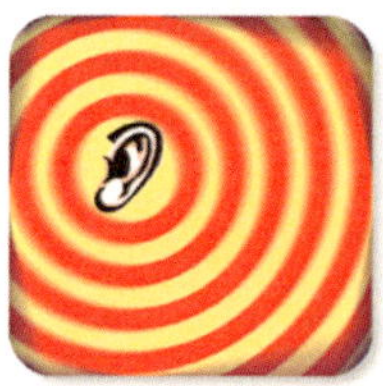

**VISIT TERMINATOR APP** Automatically scans clinic conversations for buzzword red flags, *so you don't have to!* Your smartphone will emit a deafening tone rendering conversation useless, and therefore ending the office visit, once a pre-set threshold of buzz phrases has been surpassed, saving you the time of ending the visit yourself: Example phrases include such gems as: • *"Oh, by the way . . ."* • *"What do you think about medical marijuana?"* • *"Is your nurse single?"* • *"Do you have any samples of* Viagra?" • *"I think I have chronic fatigue syndrome."*

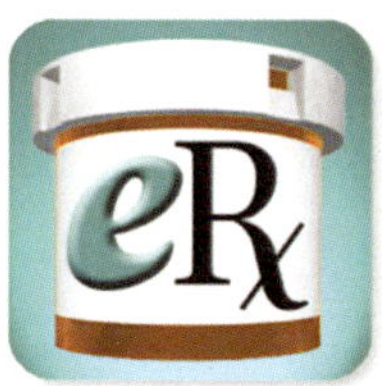

**REALISTIC E-PRESCRIBER APP** The Realistic E-Prescriber App scans the patient's past *filled* prescriptions, snake oil purchases, and internet browsing history. So if the drug you have chosen isn't on the patient's insurance formulary, is prohibitively expensive or his internet guru said that the prescription you've chosen causes autism and excessive scrotal wrinkling, a warning alarm is sent back to you before the patient leaves the office. By using complex human motivation, behavior and entitlement predictor algorithms, the Realistic E-Prescriber App changes the prescription from what you wrote to one more likely to actually be filled which most likely is . . . nothing.

**CALL 1-555-APPS-4DOCS AND ORDER YOURS TODAY!**

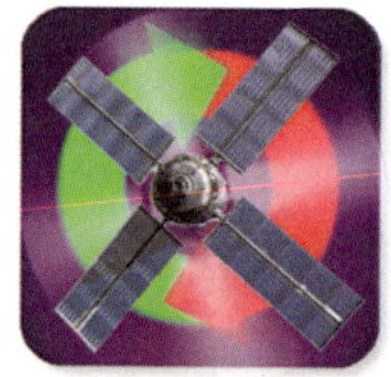

**GPS DESTINATION AUTO-CORRECTOR APP** This app re-routes you from where you think you should go to where you actually should go. *You set the level of responsibility, and it does the rest!* If you have it set to VERY RESPONSIBLE, then on a Saturday morning when you enter in the address of a country club or golf store, it instead takes you to a *Habitat for Humanity* building site. If you have it set for MILD IRRESPONSIBILITY, then on your way to work, it will take you to *Burger King*, and after work, you'll stop for a beer on your way to your kid's boring soccer game.

But the MAJOR IRRESPONSIBILITY setting is where the true value of this app lies. If you're about to go to another soul-crushing day of entitlement granting and you just can't take it, a quick change to this setting will take you on the ride of your life. After relieving several medical marijuana shops of their disgusting profits at paintball gunpoint, you'll proceed on a fugue of epic proportions, spending the cash in a excitement-packed day much like a more grown-up version of *Ferris Bueller's Day Off.* We recommend you use this setting only once a year or so, and remember to pack disguises, as much of your day may be spent breaking laws.

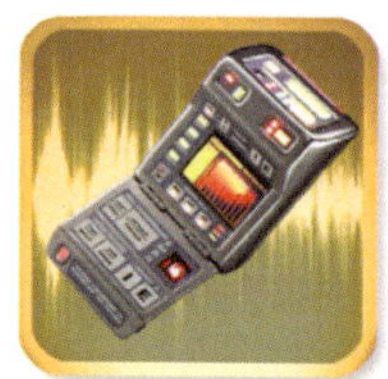

**SCI-FI MEDICAL NOISE APP** Plays sound effects from famous television shows like the tricorder – the *Star Trek* prop carried by *Dr. McCoy.* Fake images such as xrays, MRIs, and CT scans are shown on the screen while you wave it around the patients and tell them everything is just fine. Perfect for the malingerer who needs a little reassurance.

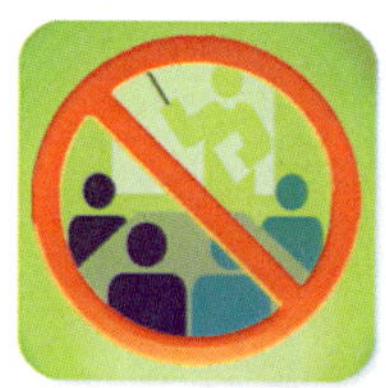

**MEETING DELETER APP** Using a database of information from over two million medical meetings, the Meeting Deleter App will calculate whether you should skip your next time waster. Just type in the words from the invite as well as the agenda. Within seconds, the Meeting Deleter App will tell you whether this is a waste of time or note.

*Note:* Almost 98% of the time the WASTE OF TIME response comes up but do not be fooled, this is not an malfunction of the app. It is a malfunction of our healthcare system. ✚

# Vagina Games

**_Being a doctor can be very enlightening._** Here are the top names patients have given their physicians when discussing their most private of parts *(as submitted through the* Placebo Journal Blog*)*:

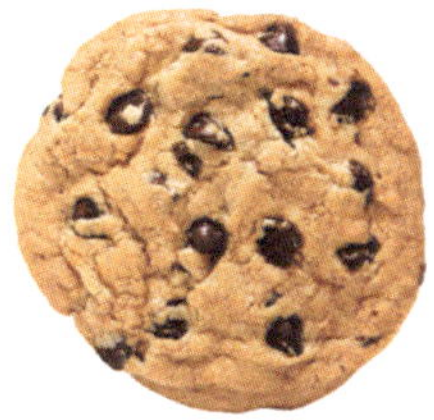

1. Hoo ha
2. Little Suzy
3. Too-too
4. Hootyhoo
5. Kitten
6. Cookie
7. Fish house
8. Fancy
9. Apparatus
10. Monkey
11. China
12. Vajanitor
13. Playpen
14. Sally
15. Coochie
16. Noony kazoo zoo
17. Cootsy
18. Biscuit

***"Really?"***

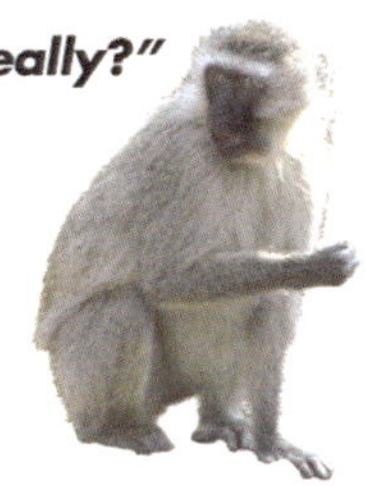

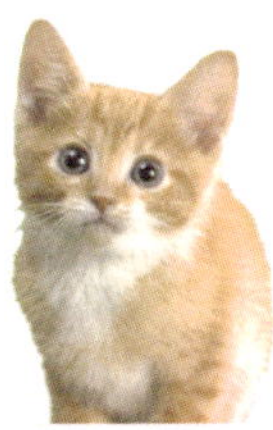

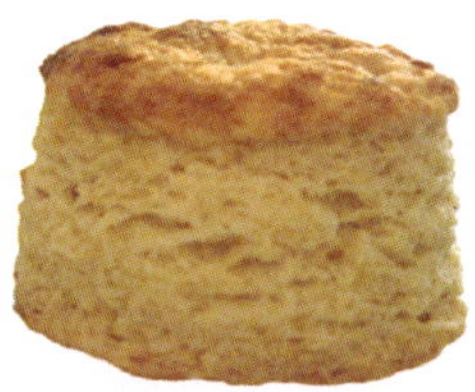

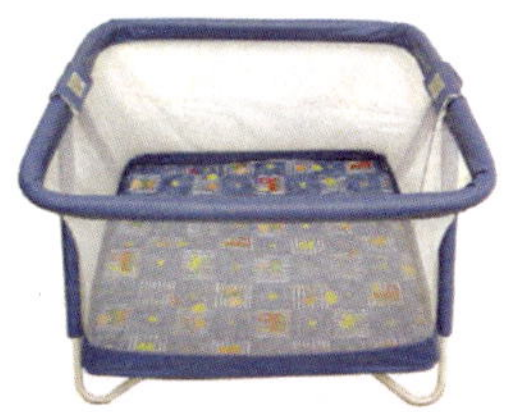

## PJ MEDICAL ALGORITHM OF REALITY

## WHAT TO DO WHEN YOU SEE A PATIENT IN PUBLIC

Do you have kids with you who can act as scouts looking for anyone who seems to recognize you?

YES – teach them to use tactical and covert military-like techniques to go out and search as much space of the venue as possible.

NO → Does the patient definitely see you?

NO – Run. Run like the wind.

YES → Are you sure?

NO – Run as if your life depended on it.

YES → Do you like the patient?

YES – Go ahead and say hello.

NO or indifferent → Could you convince the patient, via body language, that you did not see them?

YES – Keep moving, grab something and take a different direction and move as if you have a purpose.

NO → Does acting like you are in a hurry make the patient shy away?

YES – Increase your speed twofold and act stressed and uncomfortable, as if you were in a terrible emergency (good acting is important here so don't be afraid to practice at home).

NO → Is it possible to engage in a conversation with a salesperson before the patient comes over to you?

YES – Quickly grab the salesperson's attention and start asking questions; it is always smart to have three questions in mind before you go into any store to use for this purpose.

NO → Would pretending to have laryngitis work to end the conversation?

YES – Smile and point to your throat and then mouth the words, "I'm sick . . . can't talk." Once again this is good to practice at home.

NO → If you are still unable to detach from this particular patient, would you consider faking a stroke, seizure or heart attack and risk an ambulance ride in order to not talk to this particular patient?

YES – As a doctor you have seen it a million times. Slur your words, shake violently or clutch your chest. Depending on the patient, urinary or bowel incontinence may actually be worth it. You may even have a chance to make a run for it if the patient goes for help. If not, then pay the ambulance worker $100 to drop you at your house and get your car later.

NO – You are screwed. Make simple conversation. Use HIPAA to your advantage and tell them you would love to talk about their hemorrhoids but you just legally just can't do it. Even if they aren't talking about complaints or medical issues, use the HIPAA excuse. No one really knows how the law works anyway. After wrapping up, make sure you kick or punish your kids for not warning you earlier and doing their job right.

literally exploded when I plunged the #11 Bard Parker blade into it. Pure purulence – the kind that gives you a metallic taste in your mouth when you see it – was now obscuring my view.

*"Could you dab right here, Mary?"* I asked hopefully, pointing with the scalpel at the incision site. There was no dab. In my peripheral visual field, up and to my right, I saw the unmistakable swoon – her head was beginning to carve horizontal circles in the air – small ones at first, then ones of increasing circumference. The reflected light of the goose-neck lamp glistened on her damp green forehead and below it were unseeing eyes, eyes that had rolled back into their orbits. I was losing an assistant and gaining a patient. She was going down.

In a heartbeat my left leg pushed the gurney toward the wall temporarily pinning Mary at her waist in an upright position. My right hand released the clamp and placed a sterile gauze pad over the wound. At the same time my left hand cleared the instruments from Jack's abdomen. The sterile field had become the landing field.

Have you ever seen a tree fall in the forest? Slowly at first, then with increasing speed, her hands pinned at her side by the gurney, folding like a wallet at her waist, face down, she plunged toward Jack's considerable flesh. ***Kaawop!*** The sound could be likened to an egg dropped from a considerable height into a soft pillow. Her face disappeared into Jack's belly, only to reappear on the bounce, and then it settled back down, undulating as if she were on a waterbed.

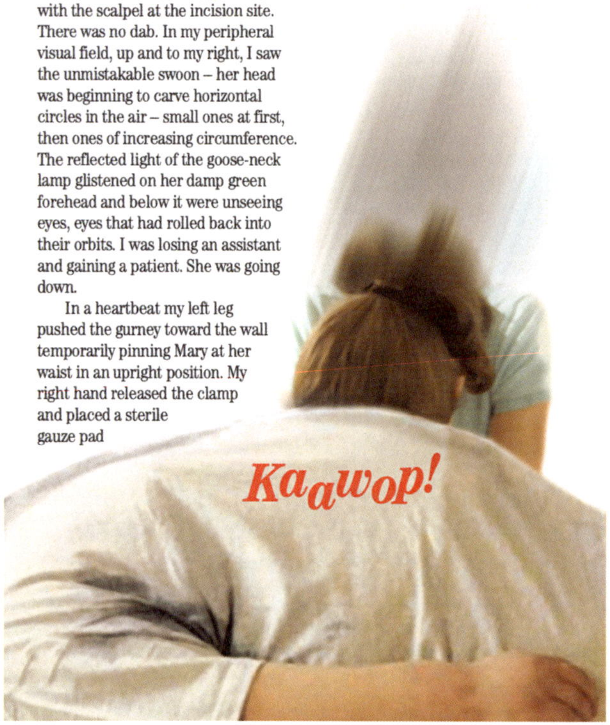


Quickly I placed Jack's finger on top of the sterile gauze and instructed him to keep pressure on it, and then I attended to my second patient. I pushed the gurney away from the wall, unfolded her, and then gently lowered her down to the floor. After elevating her feet, I reached for the ampoule of ammonia and wafted it underneath her nostrils. Mary's eyes opened widely.

*"I told you so,"* she said sadly.

*"Is she O.K. Doc?"* Jack asked from above us.

*"Yes she is,"* I replied – but privately I was thinking how perilously close to disaster we had been.

I can still recall sitting on the linoleum floor of that tiny room, my back against the door, with Mary's head in my hands and Jack lying above us on that gurney with his finger in his eye. And like much of medicine, it is funny only in retrospect. Yes, Jack's chalazion was cured. Mary switched her major. And me? Well, I never again asked another untrained person to help me. ✚

# TRUE GRIT

While working in the ED, I had a daughter bring in her 80-year-old mother due to high blood pressure. So, I took her into the ED and hooked her up to the B/P machine. It pumped up and went up to over 200 and the patient started complaining about it being tight and hurting her and could I shut it off. Her daughter told her mom *"to just grit your teeth."* Her mother states, *"I can't, they are in my purse!!"* I fell out of the cubical laughing. ✚

# OFFICE ASTRONOMER

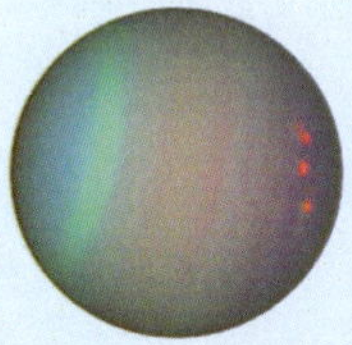

The Tuesday after a holiday Monday is always busy and this day was no exception. The waiting room was packed and there were patients lining up outside. To complicate matters, my partner was on vacation so I had the entire island practice to myself. In addition, I had overindulged on the holiday Monday so now I could work through the assembled sea of humanity with a dull hangover.

I took a deep cleansing breath and entered exam room #1. Here I found Gina, a 275-pound woman who had complaints of lower abdominal pain. I trolled for GU symptoms that might indicate a UTI and thereby preclude a pelvic exam but no such luck. So I tried to use the opposite of open-ended questions and used the power of positive suggestion. *"You are having burning when you pee, right?"*

*"No."*

*"Peeing more than normal, right?"*

*"Nope."*

With Gina failing to cooperate with my efforts to give her a UTI, I tried the power of negative suggestion. *"You DON'T have a discharge, right?"*

*"Well, maybe a little"*

*"No pain with intercourse, right?"*

*"Yeah, I guess so."*

*"You've NOT missed any periods."*

*"Well, my period has always been messed up."*

I could see this was not going my way. I could feel myself falling rapidly behind. I ordered a U/A (urinalysis) and pregnancy test and hustled off to see the febrile child in room #2.

The three-year-old child with otitis was a quick visit. Less than 10 minutes and that included handing out a sticker.

I returned to Gina's room, hoping to find an abnormal U/A. No such luck. Not only was the U/A negative, the pregnancy test was positive. I mumbled an insincere congratulation. Now there would be no hope of avoiding a pelvic exam. An ectopic pregnancy was still a potential diagnosis.

I went in search of a nurse. I tried to avoid looking at the pile of charts that was stacking up. I checked my watch. This was going to be a long day.

I returned to exam room #1 with the nurse. Gina was maneuvered into the stirrups with some difficulty. I retrieved a plastic speculum and inserted the light source.

Suddenly, Gina raised her head and peered over her sizable abdomen and said, ***"What is that Doc, a telescope?"***

The comment entered my brain like a bullet, firing synapses along the way. It seemed to awaken my hangover dulled cerebral cortex. My response was formed in a millisecond. It traveled to my mouth and escaped before I could stop it. ***"A telescope? Why yes it is a telescope because with this, I can see Uranus."***

*"Can you really?"*

Looking down at the confluence of flesh and skin folds, I realized that I was no Galileo. I was more likely to be *"Lost in Space."* ✚

## PLACEBO JOURNAL
## MEDICAL ALGORITHM OF REALITY

# Unidentified Exam Room Odor

Does smell make you cough and wheeze, or grow a lung tumor? → YES, and → Patient has bronchitis and horrific teeth → **ROOM TREATMENT 1:** Spray room and hallway liberally with citrus odor-masking spray. Keep it on hand for the other ten similar patients who will show up today.

↓ NO

Does the smell give you PTSD flashbacks to your high school boys locker room? → YES, and → Patient is wearing a well-used *Metallica* or *Korn* concert t-shirt with uber-baggy jeans and/or has dreadlocks. –OR– Patient mentions that he's been playing *World of Warcraft* for 40 straight days. → **ROOM TREATMENT 2:** Apply Room Treatment 1, AND deploy a fan to the room for one hour. Tell your nurse you can get her a date with him. This may make her vomit a little bit.

↓ NO

Does smell seem to physically slap you in the face when you open the door, and cause you to quickly back out and catch a deep breath before going back in? → YES, and → In the exam room you find a formula-fed baby, and most likely one or two other kids also, all under age three. → **ROOM TREATMENT 3:** Apply room treatments 1 & 2, and empty the trash. Look around room for the hidden diaper if odor is not controlled.

↓ NO

Does smelling this odor instantly cause you to break out in a rash? → YES, and → Patient weighs > 400 pounds, and you find an uneaten sandwich and a cheeseburger wrapper between his pannus and breasts. → **ROOM TREATMENT 4:** Apply Room Treatments 1 – 3, and abandon room use for 24 hours. Go home and shower/dispose of your clothing even if schedule is ruined. Request thorough disinfecting of room by housekeeping staff.

↓ NO

Do you vomit uncontrollably, after a valiant, but short struggle not to, and feel compelled to glance around the room in search of a decaying corpse? → YES, and → In response to your history-gathering questions, does the patient suddenly remember that she did mysteriously lose track of a tampon three months ago? → **ROOM TREATMENT 5:** Apply Room Treatments 1- 4. Close office for one week while it is fumagated and all upholstery re-done. Replace all carpet. Consider a change of career and/or some kind of memory-erasing hypnosis.

**ROOM TREATMENT 6:**
The **"perfect storm."** (This is a very rare but important room treatment. Employ it only when you experience all five smell reactions listed above, simultaneously. No other treatment will work.)
*Burn down office. Use insurance money to rebuild it, or to buy a cabin in the middle of nowhere.*

Watch million-dollar surgical robots compete to see which hospital is better.

Who care's about adequate training? A two-day course is all these surgeons need to operate on patients in the hospital and demolish the competition in our studio.

**Extreme destruction. Extreme egos. Extreme waste of money.**

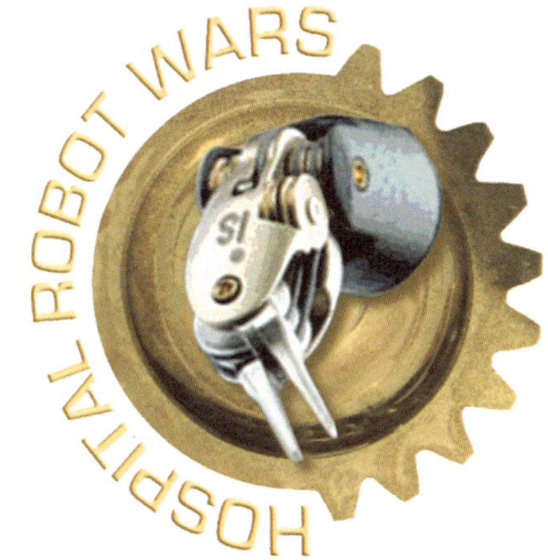


These surgical behemoths are the new weapons in the medical arms race and they are out to crush each other.

Watch as hospital CEOs try to showcase their new technological marvel regardless on whether it does any public good. See hospitals display their marketing prowess inside the death cage.

With little value, lots of cost, and tons of medical fun, the new symbol of medical progress is ready to kill for your business.

Which surgeon will get the trophy wife? Which surgeon will defend his CEO's honor? Which surgeon will cry?

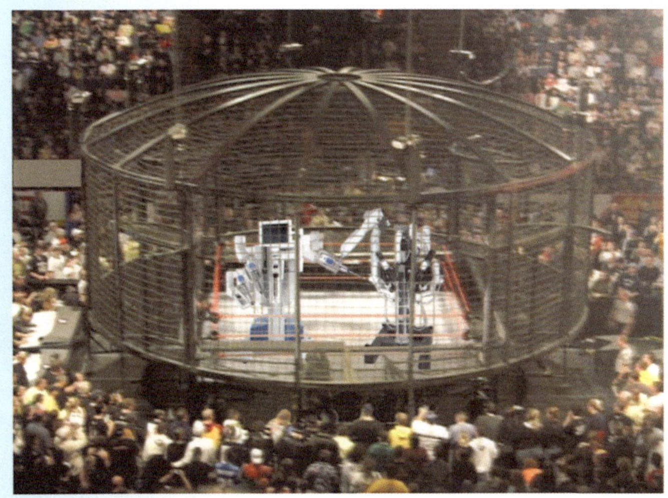

## HOSPITAL ROBOT WARS

**Good for business. Good for market share. Great for television!**

New on **POX TV**

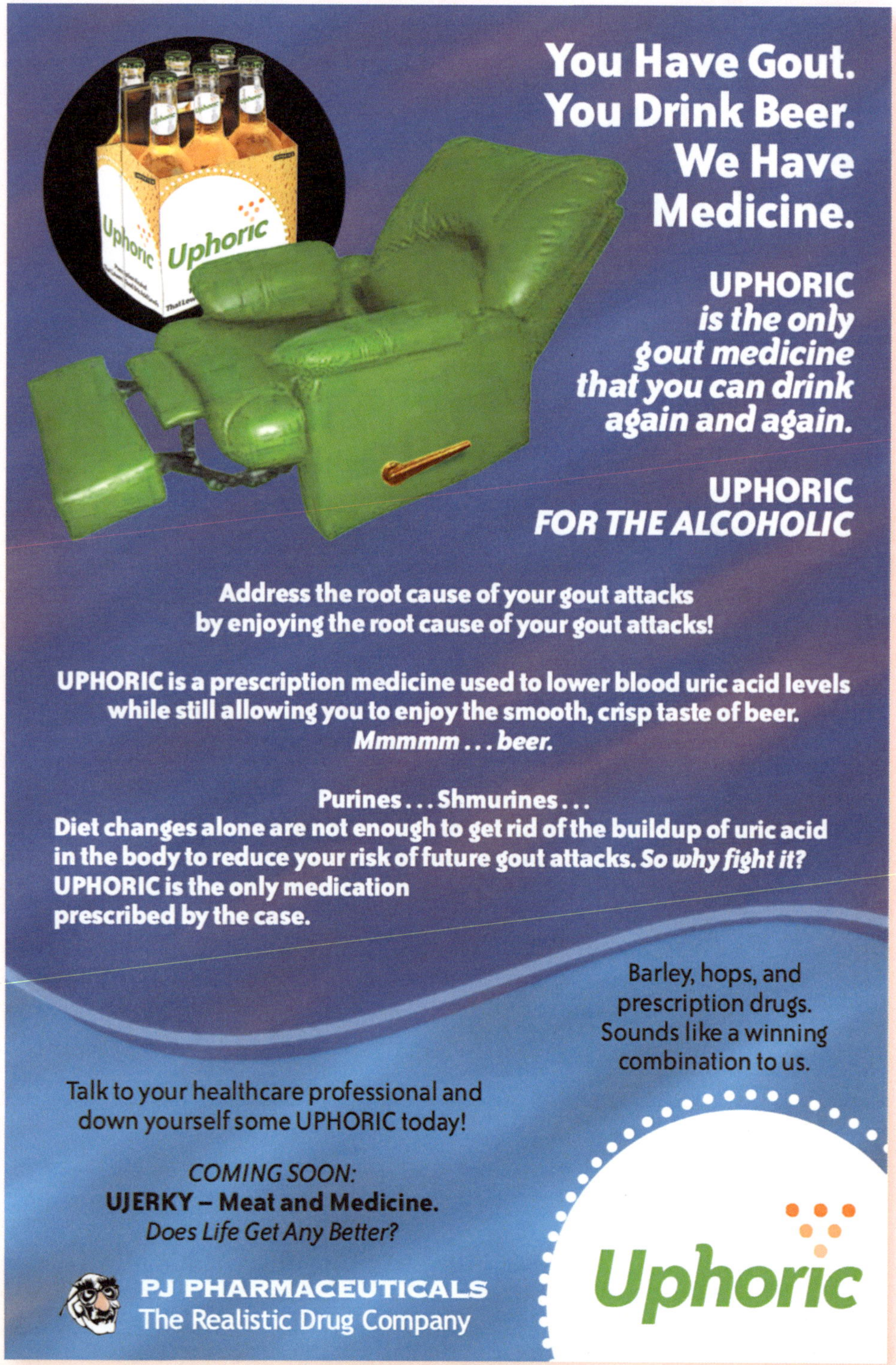
You Have Gout.
You Drink Beer.
We Have Medicine.
UPHORIC is the only gout medicine that you can drink again and again.
UPHORIC FOR THE ALCOHOLIC
Address the root cause of your gout attacks by enjoying the root cause of your gout attacks!
UPHORIC is a prescription medicine used to lower blood uric acid levels while still allowing you to enjoy the smooth, crisp taste of beer. Mmmmm . . . beer.
Purines . . . Shmurines . . .
Diet changes alone are not enough to get rid of the buildup of uric acid in the body to reduce your risk of future gout attacks. So why fight it? UPHORIC is the only medication prescribed by the case.
Barley, hops, and prescription drugs. Sounds like a winning combination to us.
Talk to your healthcare professional and down yourself some UPHORIC today!
COMING SOON:
UJERKY – Meat and Medicine.
Does Life Get Any Better?
PJ PHARMACEUTICALS
The Realistic Drug Company
Uphoric

## PJ MEDICAL ALGORITHM OF REALITY

# Doctor has to work late and misses spouse's birthday, anniversary, etc.

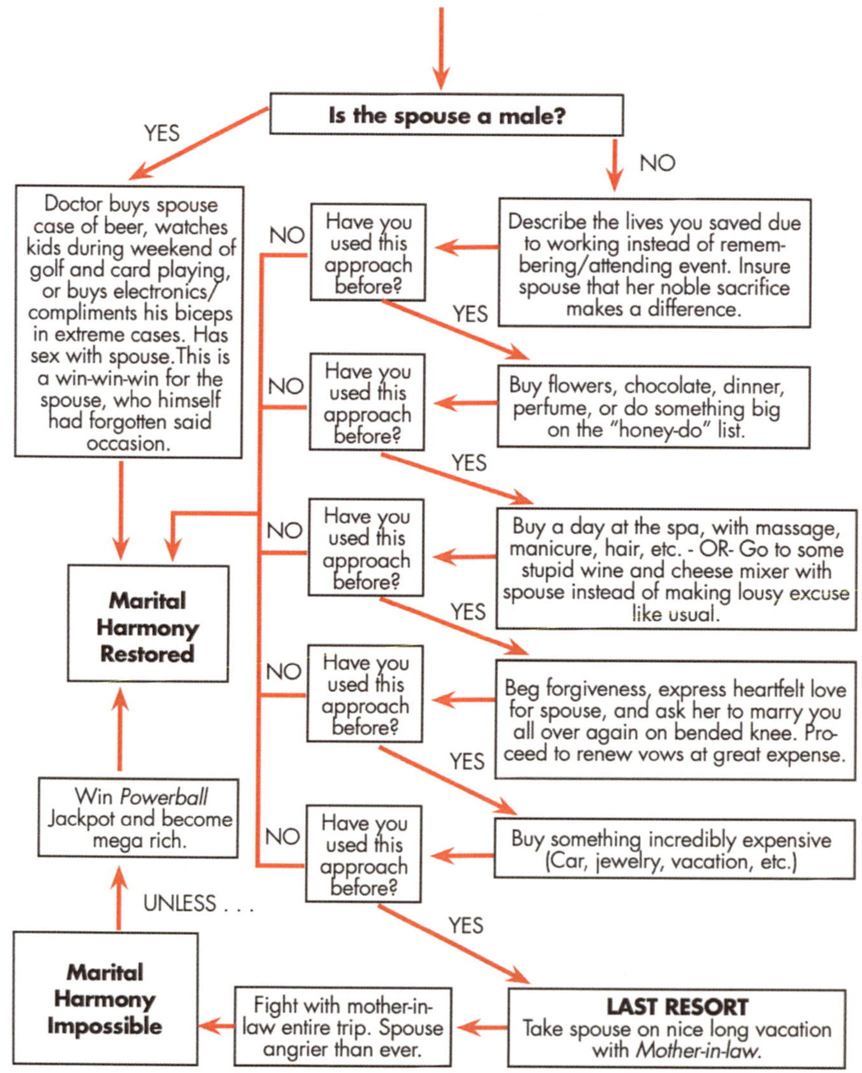

Today's times call for a new genitourinary super hero . . .

# G.U.JOE

**Able to insert foley catheters through the thickest of prostates! Can prescribe Cipro in a single electronic click of a keyboard!**

Watch G. U. JOE do battle with his nemesis . . . the evil villain, Hyde Rocele.

**Accessories**
(not included)

- Lithotripsy machine to mash painful kidney stones!

A real American medical hero,
**G.U.JOE**

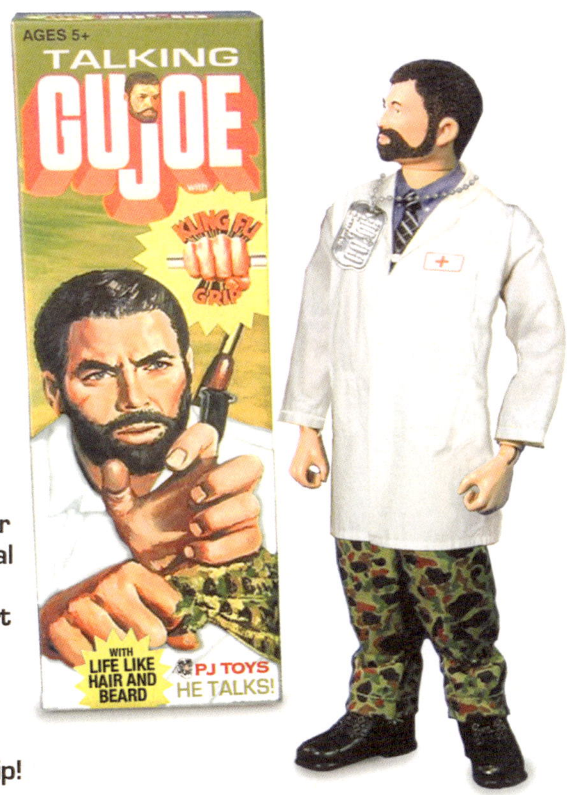


No you can pull the string and hear him say, "Transanal biopsies of the prostate don't hurt THAT much!"

Comes with new Kung Fu prostate finger grip!

From PJ TOYS +

# MY VALVE JOB

A month before the 9/11 attack I had my mitral valve replaced with an artificial one. No one warned me, including my surgeon hubby, that the thing was loud. I mean I ticked like the proverbial alligator in *Peter Pan*. Everyone explained it would quiet down in time and I would rarely notice it. That was mid-August 2001 and of course on September 11, 2001 we all know what happened.

After weeks of recovery that fall I went back to work at my large medical consulting firm that dealt almost exclusively with the *National Institute of Health* and the *CDC* in Atlanta. I was assigned to a contract and went with a colleague to the campus of the *NIH*. Our meeting was in a small room in the Library of Medicine.

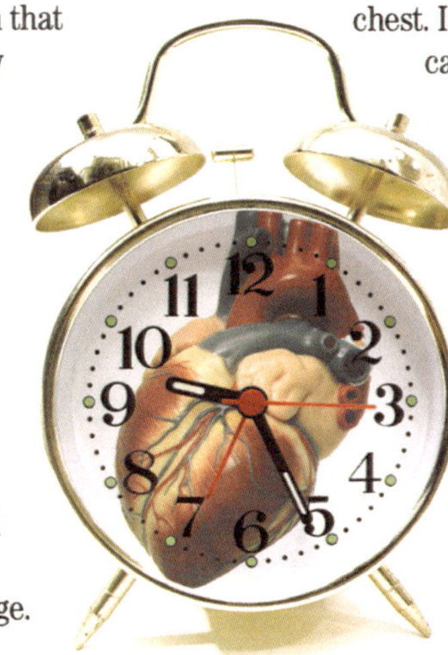

Everyone straggled in and then I began to notice something strange. Everyone was sitting well away from me and it was very very quiet. The door opened and a large uniformed guard walked over and asked me to take my belongings and follow him. I was embarrassed but did as I was told.

Outside the room the guard rushed me over to a smaller room and insisted I hand over my briefcase, purse, and to disrobe. I protested. Then the light went on! *Ah Hah!!* I started to chuckle. The guard looked puzzled.

*"Hey, put your ear on my chest and I'll introduce to my new artificial mitral heart valve,"* I explained.

Warily he moved close and listened and then began to smile at me as he heard the steady *tick, tick, tick* in my chest. I took out the card that I carry at all times explaining the St. Jude's valve, date and physician's name.

He escorted me back to the meeting and I discovered that my colleague had been explaining about the valve to the group. Several physicians and researchers apologized when they found out the source of *"the ticking bomb"* that I carried.

From then on I always managed to bring up the valve situation if I was meeting with a new group and kept this up for years. A few sharp-eared younger folks still look at me in a puzzled way but for the most part I'm good to go for now. +

## PJ PEDIATRIC MEDICAL ALGORITHM OF REALITY

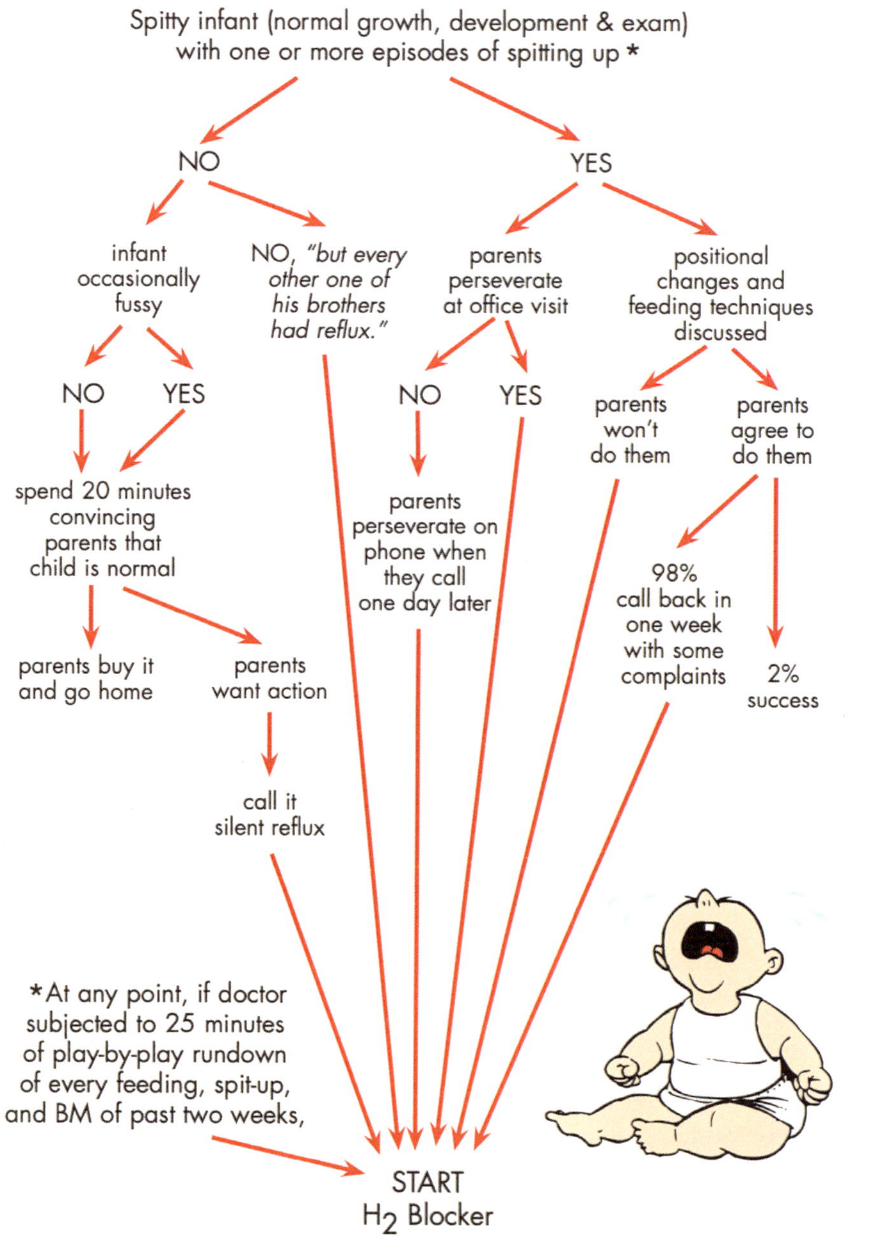


## TRUE STORIES OF MEDICINE

# WHOOPS

A patient I had seen four or five years ago returned and as we entered my office she stated, *"My, you look the same after all these years."*

I said, *"Thank you and so do you."* She quickly responded with, *"Oh, I've lost over 100 pounds."*

Bummer. ✚

# WEED HELPS ME!

"Mike" is a 21-year-old man in community college seeking treatment for ADD. He is passionate about the fact that his frequent and heavy marijuana use has NOTHING to do with his attention problems, and in fact feels like it is beneficial. He wants to take *Adderall* because he tried his friend's *Adderall* and it helped him. I continue to refuse to prescribe it until he stops smoking pot and can pass a urine drug screen. I saw him for a follow-up appointment the other day, and this was our conversation (Note: he always sounds stoned when he is in my office):

Me: *"How is school going?"*

Mike: *"Terrible! I have a test today, and I haven't studied for it . . . I don't even know what it's on!"*

Me: *"Have you had any luck being able to concentrate on your homework?"*

Mike: *"Not really . . . the ONLY thing that helps me do my homework is weed."*

Me: *"So, you're telling me that smoking weed helps you concentrate on your homework? Does that mean that you are actually completing assignments and turning them in?"*

Mike: (laughs) *"No . . . No. . . What I meant was weed helps me avoid my homework."*

Me: *"What? Say that again?"*

Mike: *"Smoking weed makes me not care that I'm not doing my homework!* (laughs) *It's awesome! It helps me play video games and watch TV and not worry about everything!"*

Needless to say, Mike will likely be failing this semester of college and returning to flipping burgers at the local fast food restaurant to pay for his habit. ✚

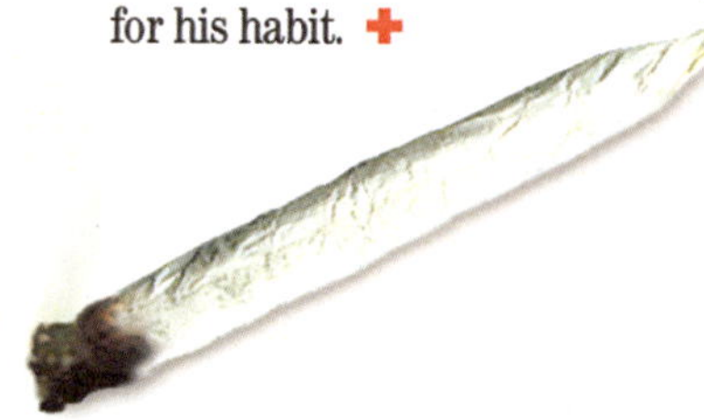

# X-Ray Files

**If we show you ours, will you show us yours?**

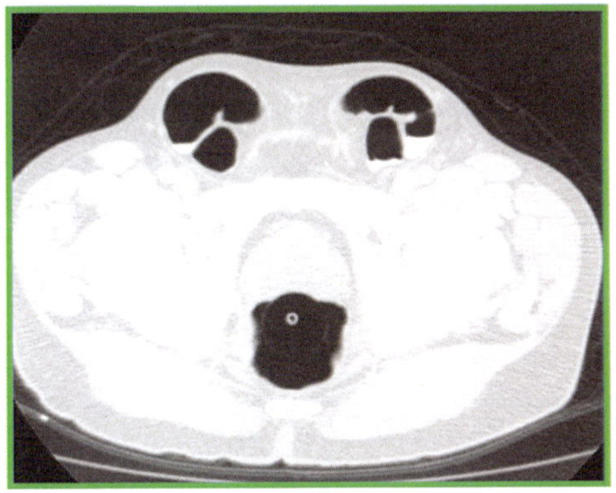

Inguinal hernias look like a certain purple dinosaur . . .

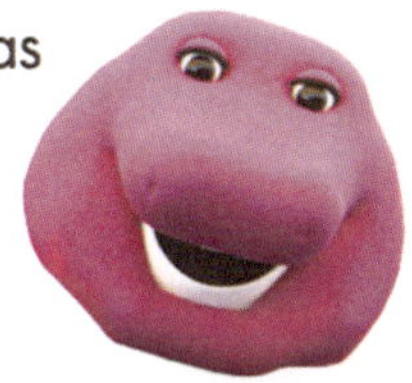

Here's a smoking pharynx on a barium swallow . . .

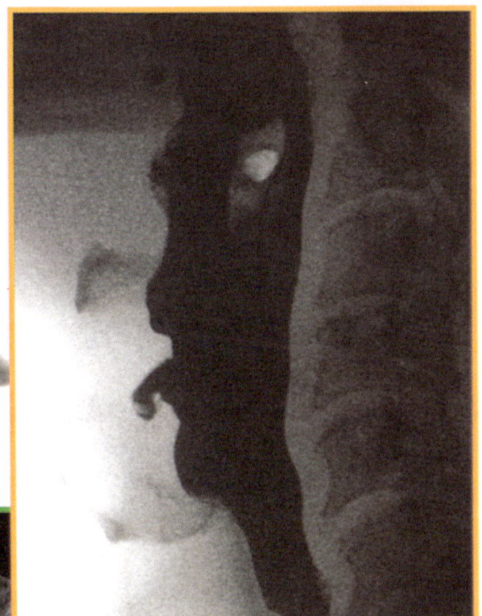

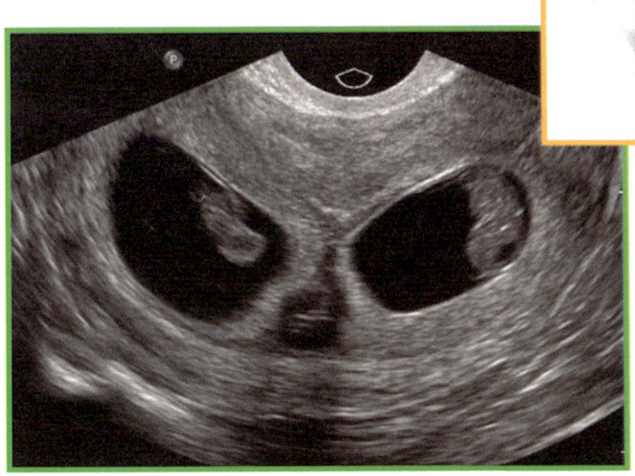

Do you suppose these twins are due on Halloween?

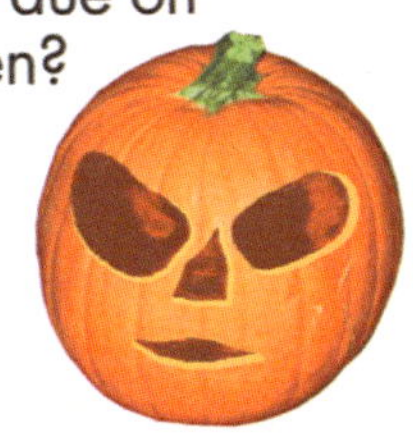

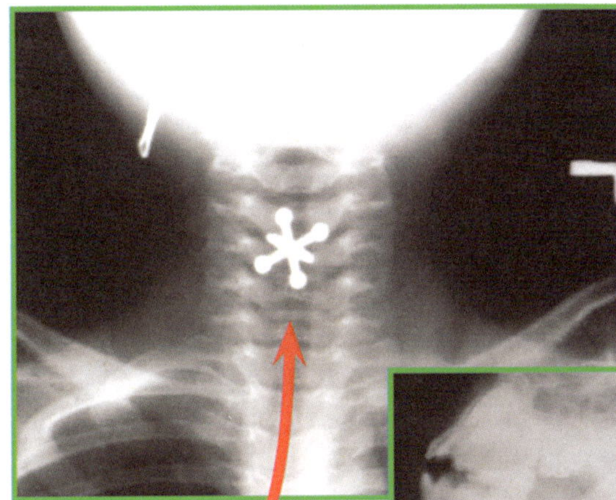

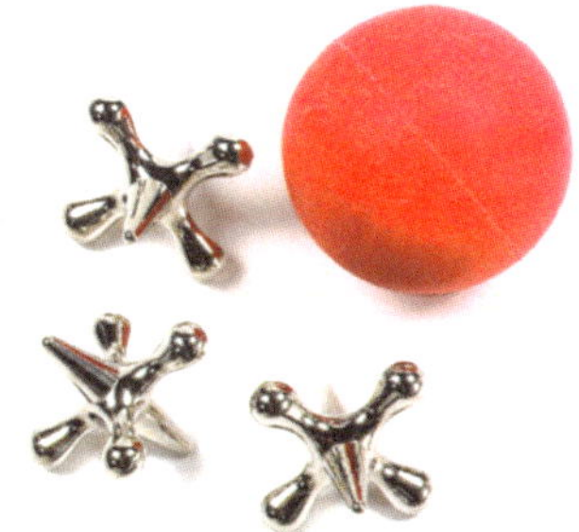

**Anyone up for a game of Jacks?**

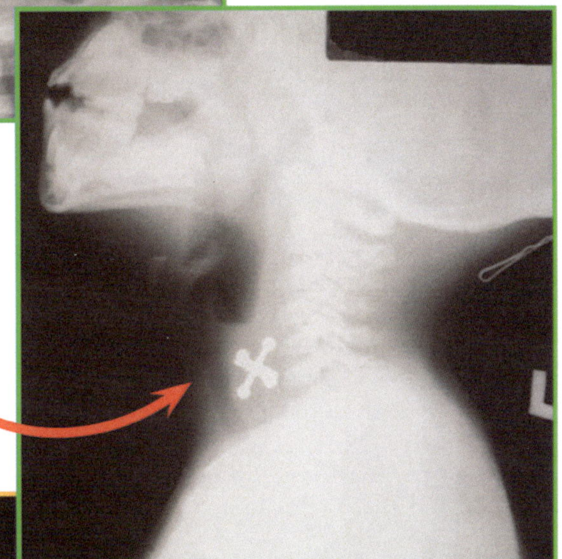

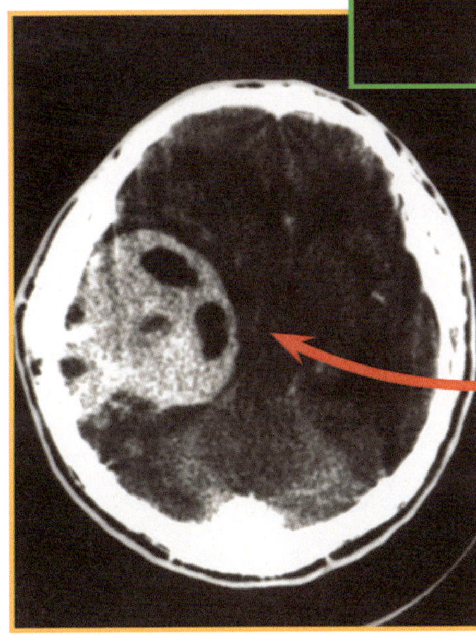

***BOO!* The haunted CAT scan** (actually it's a hemangiopericytoma).

If you're a radiologist, show us your files. If we use them, you'll get **A FREE ONE-YEAR SUBSCRIPTION!**

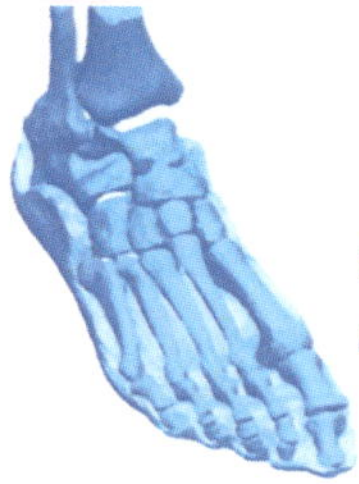

# *Welcome to the* 2010 Southwest Podiatry Conference *in beautiful Bigfoot, Texas*

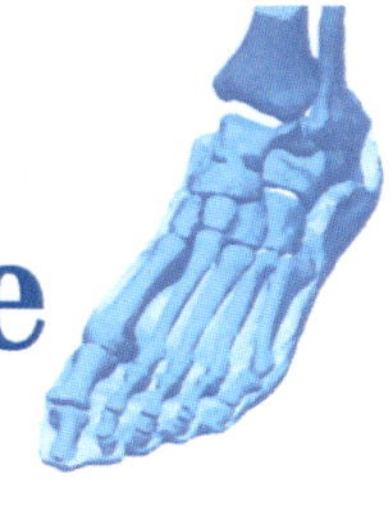

*The 2010 Southwest Podiatry Conference will take place June 18-20th, 2010 at the* Cuticle Regency *in Bigfoot, Texas. We are looking forward to presenting an exciting program that will offer a variety of sessions and workshops for all levels of skill for podiatrists, podiatric medical assistants, residents and other related healthcare specialists.*

## Friday, June 18

**9:00 AM:** Opening Remarks by President Chip Dermis DPM

**9:30 – 11:00 AM:** Keynote Speaker Kerry Tolysis DPM on *How to Repair Acute Achilles Ruptures with Fiberwire, Gum and Popsicle Sticks – The* McGuyver *Approach.*

**11:00 – 11:30 AM:** Exhibit Hall Networking Break

**11:30 AM – 12:30 PM:** *OMG, that smells! Why your patient may not be such a fungi.* Sessa Moiditis DPM

**12:45 – 2:00 PM:** Lunch

**2:30 – 3:30 PM:** *Too fat for heels; Ma'am, isn't it obvious?* Ray Nauds DPM

**3:45 – 5:00 PM:** *Cortisone Shots – How not to make them shout while not scaring your other patients away.* Phil Lanx DPM

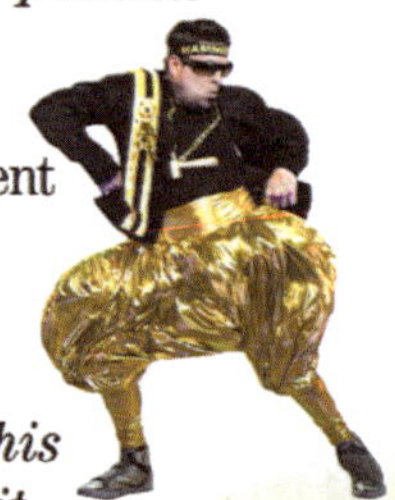

**8:00 PM:** Entertainment by ***MC Hammertoe*** who will perform his songs:

- *U Won't Touch This*
- *Too Thick To Quit*

## Saturday, June 19

**7:30 – 8:00 AM:** Breakfast Fireside Chat: *Chiropodists – Let's change our name back to confuse even more people about what we do.* Chip Dermis DPM

**8:00 – 9:00 AM:** *Biomechanical Evaluation – Watching people walk funny.* Morton Neuroma DPM

**9:15 – 10:00 AM:** *Amputation – It's not just for fun anymore.* Hal Luxvarus DPM

**10:15 – 11:00 AM:** *Ugly Feet – Is that a Charcot Foot or are you just happy to see me?* Cal Caneal DPM

**11:00 – 11:30 AM:** Exhibit Hall Networking Break

**11:30 AM – 12:30 PM:** *Fooled by Freaks: How to avoid being scammed by people with a fetish.* Arthur Ritic DPM

**12:45 – 2:00 PM:** Lunch

**2:30 – 3:15 PM:** *Podiatry and Spelling – from metatarsalgia to how many i's in fasciitis, don't be embarrased again.* Venus Statis DPM

**3:30 – 4:15 PM:** *Avoiding Vomit 101 – How to debride nasty feet without puking by focusing on your ridiculous paycheck.* Sessa Moiditis DPM

**4:30 – 5:00 PM:** *Childhood Obesity Foot Structure, Gait Characteristics & Lower Limb Pathology – Nothing we can do unless they stop eating.* Ray Nauds DPM

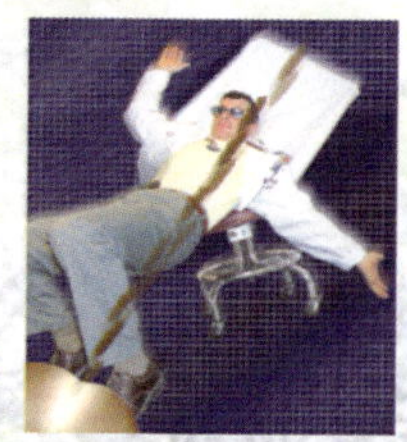

**6:00 PM:** See a sneak preview of the new movie, ***The Matrixectomy.***

## Sunday, June 20

**7:30 – 8:00 AM:** Breakfast Fireside Chat: *Orthotics: who needs evidence when you can make so much money!* Chip Dermis DPM

**8:00 – 9:00 AM:** *Peripheral Neuropathy – I can't feel you!* Phil Lanx DPM

**9:15 – 10:00 AM:** *Getting Rich by Fitting People for Diabetic Shoes – A systematic review and accounting meta-analysis.* Morton Neuroma DPM

**10:15 – 11:00 AM:** *MRSA - Damn, now we have to deal with this?!* Cal Caneal DPM

**11:30 AM – 12:30 PM:** *Difficult Foot Surgery – How to say,* "I need some help in here," *without looking ignorant.* Hal Luxvarus DPM

End Conference

## Things to Do While Attending the Southwest Podiatry Conference . . .

- Walk the local Bunion and Corn Maze
- Participate in a hands-on workshop for minimal invasive surgery on some homeless people!
- Hang out at **The Club Foot** – an after hours spot to meet and greet your peers. *Drink 'til your feet drop!*

# CONFIRMATION

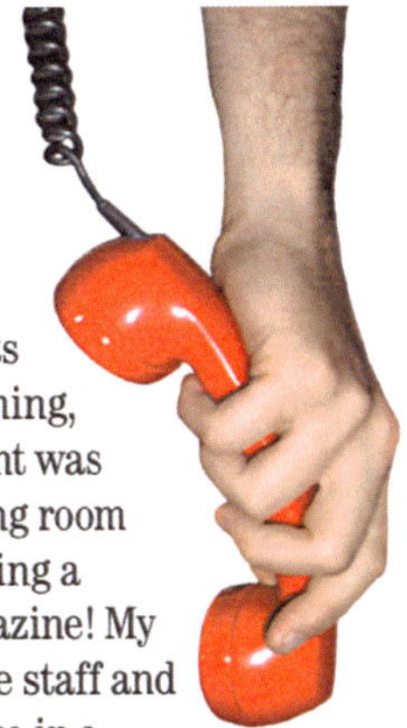

## THOSE DARN NARC SEEKERS

About three weeks ago, I got a phone call from a women I didn't know who claimed to be my patient's daughter. She said her mother had died, and she had to go up to Boston to inform her family and she needed tranquilizers to calm her nerves. I was very shocked at this news since the patient had been in my office two weeks prior and showed no signs of distress. Therefore, I willingly wrote a script for alprazolam for the daughter. The patient who died was a healthy, lovely woman who had no significant medical conditions. My office staff and I were very upset to hear of her passing. I even found myself looking through her chart to see if I had missed anything at her previous visit.

This morning, I walked out to our waiting room to bring in the patients like I do every morning, and our dead patient was sitting in the waiting room reading a magazine! My office staff and I were in a complete state of shock and I immediately brought her in to an exam room for an interview. When we told her we thought she had died, she responded, *"Oh, you should have called me!"* She in fact, never died, nor had any relation to the narc seeker who called me a few weeks earlier.

So not only did I get hit up for drugs, I also learned an important lesson. If a patient is allegedly dead, call them to confirm. ✚

# BREAKING OUT

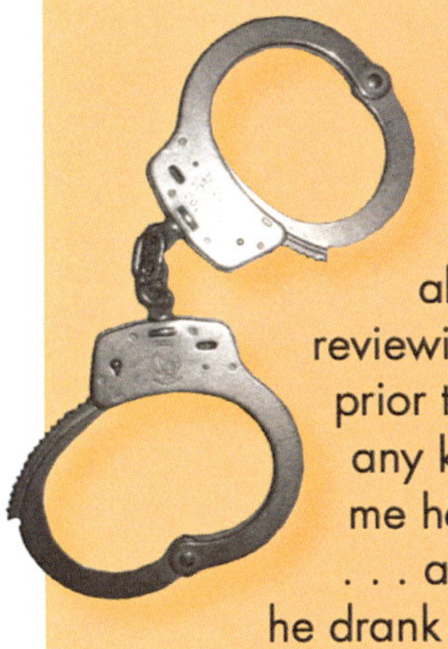

I had an emergency room patient who was brought over to Imaging for an abdomen/pelvis CT (Cat Scan). While reviewing the contrast consent form with him, prior to injection, I asked the patient if he had any known allergies. He responded by telling me he was allergic to alcohol. He paused . . . and then informed me that every time he drank he broke out in handcuffs. ✚

# SAY YES to the Pess

The only show that follows elderly women as they seek to find the perfect pessary at an upscale medical supply store in New York.

The trials and tribulations are there for all of us to see as these women scramble to find the right pessary to prevent their vaginal prolapse.

This show reveals the inner workings of a premier pessary store. *It's the ultimate shopping trip that many elderly dream about.*

- See which celebrity is on the hunt to cover up her rectocele!
- See which politician finds the perfect support for her prolapsed vaginal vault!

With the summer approaching fast it won't be long before many women are under pressure to find the perfect pessary to fit under that sun dress.

Don't miss our next episode where Helen has to have a "pess intervention" from her family.

NEW! Visit our Virtual Pessary site where you can see which style may fit you!

These women don't fret over pelvic support defects, such as uterine prolapse and vaginal prolapse. Instead, they, *"Say Yes to the Pess!"*

ONLY ON POX TV

# Medical Mash-ups

Combing classics with sinister themes is all the rage in the publishing world nowadays. We thought that the *Placebo Journal* should get in on the action. For those in the in the medical field who also enjoy gore and senseless violence, *PJ Publications* presents . . .

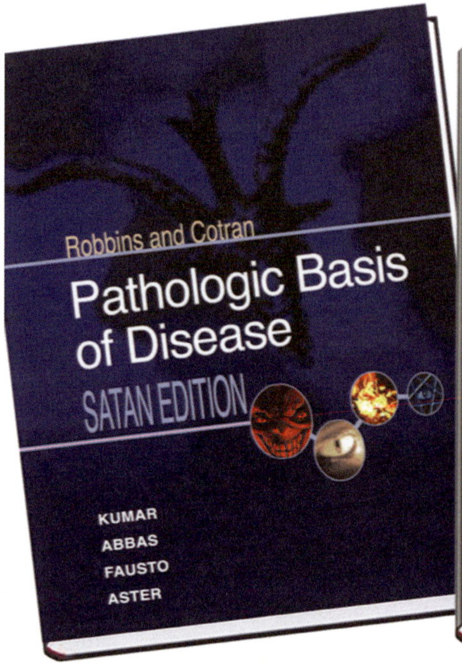


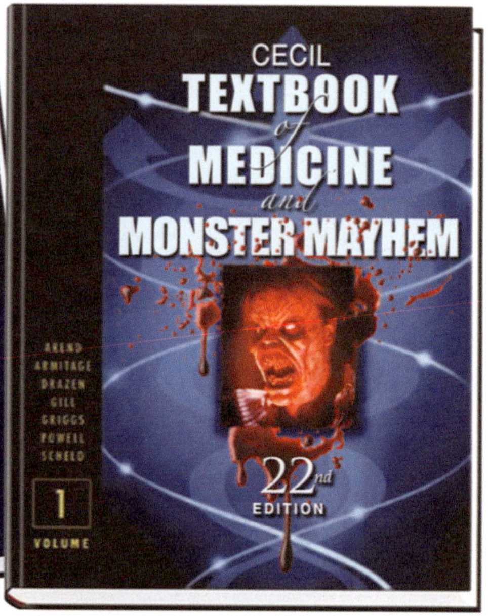


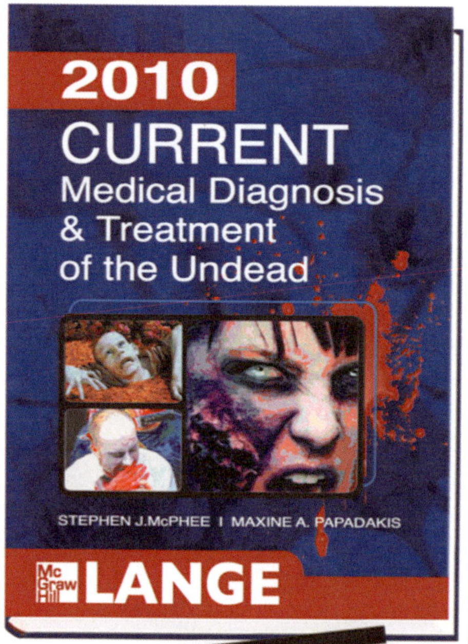


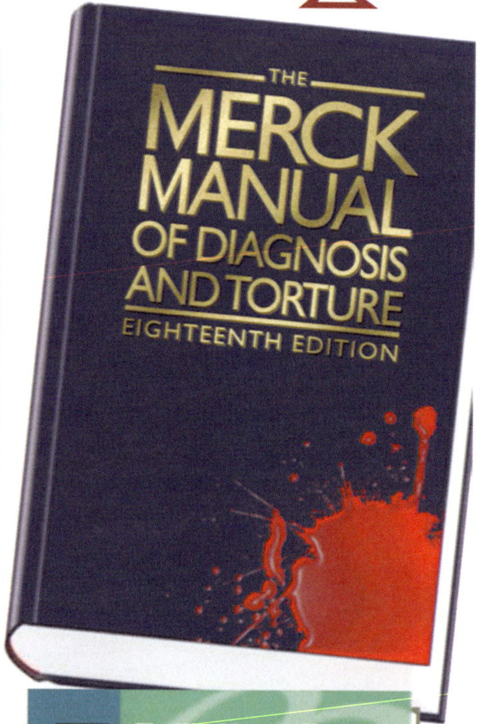


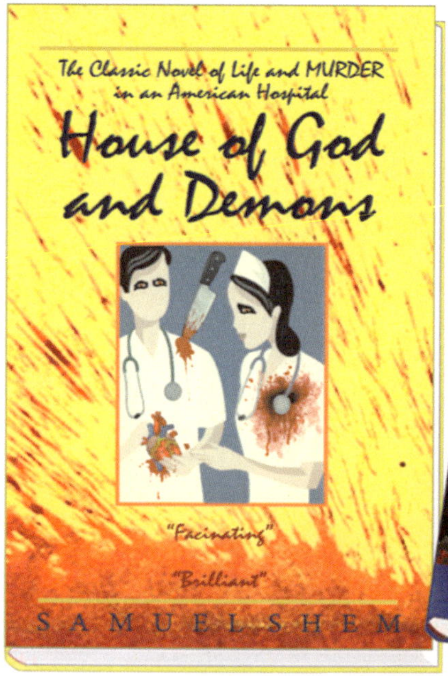


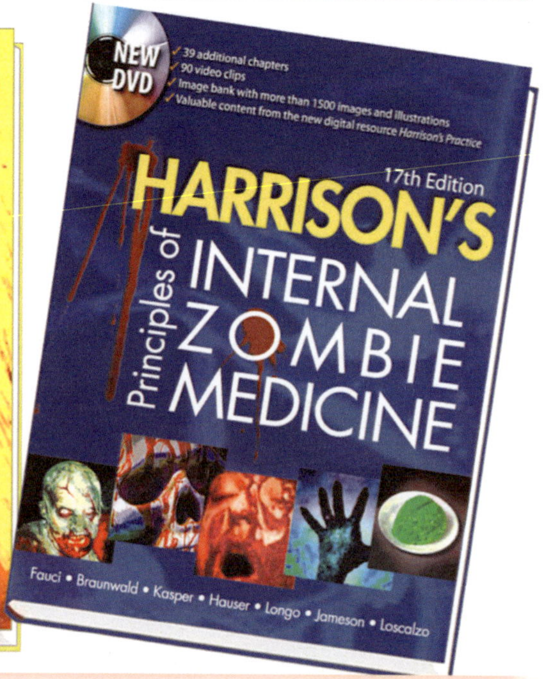


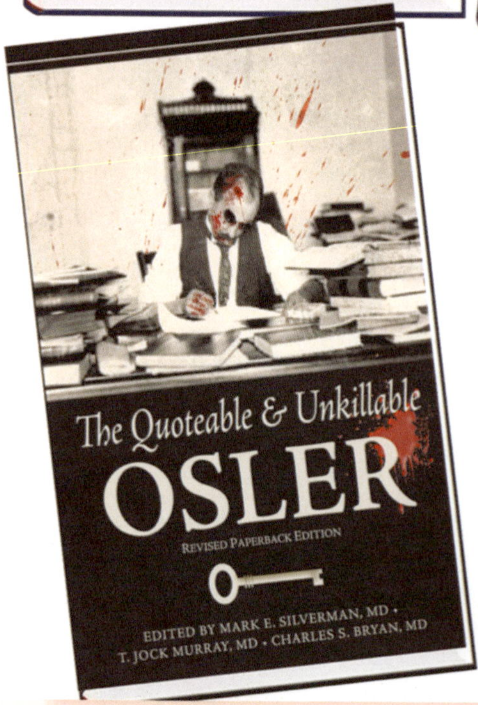


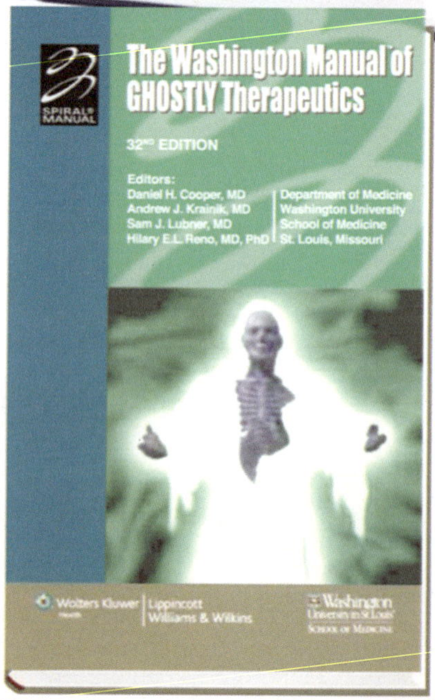

## THOSE DARN NARC SEEKERS

# Pinpointing A Problem

I had the occasion recently to care for a young woman with back pain. One of my colleagues had given her 20 *Percocet* a week earlier for the same complaint.

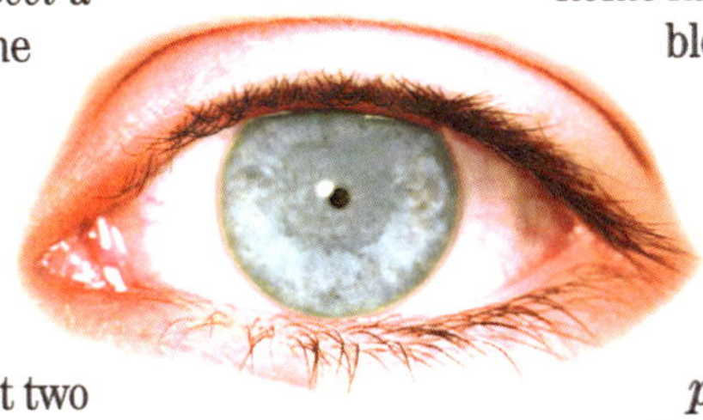

She had given birth a few months earlier and looked like she weighed about two bills. She said the back pain started after her epidural. I thought to myself, *"and had nothing to do with the 60 pounds you suddenly gained when you were pregnant and haven't lost?"*

I noticed that she had mid-dilated and reactive pupils. These should be pinpoint under the influence of *Percocet*.

I also noticed that she had a really pretty and recent French manicure that was obviously not a home hack job. Ditto with the bleached blonde hair – you can't get color that rich from a box of *nice'neasy*. *How does a teenage welfare mom afford professionally done nails and hair color?*

I asked her when she last took the *Percocet*. Said she'd run out the day before. So I checked a whiz quiz. Positive THC, negative opiates.

Looks like somebody sold their pills, bought a bag of weed, and went to the salon. ✚

## SOMEONE'S MISSING

I received a call from Dr. Brainstem, the neurologist. I had referred Sammy Seizure, a 7-month-old male, to him regarding seizure-like activity. Unfortunately, Sammy's mother arrived to the appointment without Sammy. She did not know that she needed to bring the baby to the appointment. ✚

## TOP 10 Signs That A Hospital Stay Is Not Going Well

**10.** You have trouble getting consultants to see the patient *"because I saw that $%^& the last time."*

**9.** Number of consultants on case exceeds number of grades in school completed by patient.

**8.** Number of invasive procedures performed to date exceeds patient's age in years.

**7.** Patient who has been complaining of "10 out of 10" pain is never in room for rounds because of trips to cafeteria, smoke hut, and friends who are also in the hospital.

**6.** Social worker tells you the family is refusing hospice because their only source of income is the patient's disability check.

**5.** Patient Relations calls to report family's complaint that patient is too sedated to sign paperwork changing her will.

**4.** Ethics committee and psych consultant sign off case the same day *"because we can't do anything with these crazy people."*

**3.** Case manager calls to inform you that patient has run through all his allowable Medicare days including the 60 "lifetime" days.

**2.** Sister-in-law is sitting at bedside when you come in, writing down everything that happens and the names of all hospital personnel involved in the patient's care.

**1.** Patient informs you that she is "allergic" to all analgesics except *Demerol*, then asks to have a nurse stay for a half hour after each dose *"because I tend to have seizures with it."* ✚

# THE STOLEN VAGINA

As a practicing interventional radiologist, I perform several epidural steroid injections every afternoon. The majority of these are for lower back pain, often with a radiculopathy. Our procedure is for the technologist to bring the patient into a holding area prior to my obtaining a consent. Often patients will return for a second and occasionally a third injection depending upon clinical response.

The other afternoon the technologist came to me and stated that the next patient was ready to consent. She claimed the patient stated that on her first steroid injection I had **"stolen her vagina."** I am well aware that in many patients there are supratentorial issues that quite frankly are beyond a simple radiologist. *I must admit, I had no idea what she was talking about, and certainly did not want to be openly accused of vaginal theft.* The simplest solution was to avoid this subject. However, when I was chatting with her while performing a lumbar epidural steroid injection she brought up that subject again.

With my tech in the room she clearly described that after her first epidural steroid injection she went to the bathroom when she got back in her hospital room. Only then did she realize she had **"no vagina."** *Only then did the penny drop.* Yes, I routinely inject 3-5 cc's of lidocaine with the steroid preparation. And yes, this is the same site used by anesthetists for child birth. I think what she was really trying to say was that her perineum was anesthetized.

To avoid being accused of another theft, I now routinely tell all my patients that they may experience some numbness down their legs or in their private parts (perineum) which will wear off within an hour.

In California, three epidural injections in this patient could have landed me the "three strikes and you're out" statute for theft. ✚

Tired of scrotal herpes?
Traditional condoms don't cover anything extra!

INTRODUCING

# THE C NDIE™

***THE WORLD'S FIRST FULL-BODY CONDOM***

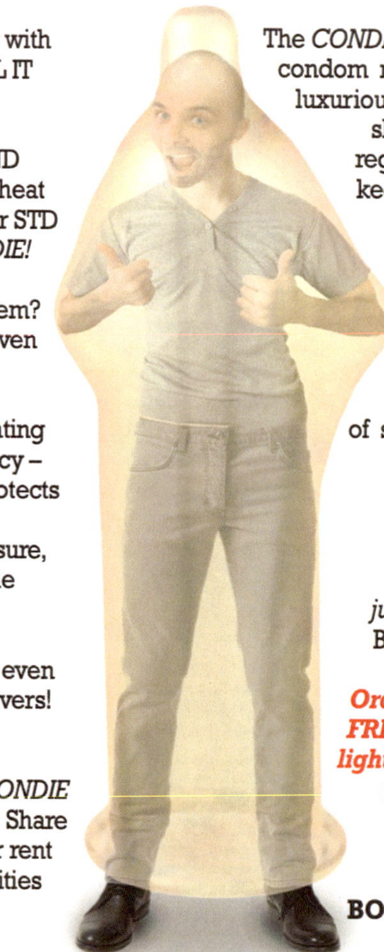

No more fumbling with application- just PULL IT OVER YOUR HEAD!

Prevents pubic AND head lice! When you heat up, you can keep your STD down with The *CONDIE!*

Body image problem? The *CONDIE* works even when fully clothed!

Go beyond preventing disease and pregnancy – The *CONDIE* even protects you from bad breath, partner's sweat exposure, and is fully compatible with menses!

Comes in all sizes, even 4XL for overweight lovers!

Use over and over again because The *CONDIE* is machine washable! Share it with your friends, or rent one out – the possibilities are endless!

The *CONDIE*™ is a super soft condom made of soft, thick, luxurious latex. It does not slip and slide like a regular condom so it keeps you protected from head to toe while allowing complete freedom of movement. Finally you can have some semblance of sex with complete peace of mind!

*"I always wear The CONDIE. Even at work. You just never know . . . "*
Brian Fruphak, MN

***Order now and get a FREE worthless LED light that you can use to get a migraine while you read!***

Available at
**BONERS, BEAVERS AND BEYOND**
or your local free clinic.

WARNING – Side effects include suffocation (by accident or on purpose) and latex sensitivity (in fact, if you use The *CONDIE* and you are allergic to latex, you can pretty much count on instantaneous death). Please use with care and supplemental oxygen. Sex is not a game.

***What do you a give a narc seeker that won't go away?***

## *PJ Pharmaceuticals* has your answer and it's called

# Vicosomething

How many times have you heard a questionable patient try to remember the drug that really worked for his pain?

Next time your patient says that he thinks the drug's name is *"vicosomething,"* now you can give him **Vicosomething!**

**Vicosomething** is pure placebo – sugar and corn fillers. It won't cure your patient's pain but it will make him happy (for now) and get him out the door.

*"I was so happy to get my pain pills. The doc didn't even blink when he wrote out my script! I'm going to tell all my peeps about him."*
John C.

## Also available: Percosomething and Oxysomething

# Vicosomething

**There's NOTHING to it!**

*PJ Pharmaceuticals* is not liable for any patient hostility caused by prescribing this **Vicosomething.** *PJ Pharmaceuticals* is also not responsible for any moral or ethical concerns you may have in regards to prescribing placebos.

**PJ PHARMACEUTICALS**
The Realistic Drug Company

# TOP 10 Phrases You Really Hate To Hear in Family Medicine

**10.** *"I'm hoping you can help me get disability."*

**9.** *"Did the CT scan show my baby?"*

**8.** *"We're waiting for my Medicaid to kick in.*

**7.** *"Don't you have any samples?"*

**6.** *"My work sent over all this paperwork for you to fill out for me."*

**5.** *"I was in a car wreck two months ago and I need to get checked out."*

**4.** *"My last eight doctors didn't help me – I'm suing them!"*

**3.** *"I need all 27 of these meds refilled. And I need a separate two-week prescription for each of them until my mail-in prescription comes back."*

**2.** *"You've got some certified letter from some lawyer."*

**1.** *"Remember that patient you saw last week?"* ✚

# Acknowledgements

I have a ton of people to thank for helping me with the Placebo Journal and now this book. My family put up with my insanity and allowed me to do it. A huge thank you to my wife, Debbie, and my kids: Jake, Luke, and Niki.

Jake was also instrumental in helping me gather, organize, and then digitize all the Placebo Journals. We lost most of the original files somehow, but I think the quality came out pretty great.

Gordon Marshall was the man behind all the illustrations. He put my ideas into picture form, and I think he did a wonderful job. Thank you, Gordon!

Vance Lassey, MD came aboard a few years into production and became a great friend of mine to this day. He was awesome to bounce ideas off of and he came up with some of the beauties in these books.

I also want to mention these contributors: Susan Summerton, MD, Michael S. Gorback, MD, Sarita Salzberg, MD, and Leonard Sharon, Esq. who acted as my wartime consigliere. You guys are awesome!

I need thank my former medical partners: Ray Stone, DO, Carolyn Pece, DO, and John Comis, DO. You guys enabled me to survive the practice of family medicine and made me laugh every day. You truly helped mold my ideas that went into the Placebo Journal.

Lastly, I want to thank my loyal readers and followers. You kept the Placebo Journal going. It never made me money, but it kept me sane and gave me a lot of fun. If you were a Knight of the Medical Roundtable then this King of Medicine salutes you.

www.ingramcontent.com/pod-product-compliance
Lightning Source LLC
LaVergne TN
LVRC080921210926
848486LV00014B/397

*9798985806212*